Leadership
in Nursing Practice

Changing the Landscape of Health Care

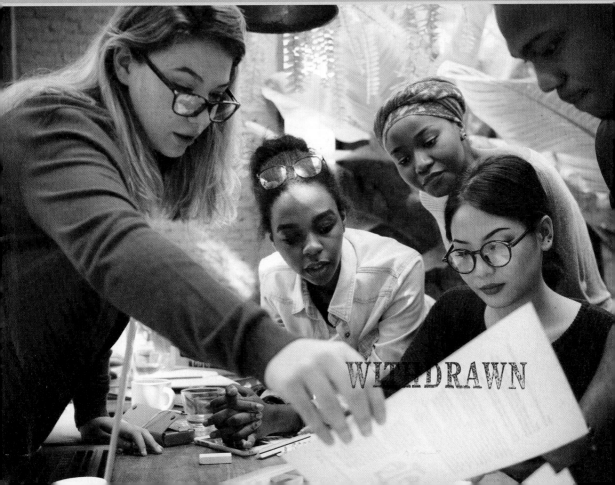

The Andragogy

Leadership in Nursing Practice: Changing the Landscape of Health Care, Third Edition drives comprehension through various strategies that meet the learning needs of students while also generating enthusiasm about the topic. This interactive approach addresses different learning styles, making this the ideal text to ensure mastery of key concepts. The andragogical aids that appear in most chapters include the following:

> I have an almost complete disregard of precedent, and a faith in the possibility of something better. It irritates me to be told how things have always been done. I defy the tyranny of precedent. I go for anything new that might improve the past. —Clara Barton

CHAPTER OBJECTIVES

Upon completion of this chapter, the reader will be able to do the following:

- » Describe the nature of change and innovation in a complex environment.
- » Compare and contrast principles of innovation and performance improvement.
- » List techniques to assist in the development of change and innovation competence.
- » Define the essential competencies and behaviors for effective change and innovation.
- » Enumerate specific strategies to embrace change.
- » Develop an understanding of the processes for overcoming obstacles to change and innovation.
- » Identify the purpose and essential elements of a contemporary business case for advancing quality using change and innovation principles.

Chapter Objectives

Chapter objectives provide instructors and students with a snapshot of the key information they will encounter in each chapter. They serve as a checklist to help guide and focus study.

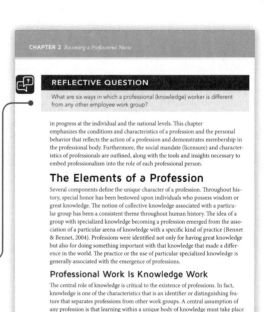

CHAPTER 2 *Becoming a Professional Nurse*

REFLECTIVE QUESTION

What are six ways in which a professional (knowledge) worker is different from any other employee work group?

in progress at the individual and the national levels. This chapter emphasizes the conditions and characteristics of a profession and the personal behavior that reflects the action of a profession and demonstrates membership in the professional body. Furthermore, the social mandate (licensure) and characteristics of professionals are outlined, along with the tools and insights necessary to embed professionalism into the role of each professional person.

The Elements of a Profession

Several components define the unique character of a profession. Throughout history, special honor has been bestowed upon individuals who possess wisdom or great knowledge. The notion of collective knowledge associated with a particular group has been a consistent theme throughout human history. The idea of a group with specialized knowledge becoming a profession emerged from the association of a particular arena of knowledge with a specific kind of practice (Bennet & Bennet, 2004). Professions were identified not only for having great knowledge but also for doing something important with that knowledge that made a difference in the world. The practice or the use of particular specialized knowledge is generally associated with the emergence of professions.

Professional Work Is Knowledge Work

The central role of knowledge is critical to the existence of professions. In fact, knowledge is one of the characteristics that is an identifier or distinguishing feature that separates professions from other work groups. A central assumption of any profession is that learning within a unique body of knowledge must take place before a person becomes a member of the profession. This body of knowledge is specific and unique to the profession and is sanctioned by the formal profession as the foundation of the expression of its work in the world. All members of the

Reflective Questions

Reflective questions, found throughout the text, prompt students to stop and reflect on what they have learned.

Critical Thoughts

Critical thought boxes, found throughout the text, summarize and expand upon what students have read.

CRITICAL THOUGHT

Leadership is about more than just changing things; it is about changing the world.

Although the political process within which transformation unfolds is noisy, messy, competitive, and challenging to work through, people of every political stripe recognize that the old system is no longer viable or relevant for the future. The design, structuring, funding, and operation of the transformed system will go through many iterations as we struggle to determine what works and what is sustainably effective. Along the way, the changes in the healthcare system will be clarified and validated through the process of experimentation, application, and evaluation.

Much of the effort to move toward a transformed generative healthcare model involves creating a system whose foundation is grounded in general access, service synthesis, critical health impact, resource and service value, impact on sustainable social health, and research-based evidence. Each of these small components of the broader dynamic shift in health care will transform the way in which the healthcare system is organized and structured and, ultimately, the way healthcare services are delivered. Although broad disagreement exists as to which strategies would best achieve this outcome, the effort to move toward that goal is clearly under way.

As the healthcare system works to recalibrate itself in a way that supports a more viable and relevant future, every clinical professional will play a role in and has a stake in both the process and the outcome of this change. Changing service means adjusting the structure needed to support that service. Building access and equity into the service framework requires that every professional role incorporate equity, ownership, and engagement as an interdisciplinary design emerges. Indeed, interprofessional teamwork will serve as one of the nonnegotiable elements that underpins all efforts at building truly effective, value-based health care (Pauly, 2010) **(Figure 9-1)**.

The structures that will best support this effort and the role characteristics of healthcare leadership that will guide its implementation focus on role clarity, autonomy with integration, professional team-based performance, shared decision making, and the means to ensure that the clinical work is resource effective, timely, value based, and works to advance the mission and vision of the healthcare system. Good clinical structure requires that leaders establish an expectation that evaluation will be ongoing, work will be continuously modified based

SCENARIO

Jane Thorton, RN, BSN, had worked on the neurology unit at Angel Hospital for a year. She was generally satisfied with her experience and had grown a great deal in terms of her clinical expertise and practice. Jane had established good relations with her colleagues and with the management of the organization and was very well liked by both. While her patients were complex, Jane had learned a great deal about care of patients with neurological concerns; she had recently successfully taken her neurological specialty examination and was certified as a neurological nurse.

Jane had taken on a number of responsibilities related to planning and improving nursing care and had agreed to participate in activities that would strengthen the evidence-based practice approach to policy and protocol development on the nursing unit. She and some of her colleagues were having a difficult time in getting general participation from other staff in these clinical activities on the unit, even though the activities were designed to improve and advance patient care. Jane had approached the manager a few times asking for support in getting more participation in clinical nursing leadership activities, but the response remained minimal on the unit.

While reviewing articles in one of her nursing journals, Jane came across an article on implementing nursing shared governance in a hospital similar to hers. The article outlined some of the challenges and processes associated with successfully implementing shared governance approaches in the hospital. Jane was especially intrigued with how empowering the staff by allocating accountability for decisions and actions had improved staff satisfaction, quality of care, and patient outcomes. The hospital that implemented this shared governance model had subsequently received Magnet recognition and presented itself as a hospital of excellence because of the exemplary work of the nursing staff.

Jane was excited and wanted to bring shared governance to Angel Hospital. But where to start? Jane realized that shared governance was a structural model that led to empowerment of the staff, increased the staff authority and accountability for decisions that affected practice, raised the professional character and behavior of the nursing staff, and

Scenarios

Scenarios in each chapter prompt students to critically apply their new knowledge to real-life situations.

CHAPTER TEST QUESTIONS

Licensure exam categories: Management of care: advocacy, evidence-based practice, professionalism, concepts of management, ethical practice

Nurse leader exam categories: Knowledge of the healthcare environment: governance; Professionalism: personal and professional accountability, ethics, advocacy

1. Nursing is a fully mature and adult profession now reflecting all of the particular characteristics of professional delineation. True or false?

2. Professionals act predominantly on principle, not simply based on their knowledge, reflecting a belief that principle drives knowledge. True or false?

3. Evidence-based practice is grounded in good policy and reflects inconsistent standardization and procedures. True or false?

4. The *Code of Ethics for Nurses* serves as a foundation for the exercise of nursing practice. True or false?

5. Shared governance is a voluntary process that invites staff to participate in decisions that affect patient care. True or false?

6. Very few professional decisions are made at the point of service or in the patient environment. Most decisions influencing nursing practice in shared governance should be made away from the patient care setting. True or false?

7. All staff must participate in shared governance activities. True or false?

8. For a professional, the identification of the profession becomes a part of personal identity such that it is impossible to separate the person from the profession. True or false?

9. Language is not nearly as important as action is. The way in which a nurse acts is the most important indicator of who the nurse is. True or false?

Chapter Tests

Review key concepts with these questions at the end of each chapter. Tests questions are linked to national licensure test categories and national leadership certification exam categories.

THIRD EDITION

Leadership in Nursing Practice

Changing the Landscape of Health Care

Dan Weberg,
PhD, MHI, BSN, RN

Kaiser Permanente
The Ohio State University

Kara Mangold,
DNP, RN-BC, CCTN, CNE

Mayo Clinic
Arizona State University

Tim Porter-O'Grady,
DM, EdD, APRN, FAAN, FAACWS

TPOG Associates, Inc.
Emory University

Kathy Malloch,
PhD, MBA, RN, FAAN

KMLS, LLC
Arizona State University
The Ohio State University

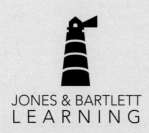

JONES & BARTLETT
LEARNING

World Headquarters
Jones & Bartlett Learning
5 Wall Street
Burlington, MA 01803
978-443-5000
info@jblearning.com
www.jblearning.com

Jones & Bartlett Learning books and products are available through most bookstores and online booksellers. To contact Jones & Bartlett Learning directly, call 800-832-0034, fax 978-443-8000, or visit our website, www.jblearning.com.

Substantial discounts on bulk quantities of Jones & Bartlett Learning publications are available to corporations, professional associations, and other qualified organizations. For details and specific discount information, contact the special sales department at Jones & Bartlett Learning via the above contact information or send an email to specialsales@jblearning.com.

14813-8

Production Credits

VP, Product Management: David D. Cella
Product Manager: Rebecca Stephenson
Product Assistant: Christina Freitas
Associate Production Editor: Alex Schab
Senior Marketing Manager: Jennifer Scherzay
Production Services Manager: Colleen Lamy
Product Fulfillment Manager: Wendy Kilborn
Composition: S4Carlisle Publishing Services
Cover Design: Kristin E. Parker
Rights & Media Specialist: Wes DeShano
Media Development Editor: Troy Liston
Cover Image (Title Page, Part Opener, Chapter Opener): © Rawpixel.com/Shutterstock
Printing and Binding: LSC Communications
Cover Printing: LSC Communications

Library of Congress Cataloging-in-Publication Data
Names: Porter-O'Grady, Timothy, author. | Weberg, Daniel Robert, author. | Mangold, Kara, author. | Malloch, Kathy, author.
Title: Leadership in nursing practice : changing the landscape of health care / Daniel Weberg, Kara Mangold, Tim Porter-O'Grady, and Kathy Malloch.
Description: Third. | Burlington, Massachusetts : Jones & Bartlett Learning, [2019] | Tim Porter-O'Grady's name appears first in previous edition. | Includes bibliographical references and index.
Identifiers: LCCN 2017044948 | ISBN 9781284146530
Subjects: | MESH: Nurse Administrators | Leadership | Nursing--organization & administration | Professional Competence
Classification: LCC RT89 | NLM WY 105 | DDC 610.73068--dc23
LC record available at https://lccn.loc.gov/2017044948

6048

Printed in the United States of America
22 21 20 19 18 10 9 8 7 6 5 4 3 2 1

Contents

Chapter 1: Change and Innovation

Chapter 2: Becoming a Professional Nurse

Chapter 3: The Person of the Leader: The Capacity to Lead

Chapter 4: Conflict Skills for Clinical Leaders

Chapter 5: Staffing, Scheduling, and Patient Care Assignments: Models, Components, and Measures of Effectiveness

Chapter 6: Principles of Ethical Decision Making

Chapter 7: Leadership: The Foundation of Practice Partnership

Chapter 8: Resources for Healthcare Excellence

Chapter 9: Navigating the Care Network: Creating the Context for Professional Practice

Chapter 10: Managing Your Career: A Lifetime of Opportunities and Obligations

Chapter 11: Policy, Legislation, Licensing, and Professional Nurse Roles

Chapter 12: Delegation and Supervision: Essential Foundations for Practice

Chapter 13: Overcoming the Uneven Table: Negotiating the White Waters of the Profession

Chapter 14: Accountability and Ownership: The Centerpiece of Professional Practice

Chapter 15: Integrating Learning: Applying the Practices of Leadership

New To This Edition

Leadership in Nursing Practice: Changing the Landscape of Health Care, Third Edition drives comprehension through various strategies that meet the needs of adult learners while also generating enthusiasm about the topic. This interactive approach addresses different learning styles, making this the ideal text to ensure mastery of key concepts. The pedagogical aids in this text are relevant to practice, experiential in nature, and engage problem-solving tactics. The organization of this text provides learners with content that is immediately relevant and applicable. New to this edition, we have linked the content within the chapters to exam categories for both initial licensure examinations and leadership certification.

Contributors

Dan Weberg, PhD, MHI, BSN, RN
Senior Director, Innovation and Leadership
Kaiser Permanente
Oakland, California
Associate Faculty
The Ohio State University College of Nursing
Columbus, Ohio
Clinical Assistant Professor, Leadership, Innovation, Interprofessional
Practice
Kaiser Permanente School of Medicine
Pasadena, California

Kara Mangold, DNP, RN-BC, CCTN, CNE
Nursing Education Specialist
Mayo Clinic
Phoenix, Arizona
Faculty
College of Nursing and Health Innovation
Arizona State University
Phoenix, Arizona

Tim Porter-O'Grady, DM, EdD, APRN, FAAN, FAACWS
Senior Partner, Health Systems
TPOG Associates, Inc.
Atlanta, GA
Clinical Professor
School of Nursing
Emory University
Atlanta, GA
Board Chair
American Nurses Foundation
Washington, DC
WOCNC Board Certified Wound Specialist
(GCNS-BC, NEA-BC, CWCN, CFCN)

Kathy Malloch, PhD, MBA, RN, FAAN
President, KMLS, LLC
Glendale, Arizona
Professor of Practice
College of Nursing and Health Innovation
Arizona State University
Phoenix, Arizona
Clinical Professor
College of Nursing
The Ohio State University
Columbus, Ohio
Hartford, Wisconsin

Foreword

I have taught courses in professional issues and leadership to prelicensure students in schools of nursing in both the United States and Canada for more than a decade. The content in these courses tends to be broad. Normally, around a dozen topics are tackled, touching on a few major themes related to the idea of nurses being citizens of their work groups, organizations, professions, and societies. It is a bit of a flyover, because whole courses could be devoted to nearly every topic. Many students start off the semester a little apathetic or even suspicious of the material; by the end, nearly everyone is clear that the course content is essential to their career success. And with good reason: On the surface, many of the topics are "high level" abstractions, but scratch beneath that surface and it becomes obvious that the themes in such courses permeate day-to-day life in healthcare settings and that an understanding of them is critical to making the most of jobs and careers in nursing, whether a titled manager or not.

Healthcare systems around the world are facing financial constraints, demographic upheavals, rising public expectations and fears, and overwhelming evidence in terms of population health measures and assessments of quality and safety of services that the status quo in health care is both unsustainable and unacceptable. Today's nurses, nursing students, and nurse educators are working in an environment that is changing much faster and in so many ways that few could have imagined even a mere decade ago—and those changes keep coming. Never has there been a greater need for nurses who have clear professional identities and the necessary habits of mind to work with colleagues and leaders in steering and reinventing health care in their communities.

What tends to help senior students make the leap to becoming well-informed, accountable professionals is a text written with a clear vision and voice that serves as a guide to new terminology and approaches to thinking about nursing work and its organizational contexts. For the diverse student body coming into nursing these days, the approach must be straightforward but challenging, clear but not oversimplified. Fantastic articles are written every year in many disciplines that touch on the core ideas in these courses, new ways of thinking about them, and current developments in the practice. Some appear in the nursing literature, while others are written in related fields. Few, however, are targeted at upper-level nursing students, and selecting and assembling them into a coherent package—let alone an up-to-date one—is a task beyond most instructors' time and resources. Moreover, while many textbooks introduce leadership and management concepts for a variety of other purposes or attempt to ease the transition of students from apprentice to professional on a very concrete plane, no texts have been written at a consistently high level, without condescension, and geared toward helping students adopt a mature professional outlook. The authors have prepared exactly such a resource.

This text will challenge and provoke. It asserts nursing's rightful legacies of social justice and service, but does not airbrush some of the past failures of nurses to assume accountability as individuals, as leaders, or as a profession. Nevertheless, the approach is forward looking and the tone is heartening and hopeful. It will help nurses, especially ones who are early in their careers, realize that leadership is their business no matter where they work now or will work in the future, and that taking social and historical context into account is critical to understanding the present and building the future of nursing. Equally vitally, it clearly shows new nurses how they are partners in the settings where they practice who need to take charge of their professional lives and engage in the improvement of their organizations as a matter of duty, rather than expecting personalized invitations to do so.

An introduction to some of the freshest and best ideas in nursing and healthcare management and leadership, prepared by some of the leading minds in our field, is in your hands. Whether you are reading it as a newcomer to the profession, picking it up later in your career, or reviewing it to prepare for guiding others into their roles as nurses, you are in for a treat. Anchored in a sense of nursing as a professional practice discipline, the authors are about to guide you through clear discussions of teamwork, leadership, staffing, and a host of other core topics. You are sure to walk away with many new ways of talking and thinking about nursing and for contributing to the future of health care.

Sean P. Clarke, PhD, RN, FAAN
Associate Dean for Undergraduate Programs and Professor, William
F. Connell School of Nursing, Boston College, Boston, Massachusetts

Preface

We are excited to offer our nursing professional leadership colleagues this newly revised *Third Edition*. We've considered this important work done on behalf of our colleagues who are leading nursing practice in the wide variety of settings where nurses work. We have worked diligently to focus this text on the vast majority of clinical nurses who do not seek to travel a management pathway yet provide leadership in any number of ways within the context of their practice. In a time of great change in health care, the critical role of the nurse leader in the practice setting is becoming increasingly clear. New models of service delivery and a growing and strengthening relationship exemplified in transdisciplinary clinical teams and the accelerating engagement of the consumer of health care in healthcare decision-making and action serve as evidence of this significant change. As a result, every professional nurse needs to be exposed to the basic concepts of leadership as applied to team-based clinical practice and to be able to provide feedback on the potential quality and effectiveness of new ideas. If such practice is to be successful and nurses are to continue to coordinate, integrate, and facilitate the continuum of health services, leadership competence is a must, and it is to those nurses that this text is directed.

We need nurses as point-of-care leaders to engage in not only the work of patient care but also the evaluation of current practices and creation of improved practices that better meet the needs of the future. New approaches to on-the-job training, new rationale for promotion for clinical competence, and digitally sound leadership development resources are essential for progress and to avoid setting health care back in its ability to adapt quickly to change. The third edition of this text is meant to provide the foundations for academia and professional organizations to facilitate the development of nurses as leaders to quickly and effectively meet the needs for the future.

The passion for this text is driven by our desire for nurses to be the best they can be and from our observations of the impact of dysfunctional or uninformed leadership behaviors. We have seen the turnover, the stress, and the care impacts that occur when leading without a foundation in the evidence. This text is an attempt to provide the critical information to better lead health care differently at the bedside and in leadership positions. This text is focused on you! As a learner, as a leader, and as a nurse.

No text can cover the vastness that is leadership, so we focused on providing you with the most impactful and relevant concepts on the topic with an eye toward application. We feel very strongly that the reader should be able to approach any chapter of this book and instantly apply what is learned to his or her work. Applying these concepts to nurses' work will enhance the ability to be a clinical leader.

Management is the application of known solutions to known problems. This is not a management text. This textbook and associated resources are meant to provide frameworks, concepts, critical thoughts, and evidence to support the behaviors of leading. Leading is the ability to create solutions to unknown and unpredictable situations. This is a leadership text.

While our work is necessarily incomplete, in this *Third Edition* we have provided the essential and foundational leadership skills necessary to thrive in a complex clinical environment. Some of the concepts covered here are simple and straightforward; others are as complex as the systems within which nurses will practice and lead. Both levels of understanding will be necessary for clinical leaders to thrive. Learning leadership content has no value if it cannot be successfully incorporated into patterns of behavior that have a meaningful impact on everyday practice. At the same time, leadership learning must challenge current thinking and confront leadership notions, practices, and behaviors that do not reflect the science and lead to expressions that may not be appropriate or effective. As leadership knowledge changes, so must leadership practices.

The chapters in this text purposely focus on foundational concepts, elements, and practices of contemporary leadership. In particular, principles of complexity leadership have guided the development of much of the content of this text. Both teachers and learners must grapple with an emerging knowledge base related to the leadership of complex systems if the expression of leadership practices is to be viable and relevant. In this text, contemporary understanding of the complexity of organizational cultures is used as a contextual framework for the discussion of leadership in each chapter. The emerging "complexity leader" must recognize that the leadership of organizations, systems, and the ways in which people work in networks and communities of practice is different from our previous understanding of the leader's role. With these newer concepts influencing complex organizational clinical and work networks, the leader applies a new framework to the expression of the leadership role. This understanding forms the backdrop of the content of each of the chapters in this text.

At the same time, it is important to integrate the obligations of the profession with the actions of the professional. Professions are a social mandate and address a significant social need. There is no greater social trust than that of nurses for the communities they serve and the health they advance. It is within this context of a social mandate that the professional nurse serves the health needs of the community. This understanding of nursing's social mandate provides the framework for meaning for each chapter. From discussion of the professional role to the incorporation of change and innovation and its application, focus remains firmly on the unique character of the professional nurse in the clinical setting. Chapters that explore foundational issues representing resource obligations provide an essential understanding of the operational mechanics of the systems within which the professional nurse will practice. Social issues related to the professional's obligation for ethical behavior and participation in policy and legislation affecting social health have also been addressed. Functional skills related to conflict, team-based leadership, negotiation, collective action, and personal relations all emphasize the individual's responsibility for effective professional behavior and relations. Given that professional practice is a lifelong pursuit, issues related to role accountability, career management, and the personal leadership learning journey have been particularly highlighted. The final chapter attempts to collate and synthesize the leadership information covered in each of the preceding chapters in a way that provides linkage and integration of leadership learning.

The content of the chapters and the learning associated with this text includes contemporary notions of development and learning practices. Relevant questions, scenarios, and online resources have all been developed in support of the learning activities associated with the leadership concepts of this text. The student of leadership is encouraged to use the full multimodal learning applications associated with this text as an opportunity to facilitate personal development and to translate concepts into leadership practices. Each of these tools reinforces learning and provides opportunities for leadership practice and personal expression of leadership skills.

Finally, this edition serves as an exemplar of the activities associated with transitioning and handing off professional work. Kathy Malloch and Tim Porter-O'Grady, the originators of this text, are in the midst of personal transition and life changes. At this point in their careers, timing and opportunity for career change, personal transition, and handing off converge. It is in this spirit of succession that Kara Mangold and Dan Weberg now become the lead authors of this text, representing that next generation of scholars and leaders continuing the tradition of strong and effective leadership and pushing the boundaries leading to new concepts and applications of leadership. This work is in good hands.

As always, the authors acknowledge that this text is a work in progress. Learning material and support associated with this *Third Edition* will be continually refined and developed, as will the content of each of the chapters during future additions, refinements, and revisions. In addition, we encourage the reader to use a wide variety of leadership learning resources to supplement the foundations laid in this text. As we are all part of the leadership learning journey, the authors likewise expect to grow and develop, with their evolution being influenced by students of leadership and other readers who challenge our own thinking and writing and participate in the improvement and advancement of leadership learning. In the final analysis, it is our hope that through this work, we will contribute in a small way to the development of future leaders in a way that provides a growing assurance of the maturation of nursing as a profession and its impact in making a difference in the health and lives of the people we serve.

Dan Weberg
Kara Mangold
Tim Porter-O'Grady
Kathy Malloch

Acknowledgments

My life and career would have never happened without the mentorship of Tim and Kathy. They have been gracious leaders, tough teachers, and amazing mentors in my journey through nursing and health care. Thank you for the opportunities. To my wife Kim and son Parker, who put up with my writing on weekends and my shenanigans in between. And to my parents for their continual support and love.

This book is also dedicated to the disruptors. Those who dare to ask "why" and are willing to challenge the status quo. These Chief Disruption Officers are the ones who create the future and build the better. Stay focused and change the world.

Dan Weberg

The foundation of servant leadership has been ever-present in my life. Starting with my grandparents and parents (Mary and Wayne), values of learning, faith, hospitality, respect, and service have been pervasive. My three brothers (Matt, Tim, and Colin) have provided a legacy of commitment and spirit of consensus, compassion, and understanding. Coupled with my supportive extended family and friends (inclusive of my canine companion Shannon), a young girl who had the support to become anything she wanted to be chose to become a nurse.

As I traversed through my nursing career, I have had the guidance of mentors at the most pivotal times. To name a few: Sandy Hart, Ruth Hamilton, Kathy Zarling, Cindy Crockett, Kathy Kenny, Dorothy Bell, Bridget Tippins, and of course Kathy Malloch and Tim Porter-O'Grady. These individuals have lived leadership through example in their varying nursing practices and along with my nursing peers and patients have influenced me daily to promote the profession of nursing. I dedicate this book to those who integrate the art and science of nursing with innovation, authenticity, and vulnerability to advance health.

Kara Mangold

As always, I am thankful for the scholarship, colleagueship, and friendship of my coauthor Kathy Malloch. She continues to challenge my own leadership learning and role with her practical wisdom and applications and serves as a role model for the caring component of the good leader for me and the profession.

My thanks to my life partner and best friend of 38 years, Mark Ponder, RN, for his lifelong support of my own learning journey, the leadership of our practice, his tolerance for my times away in the work of the profession across the globe, and his personal modeling to me of living the experience of caring for self and others.

Finally, I want to express my appreciation to the many colleagues, mentors, learners, and partners who have advanced my own learning and growth as a person, professional nurse, and leader. They have made my lifelong journey an endless joy, challenge, and exploration that has enriched me in ways both understood and reflective of the mystery that drives learning. I am in deep debt for the many gifts they have given me.

Tim Porter-O'Grady

Working with Tim Porter-O'Grady is an incredible gift that life has given to me. Tim's dedication to nursing, excellence, and advancement of the profession continues to provide me with a beacon that never dims. Most of all, I am thankful for Tim's friendship as a kindred soul in this very complex world.

I am especially grateful to my husband Bryan for his unqualified support of me and the work I have chosen to do. As we celebrate our 25 years of marriage this year, I can only hope the next 25 years are equally special and rewarding.

Finally, leadership never occurs in isolation. This work would not have been possible without all of the very special friends and colleagues who have contributed to my journey of lifelong learning. I continue to be inspired by your accomplishments, your dedication to excellence in patient care, and your never-ending challenges.

Kathy Malloch

Reviewers

Sharon E. Beck, PhD, RN
Educational Consultant

A. Maria Fisk, DNP, APRN, BC
Professor of Nursing
Piedmont College
Demorest, Georgia

Therese A. Fitzpatrick, PhD, RN
Assistant Clinical Professor
Department of Health Systems Science
University of Illinois, Chicago
Chicago, Illinois

Roy A. Herron, RN, MSN
Adjunct Faculty
University of Texas, Brownsville
San Antonio, Texas

Vonnie Pattison, MSN, RN-BC
Assistant Professor
Montana State University, Northern
Havre, Montana

Georgianna M. Thomas, EdD, MSN, RN
University Lecturer
Governors State University
University Park, Illinois

I have an almost complete disregard of precedent, and a faith in the possibility of something better. It irritates me to be told how things have always been done. I defy the tyranny of precedent. I go for anything new that might improve the past. —Clara Barton

CHAPTER OBJECTIVES

Upon completion of this chapter, the reader will be able to do the following:

» Describe the nature of change and innovation in a complex environment.

» Compare and contrast principles of innovation and performance improvement.

» List techniques to assist in the development of change and innovation competence.

» Define the essential competencies and behaviors for effective change and innovation.

» Enumerate specific strategies to embrace change.

» Develop an understanding of the processes for overcoming obstacles to change and innovation.

» Identify the purpose and essential elements of a contemporary business case for advancing quality using change and innovation principles.

Change and Innovation

For this third edition of Leadership in Nursing Practice, the authors improved the focus on the leadership of innovation and added a discussion on the differences in leading innovation versus performance improvement in health systems. The ever-present demands and expectations for all healthcare workers to be fast, flexible, and effective now require knowledge of change and innovation as a core competency. Succeeding and making progress can occur only with an evidence-driven and passionate approach to improving the quality of the healthcare experience.

At some point in time, every nurse realizes that there are better ways to provide patient care, better policies to drive patient care, and better ways to organize and lead a patient care area. These new ideas are essential to improving quality and require changes to occur frequently—and often at warp speed. Not surprisingly, the result is sometimes chaos, including both positive and negative events. Improving the processes of patient care to improve outcomes is fundamental to quality patient care and requires skills in change management. What is also important for the clinical leader is to understand the rationale for and intended impact of change proposals and processes. Changes undertaken without a supporting rationale for improvement should be seriously questioned prior to their implementation.

This chapter focuses on the nature of change and innovation, along with strategies to embrace new ideas and overcome obstacles. The role of the clinical leader in understanding the dynamics of change and innovation, as well as developing skills to challenge assumptions of practice, use innovation techniques, and communicate recommendations for improvements are discussed.

Change and innovation are widely used concepts in all sorts of industries, and these terms are often used interchangeably. Numerous descriptions and definitions of both change and innovation exist and further confound the process of gaining clarity between the two concepts. The term **innovation**, rather than *change*, is often used to gain attention and imply that something new and special is happening. One of the reasons there are significant variations in the descriptions of change and innovation can be attributed to the various underlying assumptions about the nature of change (Weberg, 2009).

Many individuals fear change and are reluctant to challenge assumptions and try something different, particularly in the work setting. A smaller number of individuals embrace change as normative and as an opportunity for new and better ways of being. What is important to remember, regardless of one's comfort with change, is that change is ever present and an inevitable attribute of being alive. There is no escaping change—except for death! Thus it makes good and prudent sense to learn as much as one can about the nature of change, including how to embrace it and how to maximize positive changes.

Most individuals and organizations see change and/or innovation as a linear process that can be managed and controlled. This perspective—that is, the view of change as a linear phenomenon—guides the processes and decisions of traditional organizations. With this perspective, it is believed that a change in one area will result in a predictable change in another specific area. It is this linear cause-and-effect assumption that most of our change processes and expectations are built upon.

Project management processes are an example of linear change that focus on predictability, equilibrium, and linear evolution while limiting flexibility, variation, and creativity so as to accomplish the goals of the change project. With this approach, deviations from the plan are viewed negatively, and the next steps focus on elimination of variances. While a linear process is helpful in providing order and structure for change processes, it also places limits on these processes.

REFLECTIVE QUESTION

Change can be considered either as a predictable linear process or as a complex, highly interrelated process. Are there advantages inherent in each view? Are there times when one approach is more or less useful? Consider a recent change in which a new policy, process, or protocol was implemented. Was the process linear or complex? Describe the areas of success and the areas identified for improvement.

Linear change does not recognize the multiple, unanticipated human actions and communications that occur and the dynamic context in which the change is occurring. As a consequence, the linear perspective often becomes rigid, control-driven, frustrating, and unsuccessful. While a project may be brought to completion, new issues and challenges emerge quickly. These unanticipated events are often viewed negatively and categorized as project shortcomings when, in fact, such events are normative and are the evolving results of complex human dynamics.

Another perspective from which to view change and innovation relies on complexity science (Fonseca, 2002). Complexity science understands the world as a dynamic phenomenon in which movement is continual and unpredictable. The world is in continual motion, and movement occurs in more than linear ways. A change in one area can result in numerous, unanticipated changes in areas not considered. As one individual or a group of individuals interacts with others, numerous actions occur spontaneously as ideas are shared and information is considered. The movement does not cease with the one interaction; instead, it continues to spread from one individual to another and so on. Interactions in a complexity perspective are characterized by creativity, interdependence, unpredictability, and collective knowledge. Change in the healthcare environment is better understood from a complexity paradigm rather than a linear paradigm, because the nature of change in this setting is seldom linear and controllable and involves and affects many individuals at many times in numerous ways. See **Box 1-1** for some common myths about change.

Dynamics of Change and Innovation

The linear and complexity perspectives of change and innovation reflect two differing dynamics underlying change processes: One is linear, while the other is highly interrelated and unpredictable. Descriptions of change and innovation are presented in **Box 1-2**.

Change has been described as an alteration of the current state. Innovation is defined as a unique type of change in which there is a novel and dramatic change that fundamentally restructures the deep social and economic value of an organization (Davidson, Weberg, Porter-O'Grady, & Malloch, 2017). Change is considered normative in a complex system, whereas it is something to be managed, controlled, and minimized in a linear system.

Innovation Versus Performance Improvement

As discussed, change processes take many forms. In health care, there is a strong attraction to the use of two methodologies, innovation and **performance improvement**. Clinical leaders should understand the difference between the two to best use the correct tool for the correct change outcome. Innovation and

BOX 1-1 MYTHS ABOUT CHANGE

- Change can be controlled. False. Change can only be facilitated; it cannot be stopped or harnessed.

- Change is painful. False. Not everyone is reluctant or resistant to change. Some individuals readily embrace change as normative and as a way of living to the fullest.

- Change is always chaotic. False. Change can be planned or unplanned. Planned change focuses on facilitating and managing the process to achieve optional outcomes.

- Strategic planning by a leader will decrease the chaos of change. False. Strategic plans serve as general guidelines that cannot by nature include all the possible outcomes.

- The environment does not affect a well-thought-out change process. False. The environment is dynamic and continually changing. Inevitably, changes in the environment, such as the economy, the climate, and political decisions, impact strategic plans.

- Change in a digital environment increases the ability of leaders to control processes and outcomes. False. The digital environment provides capacity for increased processing complexity; it does not identify which of the multiple interrelated interactions will occur, nor does a digital resource identify what will occur in the future.

performance improvement serve different purposes but are part of the same dynamic change process.

An organization needs both innovation activities and processes (it is plural in the next sentence) improvement activities to survive. Innovation efforts spark new ideas, process, and practices to be introduced into the organization, thus keeping the organization relevant in a changing environment. Performance improvement efforts refine ideas, processes, and practices to optimize them for excellence, thus making the organization more efficient and effective.

If an organization does not have innovation efforts or creates a culture that does not support innovation, then the organization will fail to keep up with changing needs of patients, employees, regulation, and technology. Even if it has a highly functioning improvement department, the organization can only optimize its current work and will eventually become irrelevant without the evolution caused by innovation. Organizations that only focus on innovation will have many new processes, but without the optimization of performance improvement, the process will remain inefficient, chaotic, and suboptimal.

BOX 1-2 CHANGE VERSUS INNOVATION

Change is . . .

- Something new or different.
- To make or become different.
- To alter; to make different; to cause to pass from one state to another, as to change the position, character, or appearance of a thing.
- To alter by substituting for something else, or by giving up for something else, as to change clothes, occupation, or one's intention.
- To give and take reciprocally with, or to exchange with, as to change places, hats, or money with another.

(*Webster's Dictionary*, 1991)

Innovation is . . .

- Anything that creates new resources, processes, or values or improves a company's existing resources, processes, or values (Christensen, Anthony, & Roth, 2004).
- The power to define the industry; the effort to create purposeful focused changed in an enterprise's economic or social potential (Drucker, 1985).
- The first practical, concrete implementation of an idea done in a way that brings broad-based extrinsic recognition to an individual or organization (Plsek, 1997).
- The slow process of accretion, building small insight upon interesting fact upon tried-and-true process.
- The new patterning of our experience of being together, as new meaning emerges from ordinary everyday work conversations; a challenging, exciting process of anticipating with others in the evolution of work (Fonseca, 2002).
- Doing new things that customers ultimately appreciate and value; not only developing new generations of products, service channels, and customer experiences but also conceiving new business processes and models (Cash, Earl, & Morison, 2008).

Clinical leaders should understand the different assumptions that drive innovation versus performance improvement to know what tool will work for the desired change and outcome. Innovation processes are founded on ideation, identifying the outliers, looking outside normal networks, and risk-taking. In essence, innovation processes look for the odd, the unrefined, and the chaotic patterns and embrace trial and error. On the other side of the dynamic, performance improvement is founded on the reduction of variation, the refinement of processes, the elimination of outliers, and the optimization of known work. Therefore, performance improvement will likely not spark radical change, and innovation may not optimize existing processes. Leaders should reflect on any perceived need for change and determine which processes would be best to achieve the desired outcome.

Understanding Change

As clinical nurse leaders embrace change, it is important to establish a common understanding of what is meant by change and innovation among team members and colleagues. Additionally, leaders and team members should be clear about the intentions of the change through the use of transparent information sharing. Poorly understood and communicated change processes only serve to start the rumor mill and disenfranchise potential innovation adopters. Clinical nurse leaders should work to perfect the communication of the who, how, and why of change. As professionals, it is our obligation to adapt our practice constantly to provide the best evidenced, safest, and relevant care. Resisting rational change conflicts with nursing's professional values and ethics.

Who, Why, What, When, and How of Change

The dynamics of change and innovation are best understood and advanced when several things are known. These include the key stakeholders of the work to be changed (who), the rationale for the change (why), the content to be changed (what), the timing for the change (when), and the techniques to change effectively (how) (**Figure 1-1**).

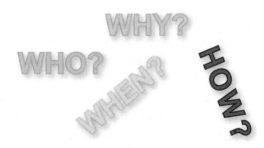

Figure 1-1 Change and Changing

Who Should Change?

Most individuals work to get others to change in hopes of improving processes and outcomes; this work is often futile and frustrating. It is nearly impossible to change or motivate others. While change is best accomplished by engagement of others to support the need and rationale for changing, the process always begins with the individual. Significant effort can be expended to create reminders, guidelines, and checklists for others that do little to advance the desired outcome. Indeed, the additional work of completing checklists may become an obstacle to change and decrease the emphasis on the real outcomes desired.

Becoming competent in understanding and thriving in today's rapidly changing world requires awareness of personal change abilities first. Individuals need to understand their personal comfort and competence with change. This understanding can be gained by first undertaking an assessment of strengths specific to the person's ability to identify critical issues for change, overcome obstacles, challenge assumptions, recognize areas for growth, provide meaningful feedback, and be resilient. The goal is for all individuals to clearly understand themselves before attempting to engage with others in advancing change in the areas of knowledge of the change process, personal comfort with change and risk-taking, relationships, conflict, and negotiation skills. When the individual's personal change competence is understood, the next step is to coach others in developing understanding and competence in change and innovation. Most importantly, the change and innovation facilitator must be comfortable with his or her personal limitations and recognize the reality that a person cannot possibly know everything there is to know about any one topic. It is the combined wisdom of the team that creates effective change. Leadership behaviors that support change and innovation emerge from multiple team members working together. There rarely is a case of a lone innovator effectively influencing entire systems. Change is a team sport.

Why Change?

Often the rationale for change is not clearly identified. When there is not a common consensus and rationale for change among the key stakeholders, the work of change can be resisted through avoidance, benign tolerance, or lack of attention. In our complex healthcare world with its limited resources, the rationale for change should be clearly linked to changes that would improve patient care outcomes and the quality of the healthcare experience. Specifically, change should be considered only when patient safety is enhanced, new evidence is available, excellence is advanced, or costs are controlled (Porter-O'Grady, 2014a, 2014b).

Change for Quality Outcomes

Value in health care is measured based on the outcomes achieved, not the volume of services delivered. Process measures, while helpful tactics, do not replace measurement of outcomes and cost. All too often, changes are made only in selected processes without logical connections to outcomes being identified. Improving processes without fully appreciating how they will change outcomes leads to misguided actions that seldom result in the desired positive change.

For example, the limited success of the national quality movement is a product of the linear process change approach. The focus on processes and completion of checklists has not impacted patient value or outcomes and continues to be problematic. In recognition of this disconnect, efforts have been made to increase the monitoring and documentation of the integration between process changes and outcomes achieved (Colevas & Rempe, 2011). Meanwhile, efforts to tightly link the desired outcomes of providing healthcare information to a patient, documentation of this process, and identifying the impact on patient health status as a result of the information are desperately needed and continue to challenge healthcare leaders. Nurses are encouraged to explore the Patient-Centered Outcomes Research Institute (PCORI) initiative to learn more about the significance of integrating patients' desired health outcomes into plans of care (Barksdale, Newhouse, & Miller, 2014). PCORI provides an evidence-driven foundation from which to determine if change is appropriate. Similarly, evidence-driven recommendations and resources are available from the federal government's Agency for Healthcare Research and Quality, including patient safety indicators appropriate for improving nursing quality (Zrelak et al., 2012). See **Box 1-3**.

As an exercise to explore these connections, consider the accompanying scenario and identify the needed linkages between processes and outcomes.

Change for Evidence

The need to implement new evidence or to meet newly identified needs of patients is driving much of current healthcare change. When there is a gap between current performance and desired performance in a facility or unit, using an evidence-based practice approach is the most logical. In an evidence-based model, patient care interventions are supported by evidence from a variety of sources and by differing strengths of research support. When there is a gap in the available evidence, patient care needs, and desired interventions, an opportunity can be identified for change and innovation to close that gap. Using the principles of evidence-based practice, linkages between clinical practice and scientific standards, the quest for consistency, minimizing idiosyncrasies, and providing a scientific basis for policy construction are the basic reasons for change in health care. Using an evidence-driven model serves to provide focus and organization of change initiatives; evidence-based practice is the platform for nurses' work. **Figure 1-2** illustrates the evidence-based practice process and the emerging gaps that provide a logical impetus for change and innovation (Porter-O'Grady & Malloch, 2010).

BOX 1-3 ONLINE RESOURCES FOR QUALITY EVALUATION

Comparative Effectiveness Research Database: https://www.nlm.nih.gov/hsrinfo/cer.html

Agency for Healthcare Research and Quality: www.ahrq.gov

Patient Safety and Quality: An Evidence-Based Handbook for Nurses: www.ahrq.gov/qual/nurseshdbk

Patient-Centered Outcomes Research Institute: www.pcori.org

National Quality Forum: www.qualityforum.org

National Patient Safety Foundation: www.npsf.org

National Institutes of Health: www.nih.gov

National Patient Advocate Foundation: www.npaf.org

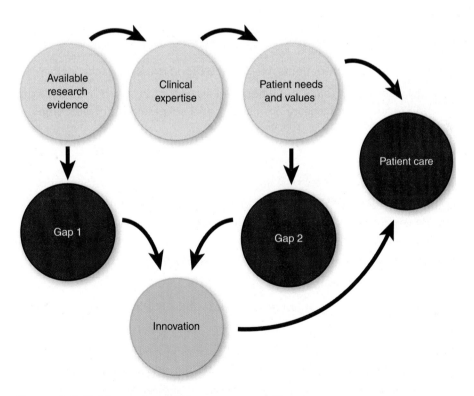

Figure 1-2 Evidence-based Processes and Gaps

SCENARIO

The following five initiatives are identified for all healthcare providers. Consider each initiative and discuss the potential patient outcomes that should occur as a result of the process changes. Discuss strategies to integrate this information into clinical processes to increase engagement of clinicians in monitoring these processes. Discuss alternative strategies to document and measure more meaningful processes to achieve improvements in patient functional health status.

Acute Myocardial Infarction

- Patients are able to take accurate 12-lead ECGs using their smartphones.
- Hospital emergency departments can see ECGs before patients arrive and can mobilize treatment teams faster.
- Primary percutaneous coronary intervention can be received within 90 minutes of the patient's arrival at the hospital.

Heart Failure

- Equip patients with digital scales and blood pressure cuffs that upload data to case managers.
- Remotely monitor patients' weight and blood pressure each week.
- Case managers reach out when vital signs trend toward unsafe ranges and reduce unnecessary admissions and adverse patient outcomes.

Pneumonia

- Assure populations receive pneumococcal vaccination.
- Collect blood cultures performed in the emergency department prior to initial antibiotic received in the hospital.
- Review initial antibiotic selection for community-associated pneumonia in an immunocompetent patient.
- Administer influenza vaccination consistently.
- Reduce healthcare-associated infections.
- Ensure prophylactic antibiotic received within one hour prior to surgical incision.

Surgeries

- Surgery teams can use CT scan images converted to 3D models to complete presurgery planning and reduce incision size.

- Surgery patients with recommended venous thromboembolism prophylaxis ordered.
- Surgery patients who received appropriate venous thromboembolism prophylaxis within 24 hours prior to surgery to 24 hours after surgery.

Hospital Consumer Assessment of Healthcare Providers and Systems (HCAHPS)

The following are nurse-sensitive indicators related to HCAHPS scoring of hospitals and health systems:

- Communication with nurses
- Responsiveness of hospital staff
- Pain management
- Communication about medicines
- Cleanliness and quietness of hospital environment
- Discharge information
- Overall rating of hospital

Data from *Federal Register*, 76(9), January 13, 2011.

Additional resource: Centers for Disease Control and Prevention, www.cdc.gov /stltpublichealth/strategy/index.html

Although there are many reasons for change and innovation, there are also reasons *not* to change, such as a lack of compelling evidence, no specific significant risk to patients and employees, isolated issues that are closely linked with individual performance rather than system performance, and indications that an intervention or change is more likely to be a fad of the moment rather than a solution that is closely linked to a probable outcome improvement. It is important to demonstrate courage by resisting the urge to move forward when the change is not appropriate for the conditions and the time.

What to Change

After a rationale for change—such as new information, patient safety, or increasing value—has been clearly established, the what of change can be determined. The what of change begins with the identification of the specific processes and policies that need to be changed, replaced, or created. In addition to specific processes or policies, relational competencies may need to be changed to fully support the transition to new processes. Specifically, individual attitudes toward the change, behaviors to support the change, an understanding of duplicate processes

CRITICAL THOUGHT

Evidence-based practice is the integration of the best research evidence with clinical expertise and clinical values. All innovation builds upon evidence and is rarely an "Aha" moment.

- *Best research evidence* refers to clinically relevant research, often from the basic health and medical sciences, but especially from patient-centered clinical research.
- *Clinical expertise* means the ability to use clinical skills and past experience to rapidly identify each patient's unique health state and diagnosis, individual risks and benefits of potential interventions, and personal values and expectations.
- *Patient values* refers to the unique preferences, concerns, and expectations that each patient brings to a clinical encounter and that must be integrated into clinical decisions if they are to serve the patient.

Reproduced from American Academy of Orthopaedic Surgeons, Evidence-Based Medicine Information, www.aaos.org/Research/. © American Academy of Orthopaedic Surgeons. Excerpted with permission.

CRITICAL THOUGHT

- *Research* is the systematic examination of an idea using rigorous principles of experimentation and measurement.
- *Research utilization* uses knowledge that is typically based on a single study.
- *Evidence-based practice* applies the relevant research and includes the expertise of the practitioner as well as patient preferences and values.

CRITICAL THOUGHT

Implementing the second-best idea now is a better strategy than doing the best thing a week from now. It is a bigger risk to delay making decisions than to make marginal ones.

that need to be eliminated, and the potential advancement of technology need to be identified as part of the desired change measures. To be sure, it is the changing of relational processes that is the most challenging aspect of this work.

When to Change

Several considerations arise in deciding when to change. When to change is best determined by taking into account the specific unit and system needs and resources. Although it has been said that timing is everything, sometimes the options for when to change are limited by the urgency of the situation. Some skeptics would ask if there is ever a good time to change or innovate.

In the healthcare environment, the pace and number of changes and new ideas for consideration are often overwhelming. Indeed, chaos is normative in health care. Given this fact, it is futile to continuously work to eliminate change or to wish for things to "stand still for just one minute." It is important not to try to eliminate all change and activity, because change is necessary for growth and sustainability of an organization. Most organizations are perpetually in the midst of change processes—new initiatives, new checklists, new electronic documentation systems, and so on. Learning to support staff with differing types of assignments with degrees of change activity provides a life skill useful in both work and personal settings. This change should occur when there is the greatest potential to positively impact outcomes with the desired individuals.

How to Change

Facilitating the change process involves much more than simply identifying what to do and when to do it. That is, facilitating change and innovation requires very specific competencies to fully engage others and advance the identified processes to achieve outcomes. The following competencies are essential for change effectiveness:

- Personal knowledge and accountability for one's own strengths and limitations specific to change and innovation, including technical capability and computer literacy
- Understanding the essence of change and innovation concepts as well as the tools of innovation
- The ability to collaborate and fully engage team members—that is, relational competencies
- Competence in embracing vulnerability and risk-taking

Personal Knowledge

Successful change and innovation agents develop a clear understanding of personal strengths specific to the work of facilitating change and innovation.

Previous experiences, the ability to overcome obstacles, engaging with others to elicit meaningful feedback, and courage and stamina to advance new ideas are all important to this effort. No one can be exceptionally competent in all areas of the change process; rather, the goal is to be comfortable in engaging and empowering team members to contribute their expertise. Thus the clinical leader needs to be comfortable in continuing to forge ahead and confront obstacles while recognizing that he or she cannot go it alone. The work of empowering others is a selfless process in which the work is always the focus and the individual facilitator becomes peripheral to the actual work.

Several assessment tools to identify communication, relationship, and conflict styles are quite useful in increasing personal understanding. For example, the Myers-Briggs (www.myersbriggs.org), DiSC profiles (www.thediscpersonalitytest.com), and Kilmann Conflict assessment tools (www.kilmann.com) are all assessment tools that can supplement self-understanding (Halvorson & Higgins, 2013).

Another important tool is peer-to-peer collegial assessment and coaching. Taking time with trusted colleagues to share feedback about communication, relationships, and conflict styles on a regular basis may, in fact, be more helpful than more formalized assessments.

Asking questions specific to behaviors supportive of change and innovation is vitally important. Examples of such questions include the following:

- Am I open to new ideas?
- Am I able to recognize my own personal limitations and understand that such limitations are reflections of reality and not of personal inadequacy?
- Am I able to clearly identify and share my strengths with others?
- Do I share my wisdom in a kind, caring, and nonthreatening manner?
- Do I trust that the motivations of others are basically goodwilled?

In contrast, asking colleagues questions specific to barriers that might impact one's ability to relate effectively with others can provide further insight into behaviors. Examples of such questions include the following:

- Can you tell me about times when I have displayed an attitude of aloofness or arrogance?
- Are there times when I always need to be right?
- Do I portray serious concern about losing control or that others are more competent than I am?
- Have I expressed fear that others might realize I do not know everything?
- Do my behaviors reflect a belief of personal immunity to anxiety, fatigue, and overwork?

Finally, personal knowledge is about understanding the expectations of a professional. Certain accountabilities, expectations, and contributions are important components of each professional and should continue to emerge throughout one's career. As a change and innovation agent, the professional nurse clearly understands that clinical practice autonomy does not imply independence. Rather, this concept focuses on practicing to the full extent of the nursing scope of practice and licensure in interdependent healthcare teams (**Box 1-4**).

Change and Innovation Knowledge

Specific knowledge about the concepts and theories of change and innovation is an essential tool for those engaged in the change process. For the nursing leader, ensuring one's own understanding of the diversity of descriptions and definitions of change and innovation is helpful in evaluating the understanding of others. Shared understandings of what change is and is not among team members serves to increase consensus and common understanding of the work being done. Finally, an understanding of the course of events in a typical change process further assists leaders in facilitating change (**Figure 1-3**).

BOX 1-4 REFLECTIONS ON PROFESSIONAL NURSING AUTONOMY

- Autonomous practice is a highly evolved clinical attribute.
- Leaders are visible, accessible, and able to communicate effectively with the staff to support decision-making processes.
- Staff leadership is about developing skills of coaching, risk-taking, and challenging the status quo.
- Leaders supporting autonomous practice are knowledgeable, strong, visionary risk takers. Their philosophy is clear and well articulated, and it guides day-to-day activities.
- A participative management style is pervasive, and staff feedback is not just welcomed but expected by leaders in making decisions about the work of patient care.
- Shared governance is a structure and process that embodies the principles of equity, partnership, accountability, and ownership, which are necessary for autonomy to flourish.
- Competent clinicians, with expertise as autonomous professionals, function most effectively in the context of a team of similarly competent professionals.

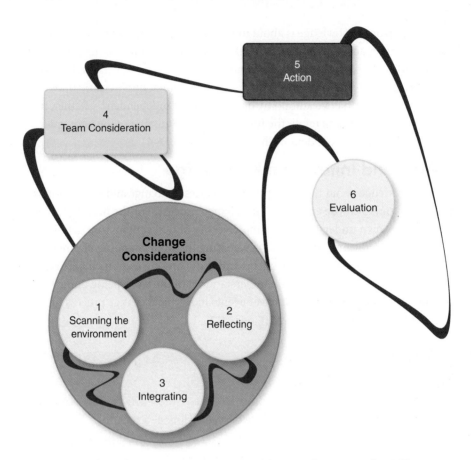

Figure 1-3 The Change Process: Essential Considerations for Effective Change and Innovation

In addition to understanding the concepts of change and innovation, basic knowledge of the tools and techniques that support change and innovation advancement is important. Tools such as **mind mapping**, brainstorming, **directed creativity**, construction of prototypes in innovation spaces, scenario planning, and **deep dive** experiences are helpful in engaging others and increasing the diversity and creativity of dialogue and change effectiveness (Endsley, 2010). See **Box 1-5**.

Collaboration

Working together effectively with wide ranges of diverse individuals is another important competency; it is necessary not only with the initiation and implementation of change but also for sustaining new processes and correcting the organization's course when appropriate. In health care, little change can be successful

BOX 1-5 SELECTED TOOLS TO ADVANCE CHANGE AND INNOVATION

Deep dive: A particular area is selected for observation in multiple ways. Workflows, photos, interviews, and observations are gathered by a team to analyze current processes and brainstorm new ways of doing the current work processes (Kelly, 2005).

Directed creativity: A situation is proposed to encourage and advance new ideas. For example, individuals are presented with the following scenario and are directed to respond: "A new unit is being designed for medical-surgical patients. If there were no limits on space, technology, resources, staff, or financial resources, how would you design the unit for the future in a way to dramatically improve the cost and quality of the healthcare experience?" (Plsek, 1997).

Mind mapping: A software tool for collecting, organizing, and synthesizing large amounts of data in layers with complex relationships. A very useful tool for documenting connectivity, interdependencies, and emerging phenomena in health care.

without the engagement of the interprofessional team. Too often, the upfront work of planning, designing, and implementing occurs with minimal challenges, and the efforts at fully integrating the new processes into the culture and operations become blurred, minimized, or marginalized. In the end, the intended change does not fully occur as planned, nor are the desired outcomes realized. Clinical nurse leaders should build change advisory teams that represent the end user of the change and that can support and challenge one another in the process. A team of blind supporters leads to failed innovation.

With the availability of digital communication, networks of communication have become critical for success (Battilana & Casciaro, 2013). Forming personal networks among colleagues—regardless of those individuals' power or position—reaching out to disconnected groups or individuals, and being close to those who are not fully committed are strategies that, when reinforced using social media, enhance the potential for success in implementing new ideas. It is the process of reaching out to multiple constituencies that increases involvement and enhances the potential for high levels of success and sustainability.

Collaboration among all team members or within a network provides the vehicle to improve numerous processes. The team becomes able to identify processes to be changed, the linkages between new processes and other organizational processes, the research evidence to support the change, technology to support the change process, anticipated policy changes needed, clear specification of the evaluation criteria, frequency of evaluation, and processes for course correction.

Embracing Vulnerability and Managing Risk

Often, change and innovation processes require individuals to take risks and to challenge long-standing status quo work processes and patterns within a strong culture. Risk-taking has not always been perceived as a positive leadership behavior, nor has it traditionally been welcomed and encouraged. Instead, risk-taking is often viewed negatively and as something that increases the organization's exposure to unforeseen hazards and to loss of net income and reputation. By comparison, playing it safe and being a hardworking employee is the more preferred behavior. The reality is that playing it safe will lead the organization nowhere; it encourages the organization and its employees to live in the past and to continue the practices that have been deemed to work yesterday, while ignoring what will work best in the future.

Taking risks in which the outcome is uncertain requires individuals to be comfortable with the reality that each person is indeed vulnerable; no one can be certain of the outcome when challenging the status quo. Despite the uncertainty and challenges encountered in day-to-day work when one takes risks, vulnerability can be a positive clinical characteristic that is vital for success. Further, the patient safety movement has created a paradoxical situation in health care: Standardization has been identified as a characteristic of high-reliability processes (Weick & Sutcliffe, 2001), yet the need to challenge long-standing processes that may not be as safe as previously believed is also a mandate.

Taking risks is inherent in healthcare work and requires skills to accept one's lack of total knowledge and develop rational risk-taking skills. Just as one uncertain situation is embraced and managed, another one is likely to appear. The feelings of vulnerability that accompany each risk-taking experience need to be recognized and

CALLOUT

Outside of health care, companies like Pixar Animations Studios, Google, and Zappos thrive on continually challenging their processes. In team meetings, individuals are incentivized to challenge assumptions and break apart processes to achieve excellence. Meeting leaders support and facilitate the process by focusing the discussion on the outcome of the change rather than on any one individual's idea. This facilitation helps remove the stigma that criticism is a personal attack and shifts the focus on achieving excellence together.

embraced willingly rather than avoided. Intentionally creating stressors in areas of vulnerability, either personal or organizational, helps build capacity and resilience for healthier functioning. (See Scenario box below.) Taking risks and acknowledging one's vulnerability is not about being irresponsible or incompetent, but rather about recognizing the reality of the ever-evolving and advancing world we live in.

Interestingly, there is no better person than the point-of-care clinical leader to identify opportunities for new ways of providing optimal patient care. The clinical leader understands the patient care need, the context in which the care is being provided, and the situations in which practices work well and do not work well. Thus the clinical leader needs to become an expert at identifying opportunities and engaging in rational risk-taking as a means to advance knowledge in the system.

Rational risk-taking is about taking risks for the right reason. Rational risk-taking is more than thrill-seeking and experience-enhancing; it is focused on and consistent with the organization's goals, values, and resources as well as consideration of others involved. This kind of risk-taking can be organized into four categories: advancing the organization, developing skills, mandatory reporting, and whistle-blowing.

Advancing the organization, the first category of rational risk-taking, is about learning to thrive and survive in the organization. Challenges in providing

SCENARIO

Trust implies that one individual is vulnerable to the actions of another. The greater the trust, the stronger the expectations are that individuals will consider others' intentions and actions based on established roles, relationships, experiences, and interdependencies.

Trust is one individual's willingness to be vulnerable to another based on the belief that the other person is competent, open, concerned, and reliable, thus rendering risk-taking more rational and realistic.

Discussion Questions

1. In a small group, discuss the level of trust among your work colleagues. Consider these topics: belief in others' promises, trust in the knowledge and data shared, and how you know when trust is lost.

2. Is there a relationship in which you can identify the behaviors that support trust and those that decrease trust levels?

3. How can you apply this information to your work team?

patient care, as well as the external introduction of new ideas, need to be considered carefully and regularly. New clinical interventions, new programs, expansion of existing services, selection of equipment, and prioritization (what comes first) are common challenges. Choices that are rational and minimize risk are those that are made on the basis of the organization's core values, respect for others, the safety of individuals, strategic goals, and available resources. The risk in proposing new ideas and challenges is that the new ideas might be rejected or dismissed. Learning to thoughtfully propose new ideas with a well-developed rationale at the right time is a basic requirement for all nurses.

Developing skills is the second rational risk-taking category. Regardless of their current competence levels, all individuals need to learn new skills to continue to be effective in the ever-changing healthcare environment. Acquiring new knowledge and skills that are rational includes learning skills specific to the job role and developing personal preferences to support the role in the most robust way. Considerations should be given to enhancing physical capability, computer skills, public speaking expertise, athletics, art, and personal protection skills. Each of these areas extends the competence and value of the individual caregiver and leader. The risk in developing new skills is that one might not be successful on the first attempt. Persistence, however, is the lifeblood of progress.

Developing teamwork expertise is vital in times of high risk and uncertainty. The greater the teamwork and support for creativity, the more new ideas that will emerge—and such ideas are ultimately the only way to accomplish this challenging and uncertain work. In addition, teamwork competence can be developed by reaching out beyond one's normal network of colleagues to others with related skills. Developing relationships beyond traditional healthcare disciplines can provide new insights and greater depth of understanding. High-functioning team collaboration also includes well-developed professional autonomy and interdependence to maximize each discipline's contribution to patient care.

The third category of rational risk-taking is mandatory reporting. Many state licensing agencies require licensees to report the unprofessional conduct of other licensees to the licensing board. The goal is to protect the public from licensees who commit repeated errors, who abuse alcohol or drug substances, or who are incompetent to do the entrusted work. Proponents of mandatory reporting believe other similarly licensed professionals are best able to identify such issues and, therefore, must speak up to protect the patient and the profession. According to most state statutes, it is not an option whether to speak up; in fact, failing to report known behaviors is itself considered an act of unprofessional conduct. Other examples of unprofessional conduct include repeated medication errors, boundary violations with patients, and theft from patients.

CRITICAL THOUGHT

Job security is truly a myth. No job is ever guaranteed forever—or even for the next month! Jobs are eliminated because of downsizing, the need for new skills, new locations, and different delivery model structures.

The workplace environment changes frequently, owing to new leaders, new colleagues, new work, and other developments. The goal for every individual is to always be employable—to always have the skills that are needed in the current and future environment.

Being employed is shortsighted; being employable is futuristic!

The fourth category of rational risk-taking is whistle-blowing. Whistle-blowing is about righting a wrong—a wrong that is believed to be dishonest and that has resulted in the mistreatment of others. The need for whistle-blower protection arises when the culture of the organization does not support open communication, honesty, differing opinions, and fairness. When individuals believe that they have not been heard on an issue and that the public interest is compromised, the federal False Claims Act provides a mechanism to report fraud and corruption while protecting those who expose information from wrongful dismissal and loss of security and benefits. Seeking the protection of this whistle-blower legislation is considered a rational and necessary risk and involves personal and professional risk, regardless of the outcome.

Embracing rational risks requires knowledge, skill, and engagement with the team to best support new ideas and changes. In contrast, avoiding irrational risks—also a learned skill—requires an understanding of the nature of irrational risks. Four categories of irrational risk are discussed next: a history of failure and oppression, poor judgment, unrealistic expectations, and lack of potential benefit for the action.

When there is a history of failed efforts, it is not prudent to attempt the same change unless new energy, new approaches, or new technology is available that would increase the potential for improvement and success. Often, education programs are provided to increase knowledge or compliance with desired practices, yet little improvement occurs. Continuing the same actions is futile without further examination of the situation and consideration of other options. Repeated notices, alerts, and education sessions to complete checklists, for example, are all poor uses of time and energy. Instead, the organization would be better served by exploring the reasons underlying the low compliance rates.

Poor judgment seems to be an obvious, irrational risk; however, it needs to be explicitly recognized. Consider the example of walking out into traffic. The risk of injury to both the pedestrian and those driving is present and probable. This type of irrational risk is similar to the leader who hires individuals without adequate depth and competence for hard-to-fill positions. It is only a matter of time until the inadequate job performance negatively impacts quality and productivity. As a result, the organization incurs additional cost and risk. When facing the challenge of a hard-to-fill position, the clinical leader must instead challenge the assumptions of that position and brainstorm other ways to consider the rational risk approach; he or she must assume some level of risk to advance the organization by creating a new role or developing another person's skills to meet the hard-to-fill position. This irrational approach further complicates a situation that is already overly complex and high risk.

Another irrational risk occurs when unrealistic expectations are embraced as the way to do business. Often, there is little potential for success when an organization attempts to implement "just one more" program or initiative in an environment in which staff are already overwhelmed. It is irrational to believe that such endeavors will be successful, even marginally.

When there is no known benefit from an action, the work can be considered an irrational risk of resources. Examples include planning education programs for which there is no audience, establishing committees for individual attendance when the work can be done electronically, and disciplining employees for outcomes over which they have no control.

In addition to rational and irrational risks, individuals often insert irrational negative fantasies into the discussion and decision-making processes for change and innovation. These negative fantasies can paralyze or hamper individuals from taking action. The irrational fears seem very real to some individuals, however, so they need to be challenged. Consider these comments and fill in the blanks:

- My dad will kill me if . . .
- I'll get fired if I say something . . .
- No one will like me if . . .
- The nurses will quit if . . .

Perhaps the most common negative fantasy in health care is the perception that one will be fired for taking risks and speaking up. Individuals worry that speaking up will have a negative impact on their reputation, their ability to communicate openly and honestly with others, and, ultimately, the security of their position. The reality is that individuals are seldom involuntarily removed from their jobs for speaking up and taking risks (see **Box 1-6**). Involuntary termination is more about incompetence, substance abuse, poor attendance, dishonesty—and *not* speaking up! Identifying and confronting negative fantasies can decrease barriers and resistance to change and innovation. See **Box 1-7**.

BOX 1-6 TAKING RISKS: TRUE AND FALSE

The more risks you take, the more secure your job is.

- This is true if with every risk, you are growing professionally and learning information that is helpful to both yourself and the organization.
- In an organization supportive of creativity and growth, this is certainly true. In a risk-averse organization, this is probably false.

The more risks you take, the greater the probability of being fired.

- This is true if taking risks compromises the organization's financial status and reputation when new approaches do not work.
- This is true in risk-averse organizations and false when rational risks are taken and the organization is supportive.

The more risks you take, the better the organization will be.

- This is true when each new attempt supports a culture dedicated to finding new and better ways to accomplish the work and more efficient ways of doing business that will increase the profitability and sustainability of the organization.
- This is false when risk-taking overshadows the ability of the organization to accomplish the work at hand. There is a need for balance between operations and stretching the limits of current processes.

BOX 1-7 CHECKLIST: DECREASING FEAR, INCREASING TRUST, AND UPWARD COMMUNICATION

- Have the right people been involved in making decisions? If not, identify who should be involved and why. Avoid the temptation to complain and mumble, "If they only had asked me."
- Are the goals and values of the organization being respected? If a decision does not seem consistent with the goals and values, take two actions. First, identify what specifically is not consistent with which value. Second, identify what you would like to see done to improve congruence with values.

(continued)

- Do not get lost in the process. If something is not working, then give it up—even if it means retreating and regrouping. Identify the fact that the work has drifted off course and a course correction is needed. It is too easy to lose sight of the original goal.

- Identify when work-arounds are created that avoid the real issue. New policies that add to all employees' workloads are often developed in response to isolated, aberrant behaviors. Challenge leaders to address the issue rather than creating another policy.

- When decisions are made on biased or impartial information, offer the additional information. Offer the information not to one-up another person, but for the purpose of achieving the best decision with all of the information.

Strategies to Minimize Risk in Change and Innovation Scenarios
Speak Up

The first strategy to minimize risk is to speak up with evidence or a rationale for action. The best safeguard to avoiding poor outcomes is using data, evidence, and a rationale. When there are significant variations in practice patterns, multiple opinions about the best solution, and little use of technology to validate the assumptions, focused communication is needed to determine the supporting evidence based on standards, experience, and values. To be sure, it is these conditions of uncertainty that precipitate evidence-based practice initiatives, thereby reducing the risks involved in attempting new strategies.

Timing and Tinkering

The second strategy is timing. As previously noted in the section on when to change or innovate, timing is always an important consideration. Not every risk needs to be or must be addressed immediately; sometimes waiting is the prudent approach. Levels of workload, the availability of key participants, and the overall climate of the organization need to be considered prior to taking risks. Classical leadership behavior encompasses strategic planning and the purposeful review of ideas. With the recent advances in information technology, however, these processes are becoming increasingly ineffective and outdated. The emphasis now includes short-term, incremental strategies that are similar to the concept of tinkering, introduced by Abramson (2000).

When this approach is embraced, tinkering becomes the expectation, the status quo—team members seriously challenge assumptions and ask questions, not out of idle curiosity but rather by looking carefully at current dogma and raising issues that open the door to substantial improvements. The values of tinkering include the following:

- It provides an opportunity to learn how to take risks.
- A little tinkering and a lot of team member experience allow a small group to make changes with big goals in mind and to evaluate the change efficiently.
- Team members' skills are stretched with little risk to the organization; support for constant tinkering minimizes the chance that the organization will drift into inertia. Rational risk becomes the norm, change is internalized as essential for survival, and employees benefit from new experiences and develop new skills.

Encourage Upward Communication

The third strategy to minimize the risk of change and innovation is about focused communication—that is, communication that gains the attention and support of decision makers. Top-down communication remains the most common type of communication in organizations today. By comparison, cultures with shared leadership structures reinforce and support vertical, horizontal, and multidirectional communication more effectively than traditional organizations; however, the need for upward communication remains a great need in organizations. Greater emphasis is needed to assure upward communication so leaders know what is going on in the organization and are able to support the best decisions.

The first step is to realize that leaders cannot and do not know everything; the second step is to learn to share the appropriate information—information that impacts the operations and reputation of the organization. Knowing which information to share and when to share it is a skill that evolves with experience and commitment to core values. Teams function based on the information they have available. The strongest tool clinical nurse leaders have is the way they gather, interpret, and craft the message related to information. This information flow can influence in powerful ways and begin to shift organizational culture.

Accelerate Personal Competence

The fourth strategy is to increase one's competence quickly as new equipment, technology, and processes become available. The more an individual can learn

CRITICAL THOUGHT

- Recognize that mistakes happen!
- Right the wrong as quickly as possible.
- Be sincere and apologize when appropriate.
- Use humor only when appropriate.
- Admit you were wrong—avoid the silent treatment.
- Do not try to rationalize and blame it on someone else.
- Say you are sorry when you are.
- Shake hands and make up!

about new approaches, the more competent that person is not only to evaluate the innovations, but also to determine if the new approach is right for the organization. Further, this approach reinforces evidence-based principles as the supportive rationale for change. Assuming a posture of risk avoidance and waiting for others to test and critique new approaches decreases the individual's ability to support an organization that stays on the cutting edge and is able to integrate processes and equipment into the work of patient care.

Further, competence can be developed by reaching out beyond the normal network of colleagues (boundary spanning) to others with related skills. Developing relationships beyond traditional healthcare disciplines can provide new insights and greater depth of understanding. Embracing environmental psychologists and human factors experts to assist in team collaboration and communication, for example, can greatly enrich work processes. Florists, musicians, and potters also give new meaning and understanding to the work of healing—and they serve to sustain the focus on healing and avoid the tendency to focus only on technology or publications.

Apologize with a Flair

The fifth strategy to minimize risk is to apologize quickly and appropriately when an error or misstep is recognized. Resiliency is the key. No patient ever expects to be harmed while under the care of a healer; further, no healer ever expects to harm a patient. Yet, unexpected events and deviations encountered in the provision of care do occur and injuries result. All healers will make mistakes, no matter how competent they are. The responsibility accepted by healers is indeed awesome, because patients entrust their care to them and give these caregivers enormous power and authority. It takes considerable spiritual and emotional

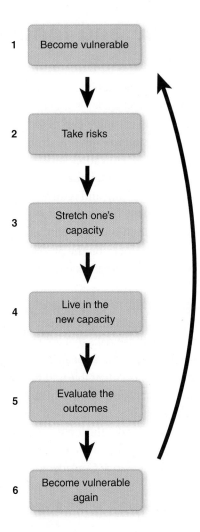

Figure 1-4 The Risk-taking Cycle

maturity to accept patient trust, understand that mistakes happen, and modify conditions when needed.

When a misstep occurs, leaders must be resilient and able to regroup and move on. Recognizing negative situations and acknowledging them with others can be therapeutic. Discussions of unsuccessful events provide an open forum in which to consider strategies to avoid similar situations in the future. It is far better to acknowledge the misstep than to ruminate endlessly. This approach avoids leaving others to wonder about the healthcare provider's competence and assists in putting everyone back on the right path (**Figure 1-4**).

Making Change and Innovation Happen

With a solid foundation in the dynamics of change and innovation, risks, and risk minimization strategies, the clinical leader is well positioned to move forward. Risk-disposed leaders develop a very high level of self-discipline that allows the processes of change and innovation to evolve. A strong sense of commitment can be more valuable than intelligence, education, luck, or talent. Clinical leaders who are adept at taking risks neither surrender nor overreact to crises or marginally successful efforts; instead, they regroup and return. They take stock of the situation, often pulling back temporarily (but not too long) while they plan their next steps. They realize that sometimes it is best to put aside personal feelings and let bygones be bygones. Finally, they focus on the present and the future, both of which offer perils and possibilities, rather than on the past, about which nothing can be done.

In the complex healthcare world, it is impossible to escape the reality of risk and the associated feelings of vulnerability. The goal for all clinicians is to examine each situation and embrace those risks that are rational and avoid or at least minimize risks that are believed to be irrational. This course of events usually begins with recognizing that one is vulnerable and then recognizes rational risks as a means to stretch one's capacity and ultimately move the work of the organization to greater quality and excellence.

Clinical leaders need to focus across the longer continuum of the change process using reflection, accountability measures, and persistence to ensure full engagement of the change. The "Change Considerations: Scanning, Reflecting, and Integrating" appendix provides specific interventions for the assessment, reflection, and integration phases of the change process. Each phase is discussed in the next section. The change process includes three major phases: assessment of the conditions, reflection with the team specific to the needed work to occur, and integration of information into a plan.

Assessment

Assessment and scanning the environment to determine current practice requires a level of consciousness that allows the leader to take in as much about the environment as possible. Data from multiple sources are involved in the activities of assessment. First and foremost, the leader must become skilled in sensing the environment, listening, and learning from the current activity. *Stilling one's mind* to be open to what is going on in the environment is essential in this process and requires discipline, practice, and commitment. To be sure, there is no template or format in which environmental scanning should occur. Each situation requires different considerations identified by the individual who best knows the organization and situation. The individual scans and assesses the environment based on previous experiences, knowledge of the current environment, and desired outcomes.

Team Reflection

The second phase is discussion with the key stakeholders about the change and innovation work. To begin the discussions, it is important to have the right individuals in the group. Team members should carefully reflect to be sure the needed stakeholders are present so the work can progress. It is equally important to exclude participants who do not add value to the processes of change and innovation.

After the environment is assessed, team members further consider past experiences, the potential impact on current events, and work to avoid negative experiences. Consideration is given to how individuals will react in new circumstances—positively or negatively. This understanding serves as critical background information in moving forward.

Integration of Ideas into a Plan

The third phase is to integrate the critical information learned in the assessment and reflection processes. The process of integration entails the assimilation of the data collected during the assessment and reflection phases—that is, all of the relevant research, values, perceptions, experiences, intuition, and the political, technological, economic, and social data. The ever-present challenge of this phase is developing skill in selecting which data to include and which data to exclude to effect the best decision. Out of necessity, effective integration is not an activity carried out by a single person; rather, full integration of work and efforts of all members of the group is required. To be sure, the preparation for change and innovation is as important as the actual work.

Integrating the data into a business plan template also provides guidance in building and documenting the rationale, plan, and expected outcomes for a change and innovation project.

REFLECTIVE QUESTION

Dare to move to a virtual world. How does one enmesh oneself in the world of technology and still retain the human touch? Moving aggressively to greater levels of technology is about advancing into uncharted territory.

Caveat: Technology, Change, and the Human Element

Much of the change in health care today involves the addition of new devices, software applications, and communication enhancements to advance the patient care experience. Clinical leaders should regularly ask what value these new technologies provide in improving patient care outcomes; in other words, they should recognize that the technology does not drive the work but rather supports the human work. Bell (2010) reminds us that when everything is digitized and connected, there can be neither stability nor genuine innovation. In particular, decisions still need to be made by humans rather than completely relegated to computer applications. The computer generates the data, and the clinical leader interprets the data within the specific patient care context.

Caveat: Measuring the Impact of Change and Innovation (What Problem Are You Fixing?)

In a world of scarce resources, the goal is to utilize resources appropriately with the expectation of success of the desired plan. In spite of the best projections and anticipated risks and benefits, precise and accurate projections of the costs of change and innovation projects are usually estimations—albeit estimates that must be constructed as carefully as possible. Creating a business case for innovation can be most helpful in identifying the many variables involved and many of the associated costs. A business case for change and innovation should become a standard practice when resources, efforts, and expertise will be expended (see **Box 1-8**). Clear and accurate business cases also provide essential information in prioritizing processes for change.

Another consideration is the challenge of benchmarking innovation work (see **Box 1-9**). Phillips (2011) identified the practice from the late 1980s through the 1990s of benchmarking against industry standards as an indication of performance compared to other companies. Interestingly, the relevance, value, and benefit of benchmarking were not determined. Benchmarking of innovation methods and processes across the industry may provide insights into practices, as well as differences in practices, which are equally important. Benchmarking of specific metrics does not provide similar value and direction.

Benchmarking innovations with other organizations is difficult for several reasons. The first reason is that innovation is closely tied to strategy and vision, which vary widely across organizations and make them difficult to compare. A second reason is that the time period over which the innovations were

BOX 1-8 BUSINESS CASE FOR INNOVATION: ESSENTIAL CONSIDERATIONS

1. Clear description of the product or service—work to be done
2. Purpose of the product or service—the goal to be accomplished
3. Projection of costs to begin and manage the project, including staff, equipment, and supplies
4. A list of costs not included and rationale for not including them
5. Estimation of benefits and evidence for the anticipated benefits
6. Timeline for development and launching of the project
7. Anticipated profit or loss for the first two years
8. Other qualitative benefits anticipated, such as community benefit, reputation, and satisfaction of staff and patients
9. Anticipated risks involved and plans to mediate the risks
10. Summary statement of short-term and long-term value to all stakeholders

Modified from Malloch, K. (2010). Innovation leadership: New perspectives for new work. *Nursing Clinics of North America, 45*(1), 1–10.

BOX 1-9 GUIDELINES FOR SELECTION OF INNOVATION METRICS

- Select metrics to assess innovation progress and costs in advance. Incremental benchmarks are especially important to track and trend progress. Different sets of funding, testing, and performance criteria for incremental, experimental, and potentially disruptive innovations are needed.
- Aim to identify early successes. Major initiatives often require significant time to realize the full benefits. Interim achievements are necessary to demonstrate progress and the likelihood of achieving the full potential of the innovation.
- Get data to back up your gut. Successful innovators begin with the gut feeling but then move quickly to develop the quantifiable, supporting data.

implemented can vary widely, from 90 days to several years. The third reason is specific to the assumptions about the customer or patient. The varying approaches to the driving force behind the innovation—namely, the company, the customer, or

SCENARIO

Often individuals state they are supportive and want to participate in change or changing; in the end, however, the change does not happen. Consider the following underlying assumptions documented by Kegan and Lahey (2001):

- Stated commitment: I want to be a team player.

- I am struggling with making this happen because I don't collaborate enough. I make unilateral decisions too often, and I really don't take people's ideas and input into account.

- Competing commitment: I am committed to being the one who gets the credit and to avoiding the frustration or conflict that comes with collaboration.

- Big underlying assumption: I assume that no one will appreciate me if I am not seen as the source of success; I assume nothing good will come of my being frustrated or in conflict.

Discussion Questions

1. Using your understanding of change and innovation, the process and dynamics, the strategies to manage resistance, and the tools of innovation, how could you and your team address this type of resistance?

2. More importantly, how could the team be proactive in minimizing the chance for this resistance in the planning phase?

the patient—provide different perspectives on consumer research and how it is integrated into the innovation work. Some believe that current customers or patients are not able to envision a radically new and better future; thus the practice of asking them to participate in the innovation process varies from organization to organization.

Managing Resistance to Change

In spite of the best preparation and planning, resistance to change and innovation occurs. In addition, the results of the anticipated change may not be optimal.

Resistance to change occurs in many formats, ranging from outspoken, verbal reactions to subtle, nonverbal, indirect avoidance of the issue. In general, individuals resist change when they perceive a threat to their safety and security or

LEADER TIP

Bringing resisters into the change process will help you understand differing viewpoints and may lead to further innovation. Leaders should know that bringing the resistant voice into the process can also derail the project if left unchecked, and leaders should plan to highly facilitate the meeting.

position. The culture of an organization or the leadership style can also impede change and innovation (Schein, 2004). Likewise, competing commitments have been identified as a source of resistance. Individuals may want to change, but other deep-seated factors may become barriers to change.

Understanding change theory can help leaders use the resistance to change as a support tool rather than a barrier. The diffusion of innovation model has been used thousands of times to study how change occurs in groups (Rogers, 2003). In any population there will be roughly 18% of people that will resist change while 82% of the population will adopt the change. Novice change leaders spend the majority of their energy and time trying to engage the 18% instead of creating a critical mass within the 82% that will eventually adopt the change. Resistance is also a point of information for the clinical leader. Resistance signals that there is disruption to the normal operating patterns of the team or organization. Not all resistance is negative. Clinical leaders should embrace the resistance, explore it, confront it, and engage it to learn how to improve the idea or process.

Course Correction

It is traditional to assign the label "failure" to those change and innovation projects that did not result in favorable outcomes. A new perspective that recognizes and values the information gained from such less-than-successful attempts is needed in health care. Embracing these situations as courageous acts that provide new insight and opportunities for further dialogue is congruent with cultures of excellence. When the less-than-optimal results are identified, the next step focuses on course correction and new attempts. The new knowledge gained from the unsuccessful effort is critical to continuing success; this information serves to inform others of a course of action that should not be repeated.

Documenting this information is essential in advancing change. Further, it is important to avoid individual employee sanctions when the outcomes involve the team and the supporting system. Punishing individuals for outcomes that involved many factors and many individuals is futile and demoralizing. Such punishment also discourages individuals from future risk-taking that could be of great benefit to the organization.

When there is an individual action of concern, remediation is the preferred option. Specifically, remediation is preferred when the potential risk of physical, emotional, or financial harm caused by the incident is low; the event is a singular event with no prior pattern of poor practice; and the individual exhibits a conscientious approach to, and accountability for, his or her practice and now appears to have the knowledge and skill to practice safely. Punitive actions are reserved for matters of last resort. These actions should be considered only when an individual has repeatedly disregarded advice and directions to modify actions, previous remediation attempts have failed, and there is evidence of incompetence that cannot be rectified.

SCENARIO

When the result is less than optimal, consider the following steps:

- Acknowledge the outcome.
- Correct negative outcomes quickly; ensure personal safety.
- Apologize to those affected by the outcome.
- Review the goal and the selected processes, and identify areas of vulnerability.
- Be sure the goals and work are still the right thing to do.
- Modify the processes to avoid further negative outcomes.
- Never be reluctant to abandon the goal if safe and effective processes cannot be determined.

Consider the scenario in which the goal is for all departments in an organization to use the SBAR (situation, background, action, recommendation) handoff method for lunch relief and shift change. Several departments, housekeeping, pharmacy, and behavioral health units are now refusing to use the SBAR process because they believe it is cumbersome and not helpful; omissions are still occurring and staff are dissatisfied.

Discussion Question

1. Which additional information do you need to determine if the SBAR should be continued or discontinued in these areas?

Leading and Managing

Clinical leaders need to be able to discern innovations that add value to the work and innovations that serve as obstacles to the work. Creating more work to streamline processes that ultimately decrease productivity and the timely achievement of quality outcomes is not a rational approach.

In times of high risk and uncertainty, the goal is to focus on effective communication through highly skilled teamwork. The greater the teamwork and the support for creativity, the more likely that new ideas will emerge as the only way to accomplish this challenging and uncertain work. Encouraging all members of the organization to share and develop their leadership skills requires passion and engagement in the richness of the collective decision-making process.

Looking to the future to support change and innovation requires a clinical leader mind-set that includes a strong personal awareness of one's strengths and vulnerability, openness to other ideas, courage to challenge the status quo, and a highly developed comfort with rational risk-taking. Innovation leadership is associated with the following characteristics:

- Self-aware
- Courageous, hopeful

CRITICAL THOUGHT

Innovation leadership is not about being an inventor; it is not about a specific leadership role. Instead, it is about envisioning a better future using the following behaviors:

- Looking outside one's immediate network (boundary spanning)
- Having the courage to challenge the status quo (risk-taking)
- Looking for resources in different places (leveraging opportunity)
- Facilitating and empowering others to be as creative as they can be (facilitation)
- Thoughtfully communicating information (coordinating information flow)
- Adapting one's work and behaviors to meet emerging needs (adaptation)
- Seeing a better future (visioning)

Modified from Weberg, D. (2016). Innovation leadership behaviors: Starting the complexity journey. In S. Davidson, D. Weberg, T. Porter-O'Grady, & K. Malloch (Eds.), *Leadership for evidence-based innovation in nursing and health professions* (1st ed., pp. 43-74). Burlington, MA: Jones & Bartlett Learning.

SCENARIO

A whistle-blower reported a nurse colleague for unethical practices. Another whistle-blower—a physician in the Veterans Administration system—reported administrators for unsafe patient care practices.

Discussion Questions

1. How do these actions qualify as rational risk?

2. Which information should be gleaned from these cases for other nurses?

- Proactive, future-oriented
- Inquisitive
- Optimistic
- Able to experiment, course correct, remediate

In contrast, management characteristics include the following:

- Focused on sustaining and strengthening the present
- Reactive
- Proof-driven
- Discipline/root cause-focused; blame-placing

Innovation leadership behaviors at the point of service are more important now than ever before as new ideas are introduced frequently and the demands for higher quality are emphasized. Shifting from a universal focus on sustaining current practices and being proof-driven before attempting new processes that support change and innovation will necessarily require time, persistence, and a different way of thinking.

The clinical leader at the point of care must necessarily continue to look for new role opportunities, improvements in decision-making structures, management of the physical space for patient care, potential partnerships, and equipment and technology needs to support the continual advancement of patient care excellence—and, of course, enjoy this very special journey of advancing healthcare excellence.

CHAPTER TEST QUESTIONS

Licensure exam categories: Management of care: performance improvement, quality improvement, concepts of management

Nurse leader exam categories: Leadership: systems thinking, change management; Patient safety: performance improvement/metrics

1. Change

   a. Is always associated with chaos.

   b. Can be controlled using project management software.

   c. Is an inevitable life process.

   d. Is best managed by an individual with expertise in change theory.

2. Innovation and change:

   a. Are similar but distinct concepts.

   b. Are the same concepts.

   c. Are based on the same assumptions.

   d. Are avoided by healthcare workers.

3. Innovation and performance improvement:

   a. Are two different change methodologies.

   b. Exist as a continuum, each informing the other.

   c. Are in direct opposition to one another.

   d. Are both required in high-performing organizations.

4. Resistance to change and innovation:

   a. Increases the chances for creativity.

   b. Is not uncommon and needs to be mediated.

   c. Provides a stopgap measure that halts inappropriate changes.

   d. Is limited to individuals with excessive workload requirements.

5. There are certain times when change is not appropriate and should not occur. Change should be avoided when:

   a. The funding to support the change is not available.

   b. The anticipated value is positive.

   c. Selected team members are resistant.

   d. There is no clear rationale or improvement anticipated.

6. Project management templates and processes:

   a. Are ideally suited for complex change and innovation.

   b. Can remove obstacles to creativity.

   c. Consider deviations from the plan to be negative.

   d. Accelerate the orderly work of change.

7. Change competencies include:

   a. Common understanding of definitions and descriptions of change.

   b. Expertise in completing checklists.

   c. Knowledge of team members' ability to create a business case.

   d. Emphasizing the limitations of other team members' competencies.

8. Which innovation leadership behaviors support building networks of people?

   a. Boundary spanning

   b. Leveraging opportunity

   c. Risk-taking

   d. Visioning

9. Measurement of change:

   a. Is best done with financial metrics.

   b. Is best done with a single quantitative or qualitative metric.

   c. Should be distinct from measurement of innovation.

   d. Requires consideration of the goals and variables involved in the change.

10. Negative fantasies about change:

   a. Are important considerations in reality checking.

   b. Encourage creativity and innovation.

   c. Can be serious obstacles to embracing change and innovation.

   d. Are more prevalent in newer employees.

11. An innovation process should start by:

   a. Brainstorming solutions.

   b. Implementing ideas.

   c. Asking colleagues about possible solutions.

   d. Understanding the evidence and literature of the problem.

12. A leader's role in change and innovation is to:

    a. Take credit for others[1] ideas.

    b. Facilitate the conditions for change and innovation to occur.

    c. Provide permission to staff to solve problems.

    d. Take suggestions but make the ultimate decision unilaterally.

13. Taking risks to advance change and innovation:

    a. Catalyzes change efforts.

    b. Disrupts change efforts.

    c. Is not recommended for nurses.

    d. Helps maintain the status quo.

14. Performance improvement and innovation cannot occur in the same organization. True or false?

15. Innovation differs from performance improvement because innovation:

    a. Uses a process to achieve an outcome.

    b. Is founded on evidence.

    c. Creates something new to the population experiencing it.

    d. Improves existing solutions.

References

Abramson, E. (2000). Change without pain. *Harvard Business Review, 78*(7), 75–79.

Barksdale, D. J., Newhouse, R., & Miller, J. A. (2014). The Patient-Centered Outcomes Research Institute: Information for academic nursing. *Nursing Outlook, 62,* 192–200.

Battilana, J., & Casciaro, T. (2013). The network secrets of great change agents. *Harvard Business Review, 91*(7/8), 62–68.

Bell, K. (2010). Will the internet destroy us? *Harvard Business Review, 88*(11), 138–139.

Cash, J. I., Earl, M. J., & Morison, R. (2008). Teaming up to crack innovation and enterprise integration. *Harvard Business Review, 86*(10), 90–99.

Christensen, C. M., Anthony, S. D., & Roth, E. A. (2004). *Seeing what's next: Using the theories of innovation to predict industry change.* Boston, MA: Harvard Business School Press.

Colevas, A. D., & Rempe, B. (2011). Nurse-sensitive indicators: Integral to the Magnet journey. *American Nurse Today, 6*(1), 39–40.

Davidson, S., Weberg, D., Porter-O'Grady, T., & Malloch, K. (2017). *Leadership for evidence-based innovation in nursing and health professions.* Burlington, MA: Jones & Bartlett Learning.

Drucker, P. (1985). The discipline of innovation. *Harvard Business Review, 63*(3), 67–72.

Endsley, S. (2010). Innovation in action: A practical system for getting results. In T. Porter-O'Grady & K. Malloch (Eds.), *Innovation leadership: Creating the landscape of health care* (pp. 59–86). Sudbury, MA: Jones and Bartlett Publishers.

Federal Register, 76(9), January 13, 2011.

Fonseca, J. (2002). *Complexity and innovation in organizations.* London, UK: Routledge.

Halvorson, H. G., & Higgins, E. T. (2013). Experience: Do you play to win? *Harvard Business Review, 113*(3), 117–120.

Kegan, R., & Lahey, L. L. (2001). The real reason people don't change. *Harvard Business Review, 102*(10), 77.

Kelly, T. (2005). *Ten faces of innovation.* New York, NY: Doubleday.

Malloch, K. (2010). Innovation leadership: New perspectives for new work. *Nursing Clinics of North America, 45*(1), 1–10.

Phillips, J. (2011). Why innovation can't be benchmarked. [Web log post]. Retrieved from innovateonpurpose.blogspot.com/2011/07/why-innovation-cant-be-benchmarked.html

Plsek, P. E. (1997). *Creativity, innovation, and quality.* Milwaukee, WI: ASQ Quality Press.

Porter-O'Grady, T. (2014a). From tradition to transformation: A revolutionary moment for nursing in the age of reform. *Nurse Leader, 12*(1), 65–69.

Porter-O'Grady, T. (2014b). Getting past widgets and digits: The fundamental transformation of the foundations of nursing practice. *Nursing Administration Quarterly, 38*(2), 113–119.

Porter-O'Grady, T., & Malloch, K. (2010). *Innovation leadership: Creating the landscape of health care.* Sudbury, MA: Jones and Bartlett Publishers.

Rogers, E. M. (2003). *Diffusion of innovations* (5th ed.). New York, NY: Free Press.

Schein, E. (2004). *Organizational culture and leadership.* San Francisco, CA: Jossey-Bass.

Weberg, D. (2009). Innovation in healthcare: A concept analysis. *Nursing Administration Quarterly, 33*(3), 227–237.

Weberg, D. (2016). Innovation leadership behaviors: Starting the complexity journey. In S. Davidson, D. Weberg, T. Porter-O'Grady, & K. Malloch (Eds.), *Leadership for evidence-based innovation in nursing and health professions* (1st ed., pp. 43–74). Burlington, MA: Jones & Bartlett Learning.

Webster's Dictionary. (1991). Change. Retrieved from www.merriam-webster.com/dictionary/change

Weick, K., & Sutcliffe, K. (2001). *Managing the unexpected: Assuring high performance in an age of complexity.* San Francisco, CA: Jossey-Bass.

Zrelak, P. A., Utter, G. H., Sadeghi, B., Cuny, J., Baron, R., & Romano, P. S. (2012). Using the Agency for Healthcare Research and Quality patient safety indicators for targeting nursing quality improvement. *Journal of Nursing Care Quality, 27*(2), 99–108.

APPENDIX A

Change Considerations: Scanning, Reflecting, and Integrating

Planning for Change

After an issue is identified, careful analysis is needed to ensure the issue is legitimate and deserving of attention. The depth and range of considerations for a change process are assessed by scanning the environment, reflecting on the current and desired state, and integrating critical information into a plan for action.

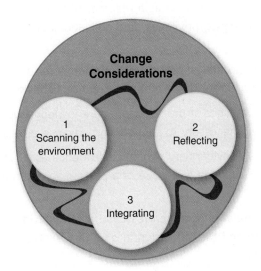

Note that these steps are deliberately detailed for illustration purposes. When an individual is familiar with these steps, they tend to occur quite quickly and more automatically. However, missing one of the steps can be problematic. A quick move to action without a comprehensive assessment of the situation and reflection with the team can lead to incomplete solutions that will ultimately need to be redone and incur unnecessary costs.

> Coming together is a beginning. Keeping together is progress. Working together is success. —Henry Ford

CHAPTER OBJECTIVES

Upon completion of this chapter, the reader will be able to do the following:

» Understand the characteristics and components of membership in a profession.

» Define the role of the professional nurse as a member of the profession with focus and emphasis on the rights, privileges, and obligations of professional membership.

» Describe the professional and ethical foundations of membership in a profession and the obligation to demonstrate those ethics in practice behaviors.

» Outline the unique characteristics of professional and knowledge workers and the environment in context necessary to support and advance professional work.

» List at least five elements of evidentiary dynamics (evidence as a system) essential to validating the meaning and value of a profession and the work it does.

» State the personal characteristics of the professional as an individual and explain how they align the person and the profession in a unitary expression of the life and work of the profession.

» Identify specific characteristics and skills of the team leader in relationship to transdisciplinary collaboration, team dynamics, team decision making, managing conflict, and achieving team outcomes.

Becoming a Professional Nurse

As a professional nurse, you are about to embark on one of the most significant careers anyone could experience. As a member of the nursing profession, there are few places in the healing community where you do not have a role to play. One of the most important realities of any career is the flexibility and opportunity it provides to fulfill meaningful goals and personal achievement. Nursing is one of the very few professional choices that meets the conditions of providing both financial value and personal meaning (Daly, 2005).

At the same time, nursing brings with it many challenges for the profession's members. While nursing is certainly one of the oldest healing practices in human history, it is one of our youngest professions (McDonald, 2010). The scientific foundations and the affirmation of the art associated with its practice have only recently been acknowledged and expanded upon, since the time of Florence Nightingale. Compared with other professions such as medicine and law, nursing is still in its formative developmental stages and is beginning to mature in a way that can be equitably compared with other disciplines (Hoeve, Jansen & Roodbol, 2014). The professional identity of nursing is evolving now more than ever. This means nurses must understand how to lead innovation in ambiguous times to shape nursing's collective future.

The journey to a **profession** and being a professional required a great deal of effort by a number of nurse leaders during the 20th century who devoted their work and lives to advancing the foundations, science, and practice of the profession. However, this effort is still considered a work in progress at the individual and the national levels. This chapter emphasizes the conditions and characteristics of a profession and the personal behavior that reflects the action of a profession and demonstrates membership in the professional body. Furthermore, the social mandate (licensure) and character-istics of professionals are outlined, along with the tools and insights necessary to embed professionalism into the role of each professional person.

The Elements of a Profession

Several components define the unique character of a profession. Throughout his-tory, special honor has been bestowed upon individuals who possess wisdom or great knowledge. The notion of collective knowledge associated with a particu-lar group has been a consistent theme throughout human history. The idea of a group with specialized knowledge becoming a profession emerged from the asso-ciation of a particular arena of knowledge with a specific kind of practice (Bennet & Bennet, 2004). Professions were identified not only for having great knowledge but also for doing something important with that knowledge that made a differ-ence in the world. The practice or the use of particular specialized knowledge is generally associated with the emergence of professions.

Professional Work Is Knowledge Work

The central role of knowledge is critical to the existence of professions. In fact, knowledge is one of the characteristics that is an identifier or distinguishing fea-ture that separates professions from other work groups. A central assumption of any profession is that learning within a unique body of knowledge must take place before a person becomes a member of the profession. This body of knowledge is specific and unique to the profession and is sanctioned by the formal profession as the foundation of the expression of its work in the world. All members of the profession are obligated to demonstrate in their own personal capacity the expres-sion of this knowledge and to demonstrate its application in all the work they do. In fact, formal membership is one of the critical elements of a profession. The spe-cialized knowledge of members is a unique professional element that grounds the profession and is one way of showcasing that special membership. Membership is earned, and all members are expected to demonstrate the ability to fully utilize this professional knowledge and participate in the life of the profession. It is also

CRITICAL THOUGHT

Being a member of a profession is not just a different way of doing work; it is a different way of being. This expression of the role and its relationship to the world represents a special contract between the person and society (called a "social contract"), and reflects the high expectations for the exercise of that role from those who will depend on it.

expected that the professional, by virtue of his or her membership and work, is committed to advancing the role and contribution of the profession.

Because knowledge is a centerpiece of the substance of a profession, the continuing relevance of the professional must be demonstrated on an ongoing basis by that person's commitment to expanding personal knowledge and his or her participation in continuing the development of knowledge over the life of membership in the profession (Steiger & Steiger, 2008). This idea that knowledge development continues for the professional and expands his or her personal knowledge base supports the profession's commitment to the people whom it serves, ensuring that they will experience the most relevant service that represents the latest state-of-the-art information or skills in a way that advances their interests and meets their needs.

SCENARIO

Freda Smith, RN, always seems to sidestep any team or group action on the unit that might improve nursing practice and patient care. Whenever asked to participate, Freda always says other demands and issues limit her availability. Freda has been heard to say, "I do 10-hour shift work; I come here to do my job, and taking care of patients is all my job requires me to do. When I'm done here, I'm done. Don't ask me to do anything more than my job; I don't have time, and I'm just not interested." Freda seems to represent the voice of others on the unit. As a result, a small percentage of nursing colleagues do most of the work related to ensuring shared governance, developing policy, defining best practices, advancing unit learning, resolving unit issues, and making practice decisions. The only problem with this model occurs when decisions are made and those nurses who did not participate in making them complain and often struggle against making recommended changes.

(continues)

(continued)

Discussion Questions

1. Name three things that are occurring in this environment that do not represent a context for professional practice.

2. Which kinds of behaviors are Freda and her colleagues representing in their attitudes?

3. Does it appear that professional behavioral expectations have been established and clarified on the unit?

4. Which kinds of professional behavioral expectations might unit staff want to establish first as terms of engagement for members on the unit?

5. After basic professional behavioral foundations are defined, which next-step actions might need to occur to establish them as the patterns of professional behavior on the unit?

6. What is the role of both the clinical leader and the manager in reinforcing these decisions and ensuring these expectations are consistently met throughout the unit?

The Profession Becomes Identified with the Person

A key element of the life of a profession is the understanding that for the professional, the role becomes closely identified with the individual, such that the profession becomes a part of the person's individual identity and the person demonstrates who he or she is through the lens of the profession. In this way the profession and the person become one and cannot be differentiated from each other (I *am* a nurse). For the professional, his or her work is not simply a job. It is, instead, an expression of the person's identity, a representation of his or her ownership of the work and life of the profession 24/7/365 at all times and in all places. For the professional, work is not codified in hourly increments and prescribed only within the context of a job category or an institutional position. Instead, the profession is a personal role the professional occupies and lives everywhere, all the time. The professional understands that members of society expect him or her to represent their best interests at all times and will respond to their call for services any time the need arises, not just when an institutional position is available.

Professional Work as a Social Mandate

One of the unique characteristics of professionals is the recognition that they provide a socially sanctioned or mandated service. Professions, in fact, often emerge as a response to a social mandate or trust that provides a social good or fulfills a social obligation for their role. As a consequence, licensing regulations usually enumerate the conditions of membership and the statutory requisites for membership and practice in the profession (U.S. Congress, House Committee on Veterans' Affairs, Subcommittee on Economic Opportunity, 2011). The language of such regulations usually specifies the nature of the social mandate and the obligations that it represents. For nurses and physicians, the mandate usually includes language about the service that is provided, the competence necessary to hold membership in the profession, and the social requisites for legitimate expression of that membership in a way that meets the demands of the license.

The social mandate may also identify penalties for nonperformance or professional wrongs. Because the expectation for personal contribution is so clearly outlined and the failure to do so causes severe social deficits, the penalties for failing to live up to the standards of the profession are usually significant. A profession is a social trust; the breach of this trust results in considerable cost to the profession and the person. Society needs to be assured that its professions do not take their obligations lightly or fail to respond to the call for service in any way; they need to know that professionals will minimizes risk to members of society and advance outcomes and fulfill the interests of those members (Roux & Halstead, 2009).

Knowledge Work Always Changes

Besides establishing a knowledge foundation for the profession, another obligation for the profession is its ability to advance and change membership and

CRITICAL THOUGHT

Professions have a social mandate; that is, they receive their authority to act from the society they serve. For nursing, as with any licensed profession, it is against the law for institutions to unilaterally control the profession. Instead, such controls are defined by state legislatures and regulated by the state's professional board. Professions and professionals are members of an international discipline that responds to a human call for care that is broad and universal. Nurses must keep in mind that this mandate responds to a greater call than is expressed in simple institutional employment. Nurses, therefore, always express their accountability to the public, which empowers them; they are not just beholden to the institutions within which they practice.

CRITICAL THOUGHT

If you are a professional, you may or may not be an employee of an institution. If your license is active, however, you are always a member of your profession.

practice expectations as new knowledge informs the actions of the professionals (Megill, 2004). This continual generation of new knowledge is so critical to all professions that they invariably have mechanisms that take the professional beyond the basics to new and higher levels of understanding and contemporary research about practice that alters expectations and changes behaviors. This knowledge generation continually assures society that the professional is fulfilling his or her obligation to advance the practices of the profession in a way that ensures the best interests of the client will always operate as the centerpiece of the work of the profession. An understanding of change and innovation is not an option for nurses but rather it is a professional obligation.

Evidence, Improvement Science, and Translation of Knowledge and Best Practices

The digitization of data in the 21st century has advanced the quality and effectiveness of the management of data and its utility in informing practice behavior (Soriano & Weberg, 2016). The fluidity, flexibility, portability, and mobility of data and data systems now make it possible to use just-in-time tools to quickly inform clinical decisions and actions. This evidence-based process has now become the fundamental expectation of clinical practice. Indeed, it serves as the frame of reference for the future of clinical professions and the work they do.

Although it is not within the scope of this text, **evidence-based practices** and the **evidentiary dynamics** (referring to evidence as a system) upon which they are based are critical characteristics of the behavior of professionals. Professionals are expected to make judgments in a way that reflects facts and truth. Because of the highly variable nature of people, conditions, and circumstances related to clinical practice, building an evidentiary foundation for deliberation and **decision making** is important to best inform clinical judgment, choices, and actions (Rapp et al., 2010).

Every contemporary knowledge-based profession, including nursing, needs to be able to demonstrate its commitment to fact- and value-based choice making and clinical action. No matter which approaches to evidence-based practice are used by the professional, the result must reflect the best evidence regarding what is both viable and effective in advancing the health and safety of the population (Melnyk & Fineout-Overholt, 2014). Evidence-based practice is both a science and a discipline. Every approach that relies on the use of evidentiary dynamics includes five components:

1. Formulating a critical clinical question using a **PICO approach** (P: patient or problem; I: intervention; C: comparison; O: outcomes).

2. Searching for, gathering, and integrating data and relevant evidence using a variety of information resources (general, filtered, and unfiltered). Officially sanctioned and integrated clinical systems databases must be used to ensure that any information used for decision making is relevant, comparable, and rigorous. **Table 2-1** identifies some of the recommended databases.

3. Determining the validity of the data. This requires critical deliberation regarding the relevance of the data to the clinical situation and the applicability of the specific data to the clinical practices being compared.

4. Using the evidence for a particular clinical scenario. It is necessary to affirm the efficacy and closeness of the relationship to the diagnosis, treatment or intervention, therapeutic impact, potential, and possible outcomes within a specific patient situation or clinical scenario in order to provide top quality care.

5. Evaluating the impact of evidence-based choice(s). Evaluation questions relate to the appropriateness of the choice for diagnosis, intervention, clinical change, practice processes, or patient condition. This critical fifth stage is what informs the most relevant up-to-date practices.

Table 2-1 Recommended Databases

Background Information	Filtered Resources	Unfiltered Resources
UpToDate	ACP Smart Medicine	OVID MEDLINE
Harrison's Online	Cochrane	PubMed
E-books	Natural Standard	CINAHL
	InfoPOEMS	PsycINFO
	ClinicalKey	BIOSIS
	Natural Medicines Comprehensive Database	
	OTseeker	
	PEDro (Physiotherapy Evidence Database)	
	National Guideline Clearinghouse	

REFLECTIVE QUESTION

What is the difference between a knowledge worker and an employee work group? Are there different performance expectations for knowledge workers and for regular employee work groups?

CRITICAL THOUGHT

Evidence-based practice suggests that practice competence is constantly in motion, reflecting the latest just-in-time information that guides patient care. Therefore, practice knowledge is always changing, and professionals change with it. The professional makes sure that every element of practice reflects the latest understanding of the best standards of patient care in everything he or she does.

When consolidated with other information related to the same clinical circumstance or scenario, this information serves to build the database and inform future practice.

Evidence-based practice principles are explained in greater detail in many other resources.

One notable characteristic of good professional reflection, interaction, and communication is the ability of professionals to base their arguments on evidence that has been well researched, clarified, and formed into a legitimate presentation or communication. The professional nurse should look at this process as a foundational framework for practice by every nurse, thereby ensuring that communication within the discipline and with other disciplines is always informed by the understanding of evidence-grounded principles. Translating these principles into specific patient applications and effectively and rationally communicating their purpose, reason, and the clear logic of nursing action, informed by good evidence, represent the very foundations of professional practice.

Regarding professional work, the professional nurse has no accidental conversations. Every opportunity for dialogue and interaction includes careful thought and planned communication. Evidentiary dynamics (the system of evidence) provides a systemic and scientific format that frames the logic that drives effective clinical decision making. Within the context of the PICO process and its faithful execution, the professional nurse relies on a consistent format within which the deliberations of practice and clinical application unfold in a confident, informed, and rational manner. The ability to express this model of communication and the disciplines embedded in it demonstrates the professional character of the nurse to everyone with whom she or he communicates. This competence generates a sense of clarity, personal confidence, accuracy, and trust in the validity of the clinical, patient-care content shared in the conversation.

The importance of this aspect of evidentiary dynamics, in which the nurse takes a systematic/scientific approach to clinical judgments and actions, cannot be understated. The professional decision-making mechanism and clinical relationship reflect a scientific manner of conversation and interaction. Furthermore, good clinical decision making is negatively affected to the extent that any of the elements of care wind up being poorly constructed, badly thought out, or not expressed in a conscious, intentional, and scientific manner (Bennet & Bennet, 2010). Ideally, the need for positive and professional communication will be addressed in the classroom during nurses' education, being explicitly recognized as a particular characteristic of competence. An evidence-based framework then becomes the tool set with which the professional nurse demonstrates great skill and accuracy in the clinical setting by projecting clarity, confidence, and understanding about practice and patient care that is palpable to those with whom he or she is communicating. Effective, clear, confident, precise, and accurate generation of information in a focused presentation leads to a more effective response, higher trust, and greater perceived value of both the informant and the information.

The Ethical Foundations of a Profession

Professions generally make an explicit statement about their trust relationship with society by developing a strong **code of ethics**. Such a code generally assures others that patients' best interests will not be jeopardized by members of the profession, that members will act within the parameters of the code and the law, that they will enforce their code with all members, and that they will update that code in ways that reflect the latest understanding of appropriate behaviors and practices.

The Nursing Code of Ethics

The nursing profession, like all professions, has a code of ethics that enumerates the expectations of members of the profession. It also defines the personal and performance standards that represent what is best in the work of the profession. The nursing code of ethics specifically spells out the role and relationship of the nurse with individual patients and addresses issues that advance the health needs of society. The code further defines the behavioral expectations of members of the nursing profession in terms that relate to who and how they serve the public and advance the social good.

The American Nurses Association (ANA) has historically created the professional code of ethics and conduct for professional nurses in the United States (Hain, 2009). This code of ethics has strong roots in ethical theory and principles and in the establishment of a culture of virtue and value. It focuses on the specific and individual role of the nurse as a professional and as a key healthcare provider. The ANA code enumerates ethical foundations of the individual and collective action taken by professionals in relation to patients' health and the health of the community. The code of ethics is grounded in the understanding that the profession as a whole and the individual nurse will use the code as the foundation for ethical analysis, decision making, and professional behavior.

The ANA's *Code of Ethics for Nurses with Interpretive Statements* includes nine specific provisions, each of which is accompanied by detailed explication of its interpretation in the application of related principles. These nine provisions are as follows:

1. The nurse, in all professional relationships, practices with compassion and respect for the inherent dignity, worth, and uniqueness of every individual, unrestricted by considerations of social or economic status, personal attributes, or the nature of health problems.

2. The nurse's primary commitment is to the patient, whether an individual, family, group, or community.

3. The nurse promotes, advocates for, and strives to protect the health, safety, and rights of the patient.

4. The nurse is responsible and accountable for individual nursing practice and determines the appropriate delegation of tasks consistent with the nurse's obligation to provide optimal patient care.

5. The nurse owes the same duties to self as to others, including the responsibility to preserve integrity and safety, to maintain competence, and to continue personal professional growth.

6. The nurse participates in establishing, maintaining, and improving healthcare environments and conditions of employment conducive to the provision of quality health care and consistent with the values of the profession through individual and collective action.

7. The nurse participates in the advancement of the profession through contributions to practice, education, administration, and knowledge development.

8. The nurse collaborates with other health professionals and the public in promoting community, national, and international efforts to meet health needs.

9. The profession of nursing, as represented by associations and their members, is responsible for articulating nursing values, for maintaining the integrity of the profession and its practice, and for shaping social policy.

(American Nurses Association, 2001)

A code of ethics is generally adopted by a profession to assist professionals in making appropriate decisions in a way that helps the individual differentiate between right and wrong and apply this understanding to critical decision making. A hallmark of a profession is that a code of ethics is considered part of the regulation of the profession. It outlines a defined framework for professional responsibility and guides **critical thinking**, especially concerning difficult decisions. The code of ethics provides as clear a framework as possible regarding which behaviors meet the criteria for ethical behavior, guiding the individual or discipline to make good decisions within a particular set of circumstances. From the perspective of the profession, failure to comply with the code of ethics for practice can result in questions regarding the appropriateness of the individual's behavior and its impact on continuing membership in the profession.

SCENARIO

A young man was admitted to your nursing unit with severe infectious complications caused by acquired immunodeficiency syndrome (AIDS). He was very sick, had many opportunistic infections, and required continuous complex medical and nursing care.

Sarah, one of the staff licensed practical nurses on the unit, had made her religious and personal feelings related to AIDS and homosexuality very clear, often stating that the disease was "a sentence from God." She was often heard to say that those who get such diseases were receiving the "wrath and punishment of God." Many on the nursing staff did not hold the same beliefs as Sarah did. They avoided scheduling Sarah as a caretaker for this patient and simply did not discuss the issue further.

Discussion Questions

1. Does the ANA *Code of Ethics for Nurses* address this clinical scenario as an ethical issue?

2. Should there be nursing code of ethics policies related to these kinds of patient care issues?

3. How should the ANA *Code of Ethics for Nurses* be implemented in the clinical environment by the professional nurse(s)?

Strong moral and ethical foundations are an essential element of the behavior of all professionals. Because the professions act within a trusting relationship forged with the society they serve, the social expectation that professionals will maintain a high level of ethical behaviors is itself considerable. Nurses' adherence to a strong code of ethics justifies the confidence placed in them by society, allowing members of society to maintain personal trust toward the professional as an individual and believe that this individual will always act in the best interests of those patients whom he or she serves. It is incumbent upon each professional nurse to be familiar with the profession's code of ethics and the ethical principles articulated by the organizations within which the nursing professional practices. Whenever questions related to ethical nursing behaviors arise in the practice environment, it is always expected that the professional nurse will explore these issues and work to resolve ethical challenges in a way that best addresses the standards of the profession and the needs of those it serves.

Shared Governance and Creation of a Professional Infrastructure

It has been more than 30 years since a professional structure of **shared governance** for nursing emerged (Allen, Calkin, & Peterson, 1988). Over that time span, many approaches have been proposed to demonstrate the appropriate applications of professional governance in a wide variety of international settings (Porter-O'Grady, 2009). Whether many of these models of professional governance (within the concept of shared governance) actually represent the principles grounding professional governance is the subject of much debate and the source of many challenges and implementation models.

The basic structures of professional governance are generally straightforward. Law, medicine, engineering, architecture, academics, and other fields have exhibited many shared characteristics of self-governance for generations, despite modifications to their models reflecting those disciplines' professional and cultural differentiation. Notions of self-governance applied to nursing and nurses, by comparison, have emerged more recently and have been approached more tentatively, with a level of reticence not generally experienced by the other professional disciplines. Although much of this uncertainty can be attributed to the relatively recent emergence of the idea of self-governance as applied to an almost completely employed profession such as nursing, the following issues also influence nursing's engagement with shared governance:

- Self-governance has historically been a masculine exercise with no prevailing mechanisms for its modification to a predominantly feminine application.

- Nursing has almost always been an employed profession; the nurse is generally an employee and, therefore, is subordinated to traditional employment conditions and legal requisites.

- Historically, power relationships in nursing have been predominantly vertically derived (hierarchical) and directed, whereas the power relationships in the major professions have traditionally been much more horizontally delineated (collateral, collaborative).

- Much of the social and legal framework for the traditional professions is designed to protect the public and the independence of the discipline—that is, the discipline's control over its right to practice with little external or regulatory constraint. Much of the social and legal language applied to nursing is also designed to protect the public. However, most regulations more carefully circumscribe nurses' practice boundaries, limiting nursing's scope in a way that keeps it fully within those defined parameters and curtailing nursing's independence.

- The requirements of professional membership in the traditional professions are clear in making succinct, crisp, and definitive statements about members' education, certification, and experience. In nursing, such statements are often diffuse, undifferentiated, and broadly described, leading to requirements that are often confusing and differ in each state.

A Profession Is as a Profession Does

The journey of nursing to professional maturity has been slow and challenging. Unbundling the historical gender challenges faced by nurses (who have traditionally been mostly female) has been a significant undertaking. Because of the social discomfort associated with working women in the past and the public challenges of institutionalized sexism and oppressed group syndrome, nursing's capacity to break out of traditional models of institutional control and to function as a viable profession has met with highly variable degrees of success. In addition, at times nurses themselves have been a significant limiting factor in gaining recognition as a fully professional discipline.

Despite certain characteristics of nursing that reflect a trade (hourly pay, shift work, unionization), the body of knowledge, social mandate, society's trust, and our ethical obligations make nursing knowledge work. The practicing nurse and the clinical leader must understand that leading and interacting with knowledge workers requires different skills from managing a production line. Shared decision making, peer review, and accountability at the point of service are structures that differ from a trade mentality and support the profession of nursing.

Constructing a Structure for Professional Practice

The initial purpose of implementing shared governance models within nursing was to provide a structural format that would enable the profession to implement the more horizontal professional relationships and practice power enablers that are so essential to professional self-governance.

The basic principles of shared governance include the following ideas:

- Ninety percent of decisions are local.
- Decisions are made where they are implemented.
- The work is knowledge work.
- Quality is achieved by the owners of the work.
- Decisional competence is required.
- Clinical decisions require ownership and investment by clinicians.

While acknowledging the social and employment structures that have long characterized the practice of nursing, shared governance provides a model where shared **accountability** serves as the framework for partnering practicing nurses with their institutions. Shared governance mechanisms provide for mutual obligation and advantage in the interest of advancing shared commitment by both nurse and institution in advancing patient care excellence. The four cornerstones of a profession's ownership and accountability—practice, quality, competence, and knowledge management—serve as the structural framework that enables nursing staff to demonstrate these professional requisites and that supports the institutional partnership necessary to incorporate resource and institutional stewardship into patient care.

Efforts to build nursing's structural forms and bylaws that state how those structures work have provided much evidence of the ability of such models to distribute ownership and instill accountability in members of the profession. Although the power balancing necessary for true professional behavior remains far from fully realized, the infrastructure for its emergence has certainly been well established. This, of course, raises an important question: Why has so little professional empowerment and transdisciplinary interdependence among nurses emerged even in organizations where significant progress toward real professional status has been evidenced?

The Four Requisites of Professional Governance

Much contemporary leadership research demonstrates the importance of differentiating the patterns of behaviors in knowledge workers from those in employee work groups (Maliszewska, 2013). Although it is considerably more difficult for nursing than for traditionally masculine professions, work has progressed to make this kind of identification possible. Since the early 1980s, considerable effort has been undertaken to challenge traditional organizational constructs and their legitimacy in light of the need to develop an organizational framework for professional behaviors identified through the structures of shared governance. As the science has broadened and experience has expanded over the past three decades, the more traditional language of shared governance has subsequently evolved into the more universal concepts of "professional governance" (Clavelle, Porter-O'Grady, Weston, & Veran, 2016). The growing body of research has suggested that professional (knowledge work) behaviors can be neither obtained nor sustained in an employee work group structure where the expectations for performance are defined and controlled by the workplace and are predominantly functional in orientation; where few peer-driven performance and evaluation processes operate; where greater value is assigned to volume (how many patients are seen), time, and motion determinants (how much work the nurse is doing); and where work is highly subordinated to others and essentially management controlled and driven (managers make the decisions about clinical work). In fact, these practices impede the occurrence of professional behaviors and prevent them from being demonstrated by practicing nurses.

These identified organizational characteristics have been entrenched in the healthcare system since its onset. Even today, medical predominance in decision making is supported by a highly vertical, tightly structured organizational construct (management and physician control) that has limited the professional growth and development of nursing in significant ways and created particular challenges to the development of a professional control framework for nursing practice. Even though contemporary nurses are academically well prepared and

CRITICAL THOUGHT

Professional delineation and functional job categories do not mix. In a professional environment, job categorization based on knowledge work is simply not an adequate framework for addressing both the requirements and the nature of professional work. Position charters and role expectations serve as better tools for defining the accountability and obligations of professionals than do job descriptions that focus on tasks and functions. It will be a continuing challenge for professional nurses to revise the language used to describe their work by adopting more professional terminology for it.

REFLECTIVE QUESTION

Does the change in the status and role of nursing parallel changes that have occurred as a result of the women's movement over the past five or six decades, or is the change specifically related to advancing women's education and its impact on nursing?

the nursing profession includes the largest number of women with bachelor of science in nursing degrees and graduate-educated women in health care, the status of professional, social, and relational equity has eluded nursing. This has largely been the product of a long-term strongly hierarchical, organizational framework woven into the fabric of the healthcare system and the rigid control exerted by the medical model over clinical decision making having served as strong impediments to nursing's ability to obtain the equity necessary to claim (and advance) the comparable professional value of nurses (Porter-O'Grady, 1992).

Yet, much has changed over the past two decades to open up the opportunity to create a stronger professional framework for nursing, thereby laying the groundwork for equity, inclusion, and leadership. Advancements in the education of nurses, the growth of nurse practitioners and their leadership in primary care, and the expansion of the nursing role in politics and policy development have all converged to enhance the credibility and status of nurses across the broad landscape of the public sector. The activities of shared governance and the research on the impact of the structures has led to a growing comprehension and demonstration of professional decision making and self-management in nursing. Many of the principles of professional governance represented in other disciplines and now applied in nursing have led to the maturation of nursing governance activities, resulting in a more accurate and contemporary governance attribution and the use of the term *professional governance* as a relevant recognition of this maturation and change (Clavelle et al., 2016). In contrast, in the hospitals and healthcare organizations where the majority of nurses still work, much of the essential structure driving organized nursing has not fundamentally changed. However, the introduction of the Magnet program for nursing excellence and the requisites of "structural empowerment" (shared governance) have done much to recalibrate the professional nurse's role in decision making affecting practice, education, quality of care, and clinical care. The construction of a professional, sustainable infrastructure that governs the nursing profession's decision making and relationship to healthcare organizations has laid the foundation for a partnership with such organizations that advances the interests of quality health care and the integrity and contribution of nursing professionals.

Personal Obligation for Participating in Governance

One of the basic obligations of members in any discipline is active participation in the life of the profession. Professions depend on the committed, concerted action of individual members who join in the collective enterprise to advance the interests of the profession and to assure the public that the profession is making its best commitment to meet the needs of the public. Professions are not amorphous bodies that do their work in an automatic or mindless manner. Because the profession is a trust held to a particularly high standard of accountability by the public, it must constantly be aware of its obligation to change and adapt to the adjusting needs of the shifting social context. Human existence never remains static. If positive and appreciative work is being undertaken, the human condition advances and improves.

Nursing has a tradition of encountering difficulty in fully engaging its members to participate in the life of the profession. Because of the long history of job and functional orientation, many, if not most, professional nurses have not always interacted with the obligations of their profession in a meaningful way to advance its interests, their role, and the practices necessary to meet changing contemporary patient needs. Yet, membership in a profession implies ownership, investment, and engagement. Nurses need to show up differently at meetings, in politics, in organizational leadership, and in advancing healthcare policy. By coming to the table prepared with evidence, supported by colleagues, and unwavering in intention for a better healthcare system, nurses will lead the innovations necessary to improve lives and systems.

When a person becomes a member of the profession, it represents a change in that individual's life circumstance, especially given that professional membership also implies social identification of the profession with each person who holds membership in the profession. This "I am a nurse" character of professional identification entails a kind of personal ownership of the life and work of the profession that is not bound by time, job, organization, or circumstance. One is a member of a profession 24/7/365; there is no respite, escape, or separation of the person from the role. If an individual seeks only job or functional work that can be dropped or forgotten when the workday ends or simply left in the workplace, then membership in a profession should not be pursued. The individual professional never really leaves the work of the profession. That is, this professional work accompanies the professional into every circumstance and activity every day he or she is a member of the profession. For true professionals, every activity they pursue represents their continuous membership in the profession. Everything the professional is and does is seen by others through the lens of the individual's membership in the profession. In every moment of action, the individual professional represents the whole profession. Often the only glimpse the patient has into what the nursing profession as a whole is or is not depends on the patient's view of the profession seen through the lens of the patient's relationship with a single nurse. At any given moment, the public's view of the nursing profession is influenced by what they see in a specific member of the profession and how that person represents the profession in the relationship between nurse and patient. For that moment, the whole of the profession rests on that professional's shoulders; he or she is, in that moment, the only window others have into the profession of nursing.

Participation in the life of the profession for the professional is not an invitation, but rather an expectation (Porter-O'Grady & Malloch, 2010). Far too often in organizations and systems where nurses work, they are invited to engage in the life of the profession where they practice. The problem with invitation is that it

SCENARIO

The nursing staff on the medical unit has noticed that numerous nursing beliefs and practices exist regarding particular approaches to preventing pressure ulcers in geriatric patients cared for over the long term. There is a wide variety of long-held clinical approaches, depending on the learning and experiential background of individual nurses. No uniform standard appears to be used on the unit. The issue has been referred to the unit practice council.

Discussion Questions

1. Does the unit practice counsel have the authority to establish clinical standards and practice for all nurses on the unit?

2. Which evidence-based approaches should the unit practice council employ in making decisions about setting a clinical standard?

3. After the clinical standard has been established for the unit, are all nursing staff required to adhere to and implement the standard in their own practice?

4. How does the unit council hold nursing staff members accountable for correctly performing the standard?

5. Should all professional staff expect to serve as members of the practice council, and how is that obligation rotated among staff members?

CRITICAL THOUGHT

All professional nurses are members of the professional nursing staff. This means they have a personal obligation to advance the profession of nursing, to fully participate and engage in professional activities that support practice, and to translate the decisions of the profession into personal practice standards that advance the delivery of high-quality nursing care. As a licensed professional, you cannot opt out of this obligation.

implies a capacity to opt out, to turn down the invitation. Too frequently, given the option implied by invitation, nurses readily reject participation in the life of their profession. Often this professional activity is seen as "extra work" or beyond the basic "call to duty." Consistent with their character, professions distinguish between the obligations of membership (expectation) and the optional elements of engagement (invitation). For example, it is optional for a professional to engage in social events and gatherings of professional members. At the same time, for example, it is an expectation that professionals will engage in quality improvement activities that demonstrate the value of their practice.

Professional membership and the structures of governance require any discipline to delineate between expectations of membership and invitational occasions. For their part, members of the nursing profession are expected to fully participate in decisions affecting practice, quality of care, education and competence, and research and the generation of knowledge. These are the fundamental activities of the nursing profession that inform the functional work of the professional nurse; they are the professional "nonnegotiables." When nurses shirk these active obligations of members in the nursing profession, it diminishes the professional character of nursing, limits the performance of its professional work, and presents an image to others of nonengagement, ultimately resulting in basic task-based, functional, process-oriented, employee workgroup behavior.

The Use of Language Characterizing Professional Dialogue

All these delineations of the professional character of nursing work suggest a critical focus on the appropriateness of language or profession. Language is a highly visible characteristic of communication that suggests to both the speaker/writer and the listener/reader a particular kind of interaction. Language communication is a specific kind of dialogue that takes into account the circumstances as well as the content of the dialogue. Language is important; others hear and perceive it in a way that represents the character and circumstances of the speaker (Zerbe, Ashkanasy, & Hartel, 2006). For good or for ill, professions have a unique framework for their dialogue that includes specific patterns of communication and interaction that represent the "personality" of the discipline. Whether the profession is law, architecture, engineering, medicine, or nursing, each has a language that uniquely frames relationships and demonstrates to the world the unique character of the discipline.

Shared decisions have the following characteristics:

- Decentralized
- Team-based
- Horizontal
- Engaging
- Accountable
- Point-of-service-based

One of the challenges for nursing is the historical language of work embedded in the traditional job-oriented categorization of organizational activity. It is easy to see why the perceptions of nurses and nursing are informed by language that demonstrates the nurse's unilateral representations and perceptions of role and function. When the nurse is heard saying, "I'm just a nurse" or "I'm a floor nurse" or "I'm just doing my job" or "I'm here for the pay," it is not surprising that those listening would assume that the individual has a more vocational or employee work group orientation. Such mistakes in identification are not supported when the professional is overheard saying, "My area of practice is . . ." or "Our standard for practice is . . ." or "I am Sandra, your professional nurse today" or "Let's change our practice plan for this patient." Such language frames serve as evidence of professional interaction and present the profession to others in a way that emphasizes the professional orientation of the nurse.

For the professional nurse, there are no accidental conversations with colleagues and patients. Every interaction has the potential to create a perceptive reaction. The professional nurse is careful to clearly reflect in her or his personal behavior and language those images that best demonstrate professional demeanor, interaction, and character.

Personal Presentation of the Professional Self

Along with language, personal behavior plays an important role in representing professional character. Personal codes of dress, conversation, action, and expression play a critical role in how people present themselves to, and are perceived by, both other members of the profession and outsiders to the profession (Samovar, Porter, & McDaniel, 2012). Professionals recognize that the codes of conduct defined by the profession and by membership in a profession operate at all times and set the parameters for behavioral and role expectations with self and others. The requisite to respect oneself and all others regardless of personal feelings or differences is an important foundation in demonstrating collateral and equitable behavior.

The personal characteristics of the leader are as follows:

- Colleague role with the staff
- Seeks to engage staff decisions
- Open to staff direction and partnership
- Uses good group process
- Models engaging, challenging decisions
- Advocates for staff leadership

Evidence indicates that the perceptual presentation an individual makes during the first three minutes of interactions with others sets the perceptual frame of reference that will linger for the longest time in the memory of others (Davidhizar, 2005). See **Box 2-1**. There is rarely an opportunity to redo these initial three minutes and recalibrate that first perceptual image obtained by others in what is essentially a flash in time. Therefore, it is important for individuals to constantly be aware of how they present themselves to their various publics and which specific image they want others to sustain about them over time.

BOX 2-1 THE FIRST THREE MINUTES LAST FOREVER

- Dress
- Grooming
- Eye engagement
- Inclusive
- Confident
- Facial features
- Posture

The intention and clarity of the professional person with regard to codes of dress, conduct, communication, competence, relationship, and interaction are critical considerations for the establishment of professional standards and guidelines for peer behavior. It is important for the professional nurse to remember that at any given moment in time, from the perspective of the patient, whatever image the individual nurse presents to the patient is the one to which the patient will consistently refer in future conversations about the nurse or the nursing profession. If the nurse's demeanor is gruff and uncaring, if an action is brusque and impatient, if the nurse's attitude is egotistical or haughty, or if the interaction is hurried and dismissive, it will contribute to the observing individual's perception and ultimately will be generalized to the profession as a whole. There are no accidental moments in the interaction between the professional nurse and others. All interaction and communication for the professional is intentional and mearningful.

Interactions with Other Disciplines

Perhaps one of the most significant barriers to full professional recognition of nursing is the perceptions that nurses create among fellow employees that influence their view of nurses (Heuer, Geisler, Kamienski, Langevin, & O'Sullivan Maillet, 2010). As psychiatric clinical studies have clearly shown, all behavior has meaning. Also, in terms of personal identity, each person is treated precisely as he or she expects to be treated and generally no different from that expectation. Although this understanding can be hotly debated, the intent here is to emphasize that how individuals express their expectations of self and others influences which behaviors toward those individuals are expressed and how others generally and consistently relate to those individuals because of those self-expectations.

Behavioral self-expectations need first to be clear to the individual before he or she can expect to see those expectations reflected in how others treat the individual. If a person is unclear about what those behavioral expectations are within his or her own role and relationship, then it should come as no surprise that others perceive mixed messages regarding which relationships and behaviors are acceptable, marginal, or completely unacceptable to the individual. Lack of clarity around expectations makes it impossible to determine correct and appropriate patterns of sustainable behavior and responses, leading to ambiguity and uncertainty that results in confusion and risk in practice and patient care.

In the absence of clearly congruent and well-defined behavioral expectations, others will often respond within the context of what they see regarding the person's behaviors. If, for example, a person is consistently angry and acting out, others' reactions to that person will be predominantly a response to the consistent anger-based behavior. This holds true if the person consistently acts passively, childishly, aggressively, or dependently or if he or she exhibits behaviors that indicate fear, anxiety, uncertainty, lack of confidence, or subordination. In each case, the individual might expect a direct response to those behaviors, not necessarily the equitable response received. When congruence is lacking between the behavior defined by the individual and the behavior exhibited by him or her, the response from others will be unclear, uncertain, and confused.

Clarity regarding professional behavior and personal behavior that demonstrates congruence is critical to ensuring consistent and appropriate interprofessional interaction. Much of a person's perception of himself or herself as a professional depends on the person having worked through his or her role and contribution within the profession. How well a person displays feelings of equity related to his or her self-perception and relationship with other professionals, and how well the person demonstrates a clear set of expectations by behaving and performing equitably, will lead, in turn, to equitable respect and behavior from others.

The issue of poor self-image within the nursing profession has some notable roots that are worth exploring, and they deserve further discussion. Indeed, it is important for nursing faculty and leadership to engage in a discussion of this issue with novice nurses prior to their beginning professional practice. Such a dialogue should address many of the impediments to equitable behavior among the professions in a frank and critical manner before new nurses begin professional practice. This frank and open class discussion or small-group dialogue between faculty and students should cover many, if not all, of the following issues affecting professional equity:

- Nurse must overcome and dismiss the notion that other disciplines (notably physicians) are better educated and more well informed; have a deeper understanding of patients' needs; are fully knowledgeable regarding the work of others in a way that informs patients' needs; are directly in control of all clinical practice; and are, in the final analysis, the captain of the clinical ship.

- Nurses must find clarity around historical gender equity issues that often persist as undercurrents in many interdisciplinary relationships. This exploration needs to include an accurate understanding of the role of women in human and workplace history; the unique contribution of women to the human experience; a full understanding of gender differentiation and its role in understanding equity; cultural gender typing, which often suggests subordinating roles for women; the unique values women contribute to knowledge management; and women's ways of critical thinking, knowledge translation, and decision processing.

- For nursing and nurses, it is important to explore traditional and originating role characteristics of the nurse; the journey from functional to professional delineations for nurses; the growing scientific foundation for nursing practice; the different foundations for clinical judgment and decision making; the centrality of nursing to the coordination, integration, and facilitation of the clinical continuum; and the health script of the nursing role forming its foundations and driving its practice.

- Nurses must consider how they present themselves to their peers and their publics. Foundational and practical issues should be explored related to dress, presentation, manner, articulation, clarity, self-acceptance, professional pride, and the dynamics of interdisciplinary interaction. Simulation or practice opportunities that clearly demonstrate appropriate patterns of behavior are critical to establishing a foundation for these behaviors upon which subsequent professional interactions can be built.

- Some dialogue should center on the sociological, ethnographic, cultural, and economic forces that influence the character of self-perception and the framework for personal expression and interdisciplinary relationships. This discussion should include mechanisms that reflect nurses' and physicians' different economic, cultural, and sociological foundations, which underpin self-perception, worldview, relational characteristics, role choices, and relational capacity. Nurse educators should suggest strategies for accommodating such differences as part of the development of behavioral patterns that will help the new nurse adopt equitable behaviors that reflect his or her personal resolution of inequitable circumstances.

There is clearly a long history of gender and cultural inequity associated with women's prevalence in the role of the nurse. It cannot be expected that individuals new to this role will automatically or "on demand" accept these prevailing realities and experientially adopt new behaviors to overcome them. Nursing as a discipline is currently grappling with fundamental issues that reflect its history as being subordinate and female-dominated and that inform contemporary challenges in building professional practice. Work devoted to resolving these ongoing issues must be intentional and incorporated into the development of the nurse. Rather than simply identifying coursework within which these contemporary issues will be implicitly embodied, it is more important for nurse educators to explicitly address them inside the curriculum and the clinical practice experience of the emerging professional nurse. In addition, faculty and practice leaders must

SCENARIO

A new inpatient delirium prevention, assessment, and treatment pathway needs to be created. The current process is totally driven by physician diagnoses and does not account for the complexity of issues surrounding delirium. Clinical leaders want to use an interdisciplinary and evidence-based approach to design the new pathway. Nurse, physician, and pharmacist teams begin posturing to be the one leader of the initiative.

Discussion Questions

1. Should there be a regular interdisciplinary meeting or council where critical cross-disciplinary clinical issues are addressed at a common table?

2. What is the nurse clinical leader's role as he or she represents nursing at the interdisciplinary table regarding participation, decision?

3. How do the nursing staff and leadership ensure continuity in collaboration and decision making within the nursing staff and between nursing and other disciplines?

4. Is participation in clinical decision making in a shared governance organization a clinical responsibility or a management responsibility? If it is a clinical responsibility, how do we ensure that the clinical representative is the most competent person to represent clinical issues at the interdisciplinary table?

represent, through their own patterns of behavior, that they have personally addressed and resolved many of these issues for themselves. As part of these efforts, they must mentor new nurses, emphasizing the continuing efforts necessary to overcome traditional inequities and to better articulate balanced and equitable behaviors inside the role and relationship of professional nurses and their interaction with the world.

CRITICAL THOUGHT

A person is always treated precisely as he or she expects to be treated, and no differently. The real question is, how do you enable or permit others to behave toward you, and how does their treatment of you closely manifest your own expectations and self-treatment?

The Public and Policy Role of the Nursing Profession

All professions work in a public forum. If a profession is to be relevant and contemporary, and to share in writing the script for its future, its members must commit to undertaking concerted and informed action in the public sector. To advance this effort, the profession must be willing to invest in those things that influence the profession to fulfill its social mandate, to achieve the ends of its work, and to make a difference in the lives of the people it serves (Finkelman, 2012).

Because nursing has been a predominantly employed profession in the past and has been generally managed and seen as an employee work group, it has proved difficult to expand nurses' presence in important roles in the public arena. Physicians and some other health professions have long recognized the critical nature of fully participating in the political and policy sector. Their willingness to actively seek out this level of engagement has advanced the medical agenda, but they often created preferred roles and circumstances for physicians that are not always in the best interests of those whom they serve and society as a whole. Because much of physicians' power and influence has not been countered by fuller, more robust participation in the public sector by nurses, much of what patients need and nurses require to advance the health of the communities they serve has gone wanting.

Public Policy

Public policy is usually defined as principled action undertaken by governments. It usually involves political decision making and legislative action. Professional involvement in public policy often demonstrates a profession's interest in advocating for those whom it serves by seeking to influence government and legislation. Public policy can occur at every level of government in the United States. Indeed, health care generally impacts all levels of government, but local entities are more heavily impacted because almost all health service is essentially local.

Shaping public policy generally comprises a multifaceted dynamic that involves the interaction and concerted contribution of a wide variety of individuals and collective groups that work in their own best interests to advance particular political or policy agendas (Cheung, Mirzaei, & Leeder, 2010). Using a variety of tactics, these individuals and groups seek to influence policy in those ways they think are best for themselves or others.

In the pursuit of favorable policy, advocacy can take many forms and can represent a variety of interests. Advocacy comprises efforts to influence public policy by educating others, lobbying for specific interests, and working within the political system to make desired or needed change. Advocates suggest that the issues on which they are speaking are critical to the quality of life of the individuals they represent. While such activity remains controversial, many professionals and knowledge workers actively advocate for those interests they feel they best represent, thereby seeking to improve the circumstances of those whom they represent and serve. Questions are often raised, however, as to whether advocates best represent those whom they serve or whether, in fact, they represent their own best interests.

Regardless of the discussion and challenges that surround advocacy and public policy involvement, it is generally assumed that professionals are interested in the welfare of those people whom they serve. Professionals often link the welfare of their profession with the greater well-being of those served by that profession. For example, they do the following:

- Illuminate the welfare of the community
- Link the profession to the community
- Meet the ethical obligation to protect the health of all people
- Ensure that the healthcare system meets the community's health needs
- Look for a fit between care and people
- Create a common vision for health

Although this can be treacherous ground to walk, this stance indicates the profession's strong ethical and moral drive to more clearly articulate the needs of those who are served and to better organize public systems to meet those needs in a more effective manner (Jaja, Gibson, & Quarles, 2013). For good or for ill, policy and political advocates have played a critical role in establishing much of the existing U.S. healthcare system, which has advanced both the quality of health and the quality of life of American citizens. Without such advocates, little would change in a democratic society.

Nurses have historically been underrepresented in public forums and in the political and legislative arena. Although nursing is the single largest health profession in the United States, nurses' per capita representation in the political and legislative arena has not demonstrated the impact that such large population numbers would suggest. While speaking out on behalf of the health interests of the community is central to the role of the nurse, it is difficult to measure that commitment with a simple headcount of nursing advocates who are active in the public forum (Jameson, 2009).

Membership in a profession assumes that a certain percentage of the member's time is spent working for the interests of the profession at some level of the public forum. Nursing professionals recognize that policy, political, and legislative action is an important vehicle for advancing improved standards of health, clinical care, and community health (Sonfield & Pollack, 2013). At least some time in the life of each professional should be devoted to addressing issues of public concern. Each professional should demonstrate the fulfillment of his or her personal obligation to make a difference in the life of the broader community and to demonstrate the value of the nursing profession in doing so. There are a number of ways in which the nursing professional can be expected to have an impact on the quality of life of the community:

- Nurses may periodically participate in the life of the profession as an active member of a professional organization and potentially as an officer of the organization. Because much of public advocacy is undertaken by professional organizations, participation in such an organization strengthens its capacity to speak out for the best interests of the population for which it advocates.
- Serving on local boards, committees, and task forces related to health and the quality of life in the community is one of the best ways to demonstrate health advocacy. These roles are generally specific, focused, and time-limited, giving the participant an opportunity to contribute at the local level in a role that can have a broad impact on the quality of health in the community.
- Testifying before boards, committees, and commissions regarding specific elements of care and service provides a notable and effective way of educating others and deepening understanding of specific issues, policies, or changes necessary to advance the health and quality-of-life issues of the community.
- Serving on specific health-related boards, committees, and commissions can enable the nurse to influence policy and support particular health causes. Such sources of collective wisdom can strongly influence changes in policy, practice, and education.
- Serving in elective office provides a more definitive and specific process for advocating and legislating advancing public policy and law. Full engagement in the political process ensures stronger ownership, direct political accountability, ability to establish law, and the capacity to drive meaningful and sustainable change.

At every level of professional life, from local agency advocacy to representation in broad-based political roles and legislation, nurses have an opportunity to significantly influence the quality of life of the community. The nurse can act as a change agent by embracing the political and social role of the profession, and

REFLECTIVE QUESTION

Does membership in the profession also imply obligation to the community? Does that mean members of the profession have an obligation to demonstrate their commitment by also serving their community in a wide range of public and personal efforts?

supporting the passage of laws and regulations that establish firm standards upon which quality, safety, and health can be advanced and assured. Each nurse should be fully aware of the personal obligation that the professional needs to address, such as issues of advocacy and public policy. Making a difference in the life of the community, individual patients, and the profession itself is a fundamental obligation of membership in the professional community (Cowen & Moorhead, 2011). This obligation should not be taken lightly. Each nurse must reflect individually on his or her level of commitment and specific role in addressing personal, professional advocacy in a way that advances the interests of those whom each nurse serves. Such advocacy need not be widely publicized; often, it may consist of taking on a quiet, normative role in making meaningful changes in health care. For example, the acts of writing letters to politicians, participating in the formulation of position papers, gathering data to support advocacy positions, and developing information materials for patients and community members all demonstrate professional participation in public policy. All nurses should see for themselves the extent to which they can participate in such activities, while recognizing their essential obligation as members of the nursing profession to have an impact on the public and the health of the community. As Florence Nightingale's life suggests, these obligations for professional nurses should not be seen as exceptional but rather as representing usual and ordinary functions congruent with the obligations of the nursing profession and representative of its commitment to expanding health in the community it serves.

CRITICAL THOUGHT

For a professional, personal identity and professional identity act together as one. When individuals become members of the profession, they become so tightly identified with the profession that their membership in it cannot be separated from their personal identity. "I am a nurse" is a statement that enumerates who I am, not just what I do.

Nursing and Transdisciplinary Partnership

As new models of clinical service and care unfold in the United States over the next decade, nursing will find itself more strongly intertwined with care partners in rendering effective patient service. The National Academy of Medicine's Health and Medicine Division (formerly the Institute of Medicine) called for nurses to lead interdisciplinary teams and coordinate the fragmented healthcare system to advance patient safety and quality outcomes (Pittman, Bass, Hargraves, Herrera, & Thompson, 2015). The movement toward accountable care, the focus on the patient's position within the healthcare continuum, and the need to demonstrate the value of healthcare services will all radically alter patient care delivery. More strongly developed team-based approaches to planning and managing a patient's care will be essential to meet the "triple aim"—advancing the patient's experience in the healthcare system, raising the quality of care using comparable metrics, and better managing affordability through good stewardship of resources. As payment for services becomes "bundled" within service categories, the partnership between healthcare disciplines will become increasingly important. Under bundled payments, one price will be paid for particular patient populations, episodes of care, or a particular continuum of care, with the single payment covering the costs of all services related to that individual patient, population, episode, or continuum.

Within this system, to assure that care is integrated, relevant, cost-effective, and demonstrates a positive impact on the health experience of the patient, nurses must work much more closely with other disciplines to coordinate, integrate, and facilitate relations among the clinical services that all practitioners provide. The professional nurse will need to clearly understand her or his contribution to the team, appreciate the value of the role of the nurse as a member of the team, and be able to plan and evaluate services and care with team members. Increasingly, practicing nurses will work independently and interdependently on clinical teams in which the majority of provider partners are not nurses. In addition, small groups of nurses will work together with other clinical partners with specific populations or categories of patients to provide the full range of services they need along their continuum of care. Many of these services—if not most—will not be offered in the hospital; rather, they will require that nurses work in smaller practice communities with other nurses and provider partners in unique, often customized models of patient care. Within this model, the new nurse may have, as her or his first clinical experiences upon licensure, service opportunities that are not hospital-based. Indeed, nurses may increasingly seek employment in settings other than hospitals, such as clinics, hospice care, home services, care management, medical homes, community clinical settings, and a range of new and emerging health service delivery settings.

The professional nurse must be aware of these emerging and growing settings for health service delivery and be prepared to ask the right questions about these opportunities and the role expectations of the nurse. Some of the issues the nurse must explore are summarized here:

1. Are clinical expectations, orientation, staff learning, and developmental opportunities available to develop and refine skills specific to success in the setting?

2. Is the documentation system seamless, integrated, and designed in a way that facilitates the management of data and information in a manner supportive of the nurse's practice and the patient's care continuum and that is relevant to both the environment and the content of clinical care?

3. Are the expectations of the nurse clearly defined in relation to those of other partners? Is the model of care designed in a way that clarifies individual roles, links individual roles to the collective role expectations, and is flexible and responds to the need for adjustment?

4. Is the physician's role as a partner clearly defined, with easy access and good communication mechanisms demonstrating availability and openness between team and physician?

5. Are patients considered as care partners and incorporated into the plan of care, in clinical communication and interaction, and in major decisions that affect the provider's role and the patient's experience?

Clinically integrated care models that include a broad range of health professionals, whose services are often coordinated within the plan of care by the nurse, are becoming more common as a foundation for clinical practice in almost every setting. The challenge for the profession is to clearly articulate the skills, knowledge, and value in these new settings. Technology and data collection are allowing nurses to demonstrate their impact to patient outcomes objectively. As practice settings continually evolve to more home- and society-based locations, the profession of nursing will need to challenge long-held assumptions, specifically state-bound licensure, hospital-based curriculum, and physician-led systems. The care of the future requires different skills and a different professional infrastructure to meet the demands of affordable and equitable care for patients.

I Am the Profession

Whatever a profession is or does depends on the contribution and commitment made by its members. How a profession is perceived by others depends on the perception generated by members of the profession who represent its interests to the public it serves. Each person who characterizes himself or herself as a member of the profession has a specific obligation to demonstrate in his or her role the characteristics of what the profession should offer. Each professional needs to demonstrate the foundations of what constitutes professional skills. These skills reflect theoretical and evidence-based foundations in knowledge, active participation in the life of the profession in ways that advance the interests of the profession such as: continuous, lifelong commitment to education and learning; peer-based competency expectations and performance measurement; meeting the ethical and moral obligations of the profession; and personal and professional behavior according to the code of ethics for the profession. At a personal level this is evidenced through personal disposition, deportment, self-confidence, personal competence, positive relationship to others, and showing the strength and character of the profession. This pattern of professional behavior is exemplified by mentoring, modeling, and contributing to the education and development of peers. Most importantly, it makes a real difference in the individual and collective lives and health of the community. Collectively, these characteristics articulate what a profession does and who a professional is. They are the nonnegotiable foundations upon which a profession is built, and they are definitive requisites that form the foundation of professional life. Without them there is no profession. In turn, without the full engagement, ownership, and investment in the activities associated with advancing these characteristics, a person cannot claim membership in a professional community. As nursing moves into the adulthood of its professional life, these characteristics become the nonnegotiable characteristics to which each professional member commits with his or her personal behavior, interactions, and clinical performance.

SCENARIO

Sandy Jones, RN, BSN, was a new nurse in the Medical Community Services division of Smith Health System. She had completed orientation and her mentorship, and was now taking on a full patient care assignment on the clinical team devoted to the treatment of patients with chronic congestive heart failure across the continuum of care. This program represented a new approach to delivering care to this at-risk population in a way that brought care services closer to the patient. Much of the design of care focused on supporting the patient in the home and providing support services to keep the patient from needing frequent hospitalizations, as had occurred in the past.

Sandy was doing well in learning the fundamentals of respiratory and cardiac care services. She established a good relationship with some of the nurses involved in the congestive heart continuum of care and was learning a great deal from their colleagueship and mentorship. She was also included as a clinical team member within a larger multidisciplinary team that involved service partners from social work, respiratory therapy, physical therapy, pharmacy, and a physician member. This team was assigned to handle the coordination and integration of services across the patient's continuum of care and was dealing with all of the issues that might arise in this population of patients. They were paid for the services provided to each patient through a capitated bundle prospective model (paid in advance with a fixed fee for all the services provided to this patient population).

Sandy saw herself as responsible for coordinating, integrating, and facilitating the efforts of the team and the relationship with the patient. Since she was a new nurse, she was unsure how to demonstrate leadership in this role. She wanted to bring the team together in a way that would more strongly define the team members' roles and their partnership and more clearly identify and distribute functions and activities, but she was not sure that she had either the permission or the skills to do so. Sandy was uncertain and needed a plan.

Discussion Questions

1. As a professional nurse, what is Sandy's specific role in relation to planning patient care?

2. What should Sandy expect regarding clarity of roles between the disciplines in planning her patient's care?

3. What is the "triple aim" and how does it apply to Sandy's work? How will it be used to measure the impact of that work on the patient's experience, quality of care, and cost of service?

4. Which skills does Sandy need to have in working with the team to clarify roles, integrate the individual efforts of the team, improve good communications among team members, and address specific challenges to the team's effectiveness in planning and delivering patient care?

5. As Sandy works through her current challenge, what concerns and issues does she need to address and resolve that are related to the nursing code of ethics and that affect the appropriate delivery of good patient care?

SCENARIO

Jane Thorton, RN, BSN, had worked on the neurology unit at Angel Hospital for a year. She was generally satisfied with her experience and had grown a great deal in terms of her clinical expertise and practice. Jane had established good relations with her colleagues and with the management of the organization and was very well liked by both. While her patients were complex, Jane had learned a great deal about care of patients with neurological concerns; she had recently successfully taken her neurological specialty examination and was certified as a neurological nurse.

Jane had taken on a number of responsibilities related to planning and improving nursing care and had agreed to participate in activities that would strengthen the evidence-based practice approach to policy and protocol development on the nursing unit. She and some of her colleagues were having a difficult time in getting general participation from other staff in these clinical activities on the unit, even though the activities were designed to improve and advance patient care. Jane had approached the manager a few times asking for support in getting more participation in clinical nursing leadership activities, but the response remained minimal on the unit.

While reviewing articles in one of her nursing journals, Jane came across an article on implementing nursing shared governance in a hospital similar to hers. The article outlined some of the challenges and processes associated with successfully implementing shared governance approaches in the hospital. Jane was especially intrigued with how empowering the staff by allocating accountability for decisions and actions had improved staff satisfaction, quality of care, and patient outcomes. The hospital that implemented this shared governance model had subsequently received Magnet recognition and presented itself as a hospital of excellence because of the exemplary work of the nursing staff.

Jane was excited and wanted to bring shared governance to Angel Hospital. But where to start? Jane realized that shared governance was a structural model that led to empowerment of the staff, increased the staff authority and accountability for decisions that affected practice, raised the professional character and behavior of the nursing staff, and advanced patient care and the patient experience. Jane was strongly encouraged by how each of those changes demonstrated significant professional value and how both the perception and the role of nursing could be transformed through the implementation of shared governance. She wondered, however, if she could start small—that is, start at the unit level and create a unique exemplar of shared governance that could grow in a way that one day could affect the whole hospital. Jane decided the time was right and began to think about how she might get started.

Discussion Questions

Respond to the following questions using information gained from this chapter related to shared governance. Expand your information base by using other references on shared governance that may be helpful in dealing with these questions.

1. As a starting point, how can Jane begin to address the possibilities of shared governance with her manager? What might you suggest would help interest her manager in supporting her?

2. Why do professions need to be self-governing when they are accountable to society and to patients? Is it enough to simply have job responsibilities as an employee? If nursing is a profession, what distinguishes it from other work groups and requires it to have a professional governance structure?

3. In implementing shared governance, how would you differentiate invitation (asking people to participate) from expectation (clearly defining which level of participation by professional members is required) so that you can make sure all professional members have a role?

4. What role would practicing staff nurses play in decision making and how does it differ from the role the unit manager would play? How do you clearly differentiate the decisions that staff can make from those decisions that the manager must make? Which decisions require partnership and engagement of both manager and staff that facilitates an effective shared governance structure?

5. When shared governance is in place, how do peers assure engagement by all nurses in the decisions made and the standards set by the professional staff when an individual challenge is issued to them? What is the role of the manager in supporting the decisions of the staff and assuring consistent engagement with them by all members of the staff?

CHAPTER TEST QUESTIONS

Licensure exam categories: Management of care: advocacy, evidence-based practice, professionalism, concepts of management, ethical practice

Nurse leader exam categories: Knowledge of the healthcare environment: governance; Professionalism: personal and professional accountability, ethics, advocacy

1. Nursing is a fully mature and adult profession now reflecting all of the particular characteristics of professional delineation. True or false?

2. Professionals act predominantly on principle, not simply based on their knowledge, reflecting a belief that principle drives knowledge. True or false?

3. Evidence-based practice is grounded in good policy and reflects inconsistent standardization and procedures. True or false?

4. The *Code of Ethics for Nurses* serves as a foundation for the exercise of nursing practice. True or false?

5. Shared governance is a voluntary process that invites staff to participate in decisions that affect patient care. True or false?

6. Very few professional decisions are made at the point of service or in the patient environment. Most decisions influencing nursing practice in shared governance should be made away from the patient care setting. True or false?

7. All staff must participate in shared governance activities. True or false?

8. For a professional, the identification of the profession becomes a part of personal identity such that it is impossible to separate the person from the profession. True or false?

9. Language is not nearly as important as action is. The way in which a nurse acts is the most important indicator of who the nurse is. True or false?

10. One of the primary roles of the nurse is to coordinate, facilitate, and integrate interdisciplinary interaction around elements of professional practice and patient care to ensure synthesis and safety for the patient. True or false?

References

Allen, D., Calkin, J., & Peterson, M. (1988). Making shared governance work: A conceptual model. *Journal of Nursing Administration, 18*(1), 37–43.

American Nurses Association. (2001). *Code of ethics for nurses with interpretive statements.* Washington, DC: ANA.

Bennet, A., & Bennet, D. (2004). *Organizational survival in the new world: The intelligent complex adaptive system.* Boston, MA: Butterworth-Heinemann.

Bennet, A., & Bennet, D. (2010). Multidimensionality: Building the mind/brain infrastructure for the next generation knowledge worker. *On the Horizon, 18*(3), 240–254.

Cheung, K., Mirzaei, M., & Leeder, S. (2010). Health policy analysis: A tool to evaluate in policy documents the alignment between policy statements and intended outcomes. *Australian Health Review, 34*(4), 405–413.

Cowen, P. S., & Moorhead, S. (2011). *Current issues in nursing.* St. Louis, MO: Mosby Elsevier.

Daly, J. (2005). *Professional nursing: Concepts, issues, and challenges.* New York, NY: Springer.

Davidhizar, R. (2005). Creating a professional image. *Journal of Practical Nursing, 55*(2), 22–24.

Finkelman, A. W. (2012). *Leadership and management for nurses: Core competencies for quality care.* Boston, MA: Pearson.

Hain, L. (2009). Guide to the Code of Ethics for nurses: Interpretation and application. *Nursing Educational Perspectives, 30*(4), 258–259.

Heuer, A., Geisler, S., Kamienski, M., Langevin, D., & O'Sullivan Maillet, J. (2010). Introducing medical students to the interdisciplinary healthcare team: Piloting a case-based approach. *Journal of Allied Health, 39*(2), 76–81.

Hoeve, Y. T., Jansen, G., & Roodbol, P. (2014). The nursing profession: Public image, self-concept and professional identity. A discussion paper. *Journal of Advanced Nursing, 70*(2), 295–309.

Jaja, C., Gibson, R., & Quarles, S. (2013). Advancing genomic research and reducing health disparities: What can nurse scholars do? *Journal of Nursing Scholarship.* doi: 10.1111/j.1547-5069.2012.01482.x

Jameson, J. (2009). Nursing policy research: Turning evidence-based research and health policy. *Choice, 46*(10), 1973–1974.

Maliszewska, J. P. (2013). *Managing knowledge workers: Value assessment, methods, and application tools.* New York, NY: Springer.

McDonald, L. (2010). *Florence Nightingale at first hand.* Waterloo, ON: Wilfred Laurier University Press.

Megill, K. A. (2004). *Thinking for a living: The coming age of knowledge work.* München, Germany: K. G. Saur.

Melnyk, B., & Fineout-Overholt, E. (2014). *Evidence-based practice in nursing and healthcare* (3rd ed.). St. Louis, MO: Lippincott Williams & Wilkins.

Pittman, P., Bass, E., Hargraves, J., Herrera, C., & Thompson, P. (2015). The future of nursing: Monitoring the progress of recommended change in hospitals, nurse-led clinics, and home health and hospice agencies. *Journal of Nursing Administration, 45*(2), 93–99.

Porter-O'Grady, T. (2009). *Interdisciplinary shared governance: Integrating practice, transforming healthcare.* Sudbury, MA: Jones and Bartlett Publishers.

Porter-O'Grady, T., & Malloch, K. (2010). *Quantum leadership: Advancing innovation, transforming health care.* Sudbury, MA: Jones and Bartlett Publishers.

Rapp, C., Etzel-Wise, D., Marty, W., Coffman, M., Carlson, L., Asher, D., . . . Whitley, R. (2010). Barriers to evidence-based practice implementation: Results of a qualitative study. *Community Mental Health Journal, 46*(2), 112–118.

Roux, G. M., & Halstead, J. A. (2009). *Issues and trends in nursing: Essential knowledge for today and tomorrow.* Sudbury, MA: Jones and Bartlett Publishers.

Samovar, L. A., Porter, R. E., & McDaniel, E. (2012*). Intercultural communication: A reader* (13th ed.). Boston, MA: Wadsworth, Cengage Learning.

Sonfield, A., & Pollack, H. A. (2013). The Affordable Care Act and reproductive health: Potential gains and serious challenges. *Journal of Health Politics, Policy and Law, 38*(2), 373–391.

Soriano, R., & Weberg, D. (2016). Incorporating new evidence from big data, emerging technology, and disruptive practices into your innovation ecosystem. In, *Leadership for Evidence-Based Innovation in Nursing and Health Professions* (pp.145). Burlington, MA: Jones and Bartlett Publishers.

Steiger, D., & Steiger, N. (2008). Instant-based cognitive mapping: A process for discovering a knowledge worker's tacit mental model. *Knowledge Management Research and Practice, 6*(4), 312–321.

U.S. Congress, House Committee on Veterans' Affairs, Subcommittee on Economic Opportunity. (2011). *Licensure and certification hearing before the Subcommittee on Economic Opportunity of the Committee on Veterans' Affairs, U.S. House of Representatives, One Hundred Eleventh Congress, second session, July 29, 2010.* Washington, DC: Government Printing Office.

Zerbe, W. J., Ashkanasy, N. M., & Hartel, C. (2006). *Individual and organizational perspectives on emotion management and display.* Boston, MA: Elsevier.

APPENDIX A

Extinguishing Childlike Behaviors in the Professional Nursing Staff

For years, the staff have been positioned as the children of the organization. Many of the control mechanisms in the organization were directed to controlling the otherwise undisciplined and misdirected energies of the workers. Because of their relative ignorance and lack of personal discipline and their willingness to escape the demands of work, it was thought necessary to develop management-derived control mechanisms to provide the frame for acceptable behaviors. Interestingly, such mechanisms proved to be a self-fulfilling prophesy for leaders, and the staff ended up behaving exactly as expected. Indeed, such behaviors have now become entrenched within the American workplace on the part of both managers and staff. The staff now exhibit the following patterns of behavior:

- No control over their own work schedules
- No full participation in the assignment of work tasks and responsibilities
- External resolution of personal problems from home or work circumstances
- Nonresolution of relationship conflicts arising out of the work relationship
- Being told what to learn and what is required for personal continuing education
- Parental disciplinary procedures that punish bad behavior and reward good behaviors

Leaders of the Profession Extinguish Parental Behaviors

Identify Ideal Leader Role	Name Gap Between Current Behavior and Ideal	State New Performance Expectations
→		→
Outline Developmental Stages for Desired Leader Behaviors	Undertake Program of Leader Development	Apply Expected Leader Behaviors
→		→
Evaluate Leader Progress Against Objectives	Enumerate Corrective Action Strategies	Apply Successful Behaviors in Constant Role Performance

Pushing the Children into Adulthood

Leaders must stop the parental patterns of behavior in their tracks if there is to be any meaningful accountability and ownership in the staff. No longer can those parental behaviors be used as a tool of control and staff management. The leader must undertake at least the following measures if that pattern is to be broken:

- We are all adults here. Staff must manage themselves and their work schedules.
- Staff must be able to problem-solve their own issues.
- Staff must fully participate in setting work goals and processes.
- Evaluation of competence is always a staff process.
- Staff must be competent enough to solve their own problems.
- Team-based approaches must be used to set direction, undertake work, and evaluate outcomes.

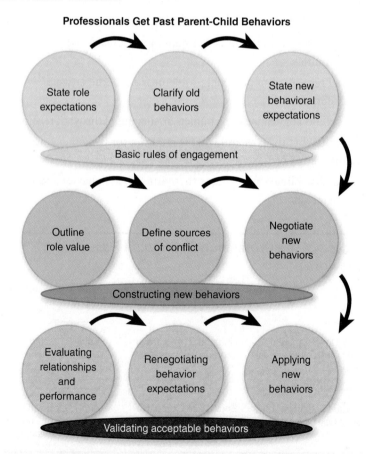

Professionals Get Past Parent-Child Behaviors

State role expectations

Clarify old behaviors

State new behavioral expectations

Basic rules of engagement

Outline role value

Define sources of conflict

Negotiate new behaviors

Constructing new behaviors

Evaluating relationships and performance

Renegotiating behavior expectations

Applying new behaviors

Validating acceptable behaviors

Expectation, Not Invitation: The Professional's Membership Obligation

In the adult workplace, all participants are expected to play the role they consented to. There are no participants who do not express an obligation to the role they occupy. Indeed, there are no invited guests to the experience of life. One either owns the role played or the role is not occupied. This seems strange at first glance, but on deeper reflection, it is an extremely important tenet of the adult-to-adult workplace.

An invitation to play the full role and engage in partnership in meeting the organization's obligations is not a subset of membership in the work community. One is engaged in work precisely to make a contribution within the skill set defined for the role. It is anticipated that the individual will commit all of his or her energies to the exercise of the role without encouragement or coercion. That commitment is a clear element of the expression of the role. Anyone not aware of that expectation as he or she begins the role will not demonstrate it, even if the person is invited to further commit to the behaviors or expectations for the role.

In the adult-to-adult equation, it is anticipated that all players are equally on board. This notion of equity is a primary centerpiece of the valuing of each role and the expression of its relationship and impact on the roles of others. The aggregated effort of all roles is necessary to create the effective interface of energy in a way that ensures good outcomes and work products. Anyone shirking any part of the role will have a clear effect on the work of others and ultimately affect the achievement of good outcomes. In such a circumstance, the effect is a negative one that reduces the net value of the work of all and pulls energy away from the collective effort to add value and produce good outcomes.

APPENDIX B

The Professional Is a Cocreator

Wise leaders recognize that innovation cannot be unilaterally driven. Ultimately, the creative act is a collective one and requires an ability to excite others and get them on board. No one person is responsible for creating the future, even if the idea was generated out of the thinking and reflecting of an individual. To translate ideas into action requires the concerted effort of a number of committed people in the dynamic act of cocreating—the transformation of an idea into reality.

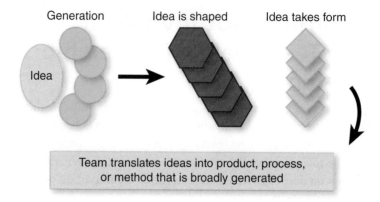

Generation   Idea is shaped   Idea takes form

Idea

Team translates ideas into product, process,
or method that is broadly generated

Creativity Demands Engagement

- Creativity can be generated by individuals or teams, but must be shared to be translated into something of value.
- The leader gathers the creative team together to feed their insight with dialogue, challenge, new thinking, and willingness to explore further.
- The leader can identify in the creative person the unique expression of creativity and make it possible to be nurtured and expressed.
- Creativity within must be regularly nourished by new thinking and exposure to other creative people; otherwise, it dies.

APPENDIX C

The Enhanced Nurse Licensure Compact (eNLC): Important Information for Nurses

Since 2000, licensed practical nurses (LPNs) and registered nurses (RNs) in the Nurse Licensure Compact (NLC) states have enjoyed the advantage of a multi-state license. Under the NLC, an eligible nurse with primary state of residence in a compact state is able to hold one multistate license issued by the home state granting the nurse the authority to practice in any of the 25 NLC states in-person or via telehealth.

In 2015, the NLC underwent a comprehensive revision that resulted in a new compact known as the enhanced NLC. The enhanced NLC will replace the origi-nal NLC, which is anticipated to be phased out in the near future. In order for a state to join the enhanced NLC, it must enact legislation.

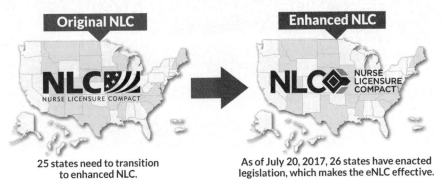

25 states need to transition to enhanced NLC.

As of July 20, 2017, 26 states have enacted legislation, which makes the eNLC effective.

Courtesy of the National Council of State Boards of Nursing.

The enhanced NLC will be implemented on January 19, 2018. To date, 26 states have enacted the enhanced NLC. Of the 25 original NLC member states, 21 states are transitioning to the eNLC and withdrawing from the original NLC, effective January 19, 2018. The four states remaining in the original NLC include New Mexico, Colorado, Wisconsin, and Rhode Island. It is important that nurses stay informed with the changes taking place at www.nursecompact.com and webpages on the National Council of State Boards of Nursing site, www.ncsbn .org/enhanced-nlc-implementation.htm.

Additional References

Clavelle, J. T., Porter-O'Grady, T., Weston, M., and Veran, J. (2016). Evolution of structural empowerment: Moving from shared to professional governance." *Journal of Nursing Administration, 46*(6), 308–312.

Porter-O'Grady, T. (1992). *Implementing shared governance: Creating a professional organization*. Rockville, MD: Aspen Systems.

Critical Thought, Leader Tip, and Scenario icons made by Freepik from www.flaticon.com; Callout icon made by Yannick from www.flaticon.com; Team Tip icon made by Chanut is Industries from www.flaticon.com

> A leader is best when people barely know he exists, when his work is done, his aim fulfilled, they will say: we did it ourselves. —Lao Tzu in the *Tao Te Ching*

CHAPTER OBJECTIVES

Upon completion of this chapter, the reader will be able to do the following:

» Understand the characteristics and components of personal leadership in a profession.

» Define the role of the professional knowledge worker as a leader in the nursing profession and its impact on the role of members.

» Enumerate the behaviors and practices of the contemporary clinical leader and the skills necessary to support them.

» Outline some of the pitfalls and challenges affecting the role of the leader, and sort truth from fiction regarding appropriate leader skills.

» List at least five critical leadership practices that are unique to the leadership role within a knowledge worker frame of reference.

» State your individual personal characteristics and identify their potential for transformation during the development of your own leadership capacity as a part of a personal leadership development plan.

The Person of the Leader: The Capacity to Lead

As a nurse and a member of the nursing profession you have accepted the call to lead in some capacity. This may manifest in formal leadership roles in organizations, the influence of patients and families, and the innovation of the profession itself. Leaders coordinate, integrate, facilitate, and provide a context for the performance of the people within an organization (Maxwell, 2010; O'Neill, 2013). They provide language used to describe the strategic direction of the organization, and in that translational capacity give real life to the work of others. Leaders really do little else other than create the context for work in a way that aligns this work to the mission and vision of the organization and ensure that this relationship is continuously played out in the activities of the people of the organization. Leaders are present in all roles of nursing because it is a professional obligation that nurses lead from where they are. If a nurse is influencing a care-team member, patient, or other part of the health system, then the nurse is leading. Being aware of the nursing professional as constantly visible and leading is an important step to growing the influence of nursing in the future of health care.

Leadership is a capacity all its own; it is a particular skill set. Although it may reflect talents gained from other focuses or activities, its expression is unique to the leader's role. Leadership requires its own time.

Cluttering the activities of leadership with responsibilities and tasks that rightfully should be assigned to others, or including the accountabilities that belong to others as a part of the role of leadership, incapacitates the leader and impedes the legitimate expression of leadership (Watkins, 2004). It is often tragic to see how leaders are subsumed by the activities of others and become overwhelmed with the day-to-day pressures of doing work and just getting things done. Although such activities are important, for the leader they are a continuous and constant impediment to the legitimate and full expression of the leadership role.

Leaders can actually lose their legitimacy and the true value of the role by becoming too personally invested for too long in the busyness, chaos, and continuous intensity of the daily activities of the workplace. For example, nurse managers must balance the obligation of influencing the work of the nurses and the tasks of running a unit. Managers that focus only on the tasks of the unit are not fully engaging with their leadership obligations. Failing to pull away from the tendency to become buried in activity and function is perhaps the greatest single impediment to fully engaging the character and function of leadership in a way that will make a difference to the organization and people to which leadership is directed (Zedeck & American Psychological Association, 2011). If the leader is overwhelmed by the intensity of daily activity, the capacity to lead is compromised and the ability of the leader to make a difference in the lives he or she leads will be extinguished.

Self-Knowledge

Over time, leaders are simply unable to hide their true leadership capacity from others. Genuine connection to the real self and the emergence of leadership out of personal genuine self-expression is a critical centerpiece to the legitimate role of the leader. Having a refined level of self-knowledge facilitates a deeper insight into the character, needs, and expression of the leader in a way that represents individual clarity, openness, and vulnerability. This vulnerability is always apparent

CRITICAL THOUGHT

Leaders end up in serious trouble when they become too personally invested for too long in busyness, chaos, and the intensity of the daily activities of work. Who will the staff depend on for seeing beyond the day's work and helping them find the meaning and sustainability in their work that can come only from rising above the daily routine and looking beyond it to discover both its purpose and direction?

in the disclosing and humane expressions associated with good leadership. The effective leader is personally available to others, to learning, and to change. He or she exhibits a continuous willingness to confront and engage the challenges of life and work head on with a level of personal enthusiasm and excitement that is palpable to others. One of the real hallmarks of leadership is the willingness to visibly display the struggles and challenges associated with grappling with problems, intractable issues, the challenges of change, and the personal struggles in adapting one's own behaviors when the demands of change call for personal adjustment.

Good leaders are many things; they also play many roles. In the 21st century, the leader must fill all of the following roles:

- A transformer
- A visionary
- A translator of direction
- Communication central
- A pursuer of truth
- A generator of creativity and innovation
- A seeker of the very next thing
- A team expert and role model
- A model of the journey to *excellence*

The Continuous Journey of Becoming

Change is a constant. People do not create change, drive change, originate change, or own and control change. Rather, change is the condition of existence. Change is a constant more than an activity. It represents the framework of existence and operates at every level throughout the universe (Hawking, 1988). Furthermore, change is not an event. It does not come and go, though it does ebb and flow. It is consistent and constant, ever present as a part of the condition of living.

Personal growth, development, and engagement of the life experience, across the continuum of one's life, collectively serve as the clearest validation of the constancy of change and the demand to continuously engage with it. This helps the individual find meaning and purpose and to express value as a member of a dynamic human community. The leader is intimately familiar with these characteristics of change. He or she is able to resonate with this dynamic so that the leader is seen as positively disposed and consistently excited about the engagement of the journey of learning and growing as it applies to the leader's role and function in the system (Werhane, 2007). In fact, this individual is so in tune with the reality of change at a personal level that this connection becomes identified with the person. This congruence between the dynamics of change and the leader, in turn,

CRITICAL THOUGHT

The leader creates a context that frames the behavior of the organization in a way that helps the organization achieve its objectives.

creates an image of availability, openness, engagement, and embracing the challenges of change as a normative part of the role of leadership. The resonance is so palpable that others who perceive the resonance and engagement of the leader in this way develop an intensity of relationships. All who share with the leader in this level of enthusiasm indicate their connection with the change dynamic and demonstrate the ability to incorporate it into their own practices and processes.

It should be evident to the emerging leader at this stage that the personal characteristics and attributes of generative leadership provide the prototype or model for personal leadership (Rondeau, 2007). See **Box 3-1**. They present it in a way that generates a community of interest and engagement from others, evidenced by people's ability to seek out, give form to, advance, and create new patterns of response to changing times and circumstances in the organization. This is the power of personal commitment and attachment to the role of leader.

The leader is able to represent within the leadership role a deeper level of understanding of life as a journey, not an event. This simply means that the view of the leader on life experiences is developed from having stood on the "balcony," translating his or her view of systems, structures, and organizations in a way that better articulates the relationship between the system and the broader context within which it operates. The wise leader is fully aware of the shifts and flows operating at the intersection between the larger social environment and the internal environment of organizations and systems. He or she knows that as those conditions and

BOX 3-1 WHO AM I AS A LEADER?

Good leaders constantly ask themselves questions that relate to their value and relevance and to the goodness of fit between their leadership practices and the changing demands of the organization:

1. Are my leadership practices consistent with the changing goals of the organization?

2. Do I focus my leadership practices on building strong relationships and creating a good fit between people and the work they do?

3. Am I aware of my own continuing developmental needs, always exposing myself to the challenges of changing developments and new learning?

circumstances adjust and change, the dynamics are altered between the external demands of the environment and the internal response of the system; the leader, in response, works to make sure that those new dynamics are sustainable (Weberg, 2013). The leader, understanding the constancy of these shifts, uses his or her predictive and adaptive capacity to translate that interface into meaningful language for the other members of the organization, explaining how these changes will affect the lives and work of the people guided by the leader. In essence, leaders influence how information is shared and interpreted in the organization. Influencing information flow is one of the critical behaviors of leadership, as it has a direct impact on team performance, organizational culture, and capacity for change.

Having a predictive and adaptive capacity simply means that the leader is able to quickly shift priorities, conversations, actions, and responses in a way that more aptly fits the present circumstances. The leader personally understands that what one knows at any given time is never permanent and does not represent a constant value. He or she understands that knowledge is mostly a utility, having value only to the extent that it is current and relevant and represents continuous growth (Wager, Wickham, & Glaser, 2005; Worren, 2012). The leader is able to surrender attachment to notions, ideas, past practices, rituals, and routines—indeed, anything that would impede the ability of people and organizations to better adapt to their work and value as the settings (the environment) within which they work change. The work of unlearning and detaching from antiquated practices to adopt new and more relevant ones is a difficult skill that requires practice by the leader. The leader understands that these shifts are driven by so-called **emergent** conditions. These emergent conditions may be driven by new sociopolitical realities, economic changes, technological advances, evidence of best practices, and a host of related changes that demonstrate that holding onto current practices is an impediment to engaging in improved work processes and better serving the interests of the organization's customers.

The Leadership Mirror

Leaders do not act in isolation. Indeed, one of the hallmarks of a leader is the ability to build and manage meaningful and sustainable relationships with a variety of others. Whether those others are executives, peers, or organizational members who depend on leadership (partners), the leader values and engages in intense relationships, recognizing that it is through this vehicle that effective work and change are accomplished. These relationships enable both the organization and its people to continue to work interactively and to achieve effective ends together. Leaders who deeply embrace and can clearly articulate the relational dynamics that drive contemporary network organizations are best able to maximize the energies that result from this knowledge (Bryman, 2011; Mackin, 2007).

The person of the leader (as witnessed through the expression of personal characteristic) serves as a mirror that reflects continuously emergent realities embedded in the leader's social relationships, in the cultural context, and in the business practices involved in the collective work of organizations. Increasingly, technology is driving much of the functional work in organizations and systems. Technology causes systems to move away from more traditional and outdated manual systems and structures that, in the contemporary world, because they are manual and functional, limit the ability of systems and people to be relevant and viable in a more just-in-time, fast-paced technological environment. The new paradigm for work includes specific characteristics and elements that directly and radically impact the role of the leader, causing him or her to reflect more deeply on the circumstances that inform effective and legitimate expression of the role. Some of these elements to consider might be the following:

- There is an acknowledgment of and an increasing and abiding dependence on both understanding and valuing collective wisdom when making decisions and setting priorities.
- Accessing the collective wisdom of diverse work partners helps discern value characteristics of sustainable work. Leaders must recognize that organizations are systems and networks. These structures serve as the foundation or context for all work and represent the interconnections that drive decision making and the actions of people in the system.
- The industrial age has long since passed; as a result, the world in which the leader operates is no longer mechanistic, linear, and vertical in its orientation. The new age represents, instead, a great relationship that is continuously dynamic, interrelated, interdependent, and continuously in motion.
- The leader remains a servant to the system and its people. The context drives the work of the leader. It is the task of creating this good fit between the context of work and the content of work that gives the leader's role focus and value. The leader coordinates, integrates, and facilitates this intersection with the intent of creating convergence between systems and people, such that the congruence and effective relations work together to sustain both the system and its people.
- Meaning is always informed by purpose. The leader is continually reminded that all people seek meaning in their lives and work, and that they want to see that purpose reflected in the character and quality of their work in a way that represents the contribution of each person to advance the sustainability and success of the organization as a whole.
- Leaders understand the constancy of change in their own lives. They are able to translate this into the lives of others and into whole systems.

Leaders seek the seamless intersection of change events and manage each stage of the change process in a way that ensures engagement of people, their movement in concert and response to meaningful change, and their collective success in advancing their own lives and the organization's interests.

- Leaders make time for self-reflection. If the leader's capacity and confidence in discerning, questioning, and translating change remain stagnant and unrefined, this inertia will be reflected in late-stage engagement, reticence, and ineffective response. Furthermore, peers who witness this incongruence will be negatively affected with regard to their own response to change. The availability to self-reflection, environmental scanning, strategizing, and translating reality is a personal leadership attribute. These reflective skills contribute to advancing the broader value of the organization and its people. This outcome happens only when the leader as an individual has engaged these practices as a personal performance expectation.

- Good leaders are transparent and become exemplars of what is valuable and right. They visibly display their own personal commitment to engagement and transformation. They recognize that they are constantly being observed, and that there are no accidental conversations, moments, or occurrences. Instead, every level of interaction has meaning, value, and impact on others. Good leadership communication is a representation of leaders' commitment, as well as their connection to others, their capacity for change, their willingness to address change, and the effectiveness of how they engage it.

Each of these components of personal leadership briefly describes the expectation of the leader in terms of self-reflection, role expression, and relationships to others. Leadership is a role, not a condition. Expressing leadership is intentional work. Leaders make a conscious choice and commitment to the work of leadership. They recognize within their own personhood certain characteristics that must converge in a way to demonstrate leadership and they make a commitment to appropriate and effective leadership behavior (see **Table 3-1**).

CRITICAL THOUGHT

If leaders want to know which kind of leaders they are, they need only look into the faces of their staff; reflected back will be the quality of their leadership.

Table 3-1 Leadership Characteristics of the 21st Century

Conceptual Competencies	Interpersonal Competencies	Participation Competencies	Leadership Competencies
Systems thinking	Receptivity and similarity	Partnership	Vulnerability and openness
Acclimation to chaos	Immediacy and equality	Equity	Systems skills
Pattern recognition	Integration	Accountability	Emotional maturity
Synthesis	Facilitation	Ownership	Self-management
Continuous learning	Coordination	Investment	Transformation skills
	Coaching	Involvement	Group process skills
	Framing new leadership language	Empowerment	Change management
			Fluidity and mobility

Leaders Versus Managers

Leadership and management are two distinct competencies. This text focuses on the development of leadership, not on functions of management. **Managers** have subordinates; leaders have partners.

By definition, management is an organizational position and function. Managers require subordinates. Managers generally have a vertical relationship to those they manage. Management is considered a particular position with vested authority given to these individuals by hierarchical organizational management. Traditional employees work for managers and largely do what the managers suggest is appropriate to their work. Management style is largely transactional or transformational, such that the manager generally informs or encourages employees regarding the nature of the work, the direction in which that work is oriented and how it impacts the organization, the functions that are critical to the activities of work, the motivation of the worker, and the training and performance expectations necessary to do the work well (Rippin, 2007; Simmons & Sharbrough, 2013).

Leadership has little to do with traditional notions of management. Leaders specifically do not have subordinates or subsequent roles. They tend to influence others by virtue of their relationship skills and by advancing the effectiveness of their relationships in a way that supports the collective work of the stakeholders and the effectiveness of their outputs (Gardner, Avolio, & Walumbwa, 2005). Leaders use well-researched principles of relationship, interaction, behavior, and communication to engage others in mutual commitment that advances the value of all and achieves the purposeful ends of their collective work. Leadership is essentially about the person rather than simply about the work. When focusing on the personal characteristics of the leader, role expectations relate to group interaction, influential characteristics between leaders and colleagues, innovation and creativity, interactional skills, team dynamics, and personal characteristics that inspire confidence, competence, commitment, engagement, and the support of others. Leadership is generally not located in a fixed position; instead, it characterizes a role. These role characteristics need to more clearly articulate leaders' ability to effectively interact, intersect, and engage with others, stimulating ownership of their contributions, coaching and developing new insights and skills, and leading others to new insights and understanding about their work system, relationships, and outcomes. Leaders can be found in both the clinical and management ranks of any organization. Indeed, as this text strongly implies, clinical leadership is as important to the success of the healthcare organization as is management leadership.

Managers direct from legitimized hierarchical positions, exercising a locus of control derived from their formal authority in the system. Leadership can be exercised from any point in the system. Indeed, if utilized appropriately, it can change the whole system regardless of where the leader may be located in it. Confidence and capacity are critical elements of the good exercise of leadership, not position. Managers do not necessarily have to be good leaders to perform their functions appropriately, but leaders do not have that same opportunity. Leaders relate by influence, not by control. Northouse (2015) distinguished management and leadership in particular ways (**Table 3-2**). The key distinction between

Table 3-2 Management Versus Leadership Competencies

Management Produces Order and Consistency	**Leadership Produces Change and Movement**
Planning and budgeting Establishing agendas Setting timetables Allocating resources	Establishing direction Creating a vision Clarifying the big picture Setting strategies
Organizing and staffing Providing structure Making job placements Establishing rules and procedures	Aligning people Communicating goals Seeking commitment Building teams and coalitions
Controlling and problem solving Developing incentives Generating creative solutions Taking corrective action	Motivating and inspiring Inspiring and energizing Empowering subordinates Satisfying unmet needs

management and leadership is that management is about function whereas leadership is about movement. The central focus of the manager's role relates specifically to functions and activities often associated with particular skills.

Another contemporary differentiation between management and leadership is that management focuses on analysis, whereas leadership focuses on synthesis. **Analysis** is often defined as breaking down the components of a problem or issue into parts or elements (Tilley, 2008). **Synthesis** works in the opposite direction: It is the act of combining and integrating numerous complex elements or components to view the system as an integrated whole (Cowen & Moorhead, 2011). Although synthesis may include analysis as a part of its infrastructure, the ultimate goal is to observe the system acting and interacting as a whole in a way that represents the desired state (Ford, Seers, & Neumann, 2013). Management tends to look at activities and functions over a short-term, sometimes immediate time frame; leadership observes longer trajectories of time and deals in broader framed circumstances related to creating conditions essential for long-term sustainability rather than short-term returns. Management often focuses on efficiency, function, and process emphasis. Leadership, in contrast, focuses on the relationship, interactions, and confluence of forces that contribute to complexity and how they can be intercepted to advance effectiveness or a trajectory of success rather than any moment of success. Leaders tend to embrace risk and experiment with trial and error. Managers tend to eliminate or reduce risk and build on the tried and tested.

The Personal Attributes of Leaders

Although leaders have many different personalities and personal characteristics, they share a consistent network of attributes that characterize leadership (Leader to Leader Institute, Hesselbein, & Goldsmith, 2006; Simmons & Sharbrough, 2013). Emerging leaders should ask some basic questions early in their career trajectory to address some of the basic attributes of leadership. Some of those questions—and the rationale for them—might be as follows:

- *Do I genuinely like people?* My leadership will bring me in contact with many people, and I may have to lead in directions others may not be interested in going at any given time. I need to be willing to relate to a wide variety of personalities, demonstrate sensitivity to their differences, be aware of their needs, and accommodate these differences in my relationships. I genuinely must like doing this work.

- *Am I able to live with a high degree of ambiguity and uncertainty?* I will be constantly working through changes. I need to be an example of willingness, openness, excitement, and engagement of change. I must be able to demonstrate a will to embrace change in my own life and demonstrate my life as a change in motion before I ask others to embrace change.

- *How well developed are my communication skills?* Communication will be the centerpiece of my leadership expression. I will be constantly communicating with others at every level of the system. I need to demonstrate competence and confidence and communicate articulately. My communication with others must show that I have been informed in my knowledge and expressions. It must be understandable, and I must be seen as competent and trustworthy.

- *Do I have the courage to have crucial conversations and confrontations when required by my leadership?* Can I be tough and disciplined regarding decisions and courses of action? Have I dealt with fear and uncertainty, and am I comfortable with my ability to cope with it and move ahead?

- *Am I able to stand alone and encourage support for a position that others are not embracing?* I must be able to be firm on a position that is evidence-based, ethical, and appropriate under the circumstances; I must defend it clearly and with firmness. I can address others' concerns and insights and develop my position as it becomes positively informed by others.

- *Am I an effective team player?* As a leader, I see my opportunity to make a contribution to the planning and implementation of critical processes. I can assume leadership in translating necessary decisions to others. I can help others refine their responses to decisions, overcome their concerns, restate their goals, and renew their direction in a way that advances integrity, effectiveness, and sustainability.

Leaders must have the ability to move others to act together. As a person, the leader must be able to connect with both heart and head. The leader helps others find a deeper purpose in their work and connect that purpose with the collective

CRITICAL THOUGHT

Leadership requires a strong sense of self. It is next to impossible for a tentative leader to influence the lives and choices of others. A context of competence and confidence can sometimes be the only difference between encouragement and failure.

energy necessary to advance their work and the system to which it is directed. The leader understands the value of emotional and psychodynamic connection to work, to others, and to a cause greater than oneself. Leaders create a culture of ownership and investment in the collective action of work, helping to build a community around the purposes of work and deepening the understanding of the relationship among individual work activities, the collective convergence of that effort, and its power to make a difference (Miner, 2005; Sohmen, 2013).

The leader constantly dances with credibility. To maintain long-term viability and relationships with others, the leader must be able to reflect values of honesty, transparency, personal integrity, and leadership discipline. These values form the foundation of lasting relationships with others in the workplace. Through the exercise of these values, each person to whom the leader relates develops a special connection to the leader through his or her own efforts and personal representation of those same values. In the struggle to act consonant with those values, individuals look to the leader as a mentor and validator in a way that keeps them in touch with their own needs and struggles to keep these values at the forefront of their own lives. The leader models these behaviors by demonstrating personal integrity and living his or her values, using them as the vehicle for self-expression and presentation to others. The leader best communicates these values by maintaining consistency in personal behavior, thereby generating the understanding that integrity is a way of being, not simply a reaction to a single circumstance or event.

SCENARIO

Many leaders are promoted into a leadership role from staff positions. Often, their selection is a reflection of the good work that the individual did as a staff person. In the staff role, this individual became an expert at his or her work. This expertise and effectiveness then ultimately led this individual into the role of new leader. The greatest problem with this process relates to the conflict between really great preparation in the work process and the demands of a good leader: Often they are not aligned. Leadership skills are unique to the role. Staff expertise may be an indicator of potential competence, but there is no guarantee it will be transferred into the leader role. The emerging leader must understand this differentiation from the outset. Failure to do so skews the new leader's understanding of the role and affects the quality of how the role is applied.

You have been selected to lead the development of the practice council in your clinical department. Your manager saw strong leadership potential in you as evidenced by your commitment to care, your ability to influence your colleagues, and your willingness to help make decisions on the unit. You have never been asked to be the leader before or to organize something as important as a practice council. You are eager to perform this role well but are a little concerned about your ability to carry it off.

In an effort to get ready for your role, you have gathered some of your colleagues together to help you with some initial questions. How might you respond to the following questions?

Discussion Questions

1. How many and what range of diversity of staff members do you want to gather for the initial council?

2. What are the first personal activities related to your leadership that you need to address before establishing a council meeting time?

3. Which specific types of mentorship would you look for from your manager to guide you through your initial leadership experiences with the council?

4. Which kinds of reactions from your colleagues on the staff should you anticipate and plan for as you assume this important role?

5. As you prepare for the first council meeting, what might be some of the first agenda items to establish a firm foundation from which the council can launch its work?

Courage and Leadership

Leadership is not easy work. Invested and committed leaders see themselves as though leadership and their own person are one and the same thing. Leadership is intentional work, and leaders are fully conscious of the implications, meaning, and value of their personal actions. Without this awareness of intentionality and the requisite clarity around the impact of the role in the organization and on others, the leader can slip into a sort of passive functionalism that reflects more the characteristics of the management of functions and processes than the leadership characteristics of vision and direction (Kellough, 2008).

Often in nursing, leaders are promoted into management roles out of need rather than because they have clearly demonstrated the skills and capacity necessary for managers. Just as often, the individuals promoted into roles of management leadership are excellent practitioners who are tapped for these roles because of their quality of and passion for patient care. The problem inherent in this process is that clinical work excellence is a poor predictor of management or leadership success (Winkler, 2010). This statement is not meant to imply that excellent clinical practitioners cannot be good leaders. If they are good leaders, however, it is often the result of other circumstances not directly aligned with their excellence in clinical practice. Leadership comprises a specific set of competencies with unique characteristics and content. The evaluation of the elements and components of leadership suggests different characteristics are needed for success in this role than for success as a clinical practitioner. Whether an individual is a clinical leader or a management leader, the leadership characteristics and skill sets are precisely the same:

- Solid self-perception
- Strongly self-directed
- Ability to relate to others well
- Effective verbal skills
- Willingness to interact
- Able to clarify issues
- Unafraid of ambiguity
- Willing to face conflict head on and early
- Embraces the noise of creativity
- Allows others to be innovative and to break the rules
- Not good at avoiding anything
- Lands running
- Can live in the reflected glory of others' accomplishments
- Does not mind a little chaos
- Demonstrates empathy
- Loves to celebrate others' successes

One of the unique ingredients to effective and sustainable leadership is the leader's ability to demonstrate reasoned and careful judgment when making especially difficult and challenging decisions. The leader's relationship with colleagues is often complicated and involves a myriad of patterns of interaction and communication. Sometimes decisions that are appropriate and correct are not universally acceptable or agreed to. It is at this point where leadership courage becomes especially important. Those times when the current runs counter to the correct or most appropriate decision become the true test of one of the leader's most critical skills. Good leaders are calculated risk takers, are comfortable with failing, and transparent in their interpretation of information and decision making. These behaviors require courage. There are elements related to courage that are important to manifest in the personal exercise of the leadership role, as discussed next.

The Courage to Initiate and Act

Often the leader will need to push the walls of current practices, rituals, and routines of work in favor of implementing new evidence-based processes, practices, or initiatives. Some of these changes will not be popular. Yet, the leader must act consistently with the obligation to make sure that clinical action is evidence-based and state of the art. This will often mean challenging colleagues and raising the bar for performance and impact. If the leader has a need for a great number of personal friendships at work, that individual should not seek the role of leadership because it will often call into question these more personal relationships in the interests of making right decisions, creating the perception of conflicts of interest.

The Courage to Stand up for What Is Right in Others

Occasionally in the work setting, relationships among colleagues may be stressed, stretched, or otherwise subjected to a high level of tension. The leader must be willing to enter the intensity and fray of challenged relationships, and with courage and clarity sort through them to identify common ground and to build essential partnerships. The work of the leader focuses on the integrity and effectiveness of the team. To ensure that team-based processes and practices remain fluid and consistent, the leader often will need to confront barriers, boundaries, and perceptual relational differences between members of the team. It is here where skill, courage, and the energy necessary to work through differences become critical in the role of the leader. Establishing group norms, clarifying challenges among individuals, building effective relationships, and confronting issues and concerns head on are acts of personal courage evident in the day-to-day leadership of every system.

The Courage to Trust

Often leaders are seen in terms of their capacity to control things. This notion of control is a viable constituent of leadership capacity, but is frequently overrated. In fact, the effective leader often is the one who is best able to let go of personal control and to trust in colleagues that they will act in the best interests of the profession, the organization, and those whom they serve. Trust is evidence of the quality of the relationship between members of the team. A significant role of the leader is to ensure that expectations, accountability, relationships, and performance are clear for team members, so that each person understands his or her role's obligations in terms of contributing to an effective work environment, exemplary practice, and improved patient outcomes. Showing confidence and trust in colleagues and team members best demonstrates the effectiveness and positive characteristics of the application of the leadership role. Trust reflects the existence of effective relationships, clearly understood expectations, consistent and well-articulated accountabilities, and performance results that reveal the best in clinical practice.

A Personal Connection to Leadership Courage

Courage is palpable and visible. Through all the small, daily activities of the expression of leadership, the personal courage of the leader becomes evident. The way that the leader interacts with others, the voice the leader gives to issues, the leader's personal pattern of behavior, and the critical choices the leader makes in times of challenge or difficulty all express the leader's courage. It is in these small daily events where courage becomes most visible. Some exemplars of daily personal courage include the following:

- Speaking up when the individual knows his or her views will not be popular
- Receiving critical feedback from others regarding personal behavior, positions, or expression
- Saying no when it is easier and more acceptable to say yes
- Publicly accepting responsibility for one's own behavior and for the behavior and outcomes of the team
- Walking away when passions generate childishness, create polarization, or lead to unprincipled language or behaviors
- Speaking with firmness and commitment on issues of principle, best practice, personal rights, and integrity, and in the interests of the patient
- Seeking reflective time when precipitous action may be more expedient or acceptable
- Defending disadvantaged, discriminated-against, aggrieved, or repressed individuals and groups, especially when it is not popular to do so
- Giving passion and language to vision, innovation, and creativity, especially at points where it is not universally acceptable
- Admitting error and personal failing with full ownership and accountability

- Listening deeply when one wants to talk and asking when one wants to tell
- Easily giving credit to others, especially when it is easier to take it oneself
- Finding potential in others and working diligently to develop it

Courage is not reserved solely for those times of great significance or importance where the gestures of courage can be grand or sweeping. In fact, courage is most often evident in the small and unrecognizable daily acts of integrity, honesty, and commitment to truth. Effective leaders see courage simply as one of the elements present in their exercise of the leadership role. Courageous behavior for the effective leader is no big deal, and it is evident in the usual and ordinary behavior of daily leadership. It is the leader who can make courage ordinary and reflect it in every decision and action who best exemplifies the meaning, value, and impact of courage in the act of leading (Harbour & Kisfalvi, 2014).

Leaders Engage Stakeholders

Good leaders know that they are not the center of their organizations and that they do not have all the answers to the myriad questions generated by organizational work. They recognize that they are agents in complex organizational systems (Bergmann & Brough, 2007). While there are many agents in the system, the leader is an unintentional agent located at the intersection of various levels in the system and serves to create opportunities for linkage, interface, and synthesis in the system. In essence, the intentional leader is a catalyst for action rather than the action itself.

The leader as organizational agent recognizes some fundamental elements in the leadership role that are necessary to incorporate to best exercise the role of the leader. Some central themes of the leader's role in the work community are as follows:

- Instead of looking for answers, the leader seeks the right question. This quest ensures that subsequent activity undertaken by organizational members will address the issues that best align with the critical requisites of goodness of fit between the organization and its environment.
- Leaders create the circumstances that make it possible to fully engage all stakeholders regarding issues, processes, and problem resolution. The leader does not so much seek the resolution of the problem as he or she directs the problem to those who have ownership for its solution.
- The leader as agent does not try to be the locus of control for decisions, processes, or actions. Instead, the leader attempts to find the legitimate

locus of control for a decision or action to ensure that the right stakeholders who have direct ownership of the issue are invested in leading the response to it.

- The leader continually questions who the stakeholders are, to shape the focus on particular issues, concerns, processes, or problem solving. The leader's primary role in this scenario is to set the table with the right players who have ownership and competence in addressing the issue or resolving the problem.

- The leader seeks to use the correct language to describe a priority, issue, or concern of the organization. The goal is that, through appropriate dialogue, stakeholders will align the right effort to the right issue and devote the right resources to addressing it.

- The leader serves primarily as a catalyst for issue owners to address and resolve problems, processes, or concerns. The leader makes sure that the right players, tools, processes, and expertise are appropriately aligned to support decision makers in a way that facilitates the best possible problem solving.

- The leader acts as circuit rider to the deliberation and decisional process, ensuring that the right people, processes, tools, and data are available in a format that best supports arriving at the right solution and undertaking the best action.

Wise leaders never put themselves at the center of the deliberative or decisional activities of stakeholders. Instead, they see that the stakeholders have what they need to exercise full ownership of their issues and to fully invest resources and effort in the appropriate deliberation and decisions necessary to address particular issues and concerns (Winkler, 2010). In this way, a leader ensures that ownership of the resolution of issues remains in the hands of those people who will be most strongly impacted by those solutions. As part of this effort, the leader ensures that stakeholders develop the right skills, talents, insights, and applications necessary to address the issues of concern over which they exercise ownership. Although it might be easier for the leader to undertake these activities unilaterally and to be the center of problem solving in his or her area of accountability, that is not always the wisest course of action. Research has shown that the closer to the point of service a problem is dealt with and resolved by those who have direct ownership for it, the better the process and the better the solution (Barker, 1990; Edwards & Elwyn, 2009). However, it is important to the leader that those who have ownership of problems and issues undertake the processes directed toward addressing those problems and issues, and that they have the essential tools necessary to do so. The leader is responsible for seeing that needs and resources converge in a meaningful way, and that through the application of these resources, issues are addressed, problems are solved, and change is advanced.

The Leader Stays in the Question

Wise leaders know that given any opportunity, the locus of control for an issue or concern will always seek to move from the higher intensity and more volatile environment from which it emerged to a level in the system where the volatility, intensity, and anxiety are less concentrated. This basic law of entropy also applies to human dynamics and behavior. If they are left intentionally unaddressed, most problems will arrive at the manager's desk or in the leader's hands, whether they belong there or not.

While solving problems for others might offer a temporary sense of satisfaction for the leader, it serves to create a culture of dysfunctional reliance in the team. Over time, teams will stop trying to solve issues on their own, thus further burdening the leader. The leader recognizes that virtually all problems belong where they originated and seeks to return them there to ensure the problems' legitimate and effective resolutions. Because the leader does not own the problem, if he or she attempts to resolve it, the resolution is likely to address only the symptoms—not the root cause—and the problem is likely to recur. If a permanent solution is to be sought and obtained, the problem must return to its point of origin, where those who own it can resolve it in a way that permanently addresses the issue. It is the leader's obligation to see that the issue returns to its legitimate locus of control and is handled by those who own it (Malloch, 2010).

Good leaders know that they are not the answer to all the questions that others raise. Indeed, they must recognize that accountability for answers always rests with the questioner. The minute the leader answers the question, a transfer of the locus of control for the answer moves to the leader, essentially absolving the questioner of any ownership of the solution to his or her own questions. This transfer occurs thousands of times every day in the life and role of the leader.

The wise leader recognizes that the accountable answer to any question is the next question. He or she recognizes that ownership of the issue should remain with the person who brings it, and that person must be encouraged and enabled to respond and seek the best, most sustainable solution. The leader seeks to have the questioner do the following:

- Retain ownership and control over the issue.
- Identify the resources necessary to pursue a solution.
- Name the barriers impeding a solution.
- Identify the best deliverables related to a sustainable solution.
- Enumerate a mechanism for selecting the best alternative.

- Outline the process steps necessary to address the issue.
- Indicate the impact of the selected approach.
- Evaluate the results of the approaches selected.
- Undertake corrective action related to an effective solution.
- Validate the action of the staff.
- Celebrate the success for the staff in resolving their own issues.

To make sure that a legitimate locus of control is maintained in problem solving, the leader takes a step back when issues that belong to others arise. The leader sees that he or she is not the source of the solution of the problem. Although the leader can access resources, support decision making, provide skill opportunities, and gather the right stakeholders, the leader cannot resolve the problem in any sustainable way on behalf of those who own it. Instead, those parties must resolve it themselves.

In the interests of ensuring this appropriate alignment, the leader stays in the question. This means raising the right issues, engaging appropriate stakeholders, helping others to find the core of the issue or problem, discerning the right agents for problem resolution, and creating the right format and forum for addressing the issue in a way that produces viable and sustainable solutions. In short, the leader stays focused on the *context* of problem solving; the staff stays focused on the *content* of problem solving. This context–content set of parameters helps clarify and distinguish between the elements of the role of the leader and those of the stakeholder. Leaders firmly stay within the context obligations of their role and support stakeholders in addressing their ownership of the content of their issue or concern.

Leaders who stay in the question will find the personal skill set needed for this role to be challenging at best. Put simply, leaders must develop personal attributes that make it comfortable for them to refrain from being the centerpiece or the control point for managing, deciding, and directing resolution of issues that belong to the staff. People who express leadership potential, however, are not often shy, passive, or wilting lily personalities. The unique leadership characteristics evidenced by high energy, strong sense of ownership, creativity and innovation, clear direction, and desire to problem solve, therefore, often trip up these individuals when they need to transfer the locus of control for the answer. Often, they assume that the sometimes much more effective leadership characteristics that remove them as the centerpiece of the action and move them to the side are less meaningful and valuable than being at the "center of the action" (Porter-O'Grady & Malloch, 2010a).

Some self-reflection on leadership capacity is critical for leaders to remain in touch with and to assess the competence required for any particular leadership action. Understanding motive, leadership role content, and personal attributes is important to the appropriate self-development of the leader in leading a team of equals (knowledge workers/professionals) in ways that best engage them, prevent the illegitimate transfer of ownership, and create the conditions for effective problem solving. Some of these self-characteristics are as follows:

- Self-confidence and clear awareness of personal ego challenges and reward needs
- A sense of self-direction and the ability to meet one's own needs without depending on the reflected praise of others
- Assertive skills that make it clear to others where the locus of control is for obligations and accountability
- A strong ability to articulate and clarify issues in a language that can clearly be understood by others, especially those who may own the issues
- A capacity to face the potential for conflict head on and early enough to help people engage it and translate it into purposeful action
- An ability to embrace the noise of initially chaotic, often creative efforts at aligning stakeholders and undertaking deliberations resulting in creative solutions
- An ability to obtain equal satisfaction and personal reward in the reflected light of the team's accomplishment and in colleagues' recognition of the leader's contribution to creativity or effective solutions
- A capability to celebrate others' success and to make celebration a consistent part of the life of the unit or department in ways that acknowledge successes and other individual contributions toward attaining success

Recognizing Personal Needs for Self-Development

Effective leaders appreciate the value associated with being an effective leader. They believe that through the development of their effective leadership skills, they will themselves become better leaders. Leaders also believe that they can develop and, through personal self-development, can grow and become even more effective. They also know that a good foundation in self-awareness is essential to anchor the foundations of this leadership development.

Every leader, no matter how experienced, must be aware of the need to continually develop and grow in this role. Competence in the leadership role is neither static nor ensured. Each leader must recognize how dynamic change is, constantly shifting the work landscape and calling all who work to continually reflect on the value of their contribution and the currency of their skills. This means participating in an endless assessment of competence and the need to adjust and grow in the role as it responds to new demands. Such a self-assessment includes questions such as the following:

- Am I able to see the whole picture, not just the part that applies to me?
- Do I focus on systems models and not merely reflect a process orientation?
- Am I able to look past the current issues and see where I am?
- Can I envision the journey and reflect on where I am in it?
- Am I good at translating reality and change so that others understand?
- Am I willing to face issues first before others must contend with them?
- Do I anticipate the needs of the system and of others in it?
- Do I explore different ways of seeing things and expand my thinking?
- Will I experiment with and evaluate options to current routines?
- Is there a place in my life for the uncertain and the chaotic?
- Can I find the energy in stress and use it to good advantage?
- Am I disciplined in my work and my life without being limited by it?
- Can I see the pain and noise in others and respond with empathy?
- Do I push others into their own challenges and support them in it?

Awareness of some of the common pitfalls that prevent leaders from developing their skills is in the person's own best interest in developing a stronger capacity for leadership. Many simple situations and occurrences contribute to the incapacitating or early destruction of leadership effectiveness. Developing leadership skills is a lifelong process that demands a continuous level of awareness of the leadership journey, its pitfalls and promises, and the individual hooks and traps that impede one's movement along the leadership trajectory. Some of the more common issues related to effective leadership are ones that are most frequently overlooked; here they are italicized.

Some new leaders have an early tendency to self-destruct. Sometimes egos are fragile, and new leaders can often come to believe in their own sense of self-importance and thereby lose perspective of their leadership role and impact on the organization. It is not uncommon to see leaders begin to believe that they are more important, capable, and valuable than is truly the case. Often this occurs when they receive recognition or praise for a singular accomplishment. The individual gets lost in the praise, begins to lose his or her center, and starts to believe his or her value is far more than it actually is. Allowing his or her personal ego to run rampant creates a condition that threatens the value and viability of the leader's role; it also tends to make the leader as much of a problem as the issues to which he or she directs attention. When the leader fails to exercise the same restraint of his or her ego that the leader demands of others, the leader actually tends to stop the very activities that made him or her successful. A humble but balanced recognition of the leader's contribution to creating a positive context for good team relationships, effective problem solving, and advancing creativity is the best countermeasure to an uncontrolled ego and to misappropriation of the leader's role in making meaningful change in attaining sustainable success.

Some leaders fail to accommodate and manage the stress that inevitably accompanies the leadership role. Burnout is the most common occurrence in leaders. Burnout reflects the loss of personal balance, an eroding support system, too much emphasis on the role of the leader, and the diminishment of the moral and ethical center to leadership expression. Often these leaders failed to pay attention to their personal and family supports and the development of close friendships. They lose the ability to manage their time effectively, become overwhelmed with work, and have an inflated sense of their own value to others. Failure to obtain appropriate leadership peer support and mentorship often contributes to growing leadership stress. If these issues are left unaddressed long enough, they can lead to a lack of self-awareness that directly increases impending levels of personal burnout.

Excessive focus on task and function diminishes leadership effectiveness. Because of the pressures to perform and to achieve outcomes, leaders can become overly focused on short-term functions and results at the expense of long-term viability and sustainability. Leadership over the long term is about more than achieving short-term goals; it emphasizes maintaining continuous levels of satisfaction and performance. The task-focused leader descends into the middle of the fray and becomes a part of the problems that ensue. The distance, objectivity, and long-range view expected of the leader diminish, and the individual fails to maintain the context or environment necessary to advance creativity and to recognize value in others.

CRITICAL THOUGHT

Self-awareness ensures that a leader is able to confront the challenges that lie within and to adjust for the conflicts and challenges that will move the individual to grow and develop in a way that takes the person beyond his or her limitations and into the arena of true innovation and creativity. Today most organizations are hungry for just such people.

Treating everyone the same can lead to problems for the leader. **Equity** does not mean **equality**: One is a measure of value; the other is a measure of condition. Everyone should be treated equally; that is beyond question. However, equity indicates that different roles contribute different kinds of value to the organization, such that each role must be respected within the context of its unique value contribution. Simply treating everyone the same ignores the uniqueness that each person brings to his or her role, confuses the specific contribution that each role makes, and eliminates the value of diversity to the mosaic of contributions necessary to the life and energy of the workplace. Recognizing and honoring role differences and individual contributions also advance the life and vitality of the leader.

Admitting personal error does not lead to a lack of credibility; in fact, it advances personal credibility. Regularly making mistakes as a leader is a problem, and it must be addressed as such. However, effective leaders do not generally make frequent and significant errors. When errors or mistakes have been made, the wise leader owns up to his or her part in the error and demonstrates personal transparency with regard to its disclosure. By so doing, disclosure of errors becomes a safe and credible step for everyone, which in turn reduces the intensity and pressure that often accompany the discovery of errors. Setting the example of self-disclosure creates a safe space for those behaviors and helps eliminate the personal stress of hiding inadequacy, failure, and personal error.

The desire to be liked and to be a friend to staff can create significant leadership trauma. In the unique exercise of leadership, friendship is not a part of the quotient. With tongue firmly in cheek, one can say, "Leaders have no friends." Although this is potentially an overstatement, the truth of this principle lies in the fact that leadership is not a constituent of friendship, and friendship is often an impediment to the exercise of good leadership. Leaders need to be honored, respected, and even loved for their excellent exercise of leadership. However, this should not be mistaken for personal friendship with respect to role and performance excellence. Leaders who develop friendships within the context of the team format encourage stress, crisis, inequity, and personal problem generation. The wise leader develops a balanced view of the role requirements of leadership as distinguished from the personal requirements of friendship. Failure to work through this misalignment and set clearly demarcated boundaries in this arena creates a volatile mix that results in diminishing leadership effectiveness and leads to considerable personal harm to both leaders and colleagues.

Leaders need to be available to each other and to their staff. Leaders who isolate themselves or wall themselves off from communication with other leaders and their own staff or colleagues create conditions that facilitate the development of self-harm. Leaders need to be visible and available to one another and to staff in ways that advance communication, dialogue, interaction, and problem solving. A valuable skill for new leaders is to build a network of peers and mentors. The leader's exposure to other leaders and the constant interaction that this person maintains with other leaders helps keep the leader centered, expands the opportunities for new insights, encourages sharing of new tools and resources for self-development, and provides opportunities for mentorship and role clarification. Leadership isolation creates the exact opposite scenario and diminishes both the support and the effectiveness of the leader's role, increasing stress and limiting the leader's viability.

Staying out of touch with the personal and professional issues of colleagues and staff can create emotional isolation for the leader. If the leader becomes so enmeshed in his or her own management or functional activities and becomes captured by them, boundaries between the functional activities of the leader and the relational demands of the staff can accelerate into leadership isolation and stress. Becoming overwhelmed with function and activity is a common condition for leaders. Although many leaders use this condition as a vehicle for identifying with staff concerns, they fail to recognize the part they played in creating staff concerns; thus they do not have the objectivity essential to helping staff deal with their concerns. Availability to problem solve with the staff is critical to building effective staff relationships and preventing leadership isolation. However, the gift the leader brings to the staff and colleagues is a balanced attitude toward problems and issues that often cannot be attained while being inside the problems or issues themselves. Staying in touch with the issues and the staff connects the leader to the staff's concerns, while enabling the leader to maintain some measure of objectivity and lend insight from a new perspective—that is, from the outside looking in—to support the staff's resolution of issues and concerns.

This sample of common pitfalls that impact leadership effectiveness suggests that the leader must understand his or her own personal needs and attributes and develop a deeper awareness of those boundaries and traps that can limit leadership effectiveness and weaken relationships with colleagues. Leadership development builds on a continuous awareness of the needs for individual growth and the range of competencies embedded in the role of each leader (**Figure 3-1**). Leadership self-development is a lifelong process that becomes deeper and more enriching as the individual leader increasingly commits to and expands self-awareness and continuous need for growth and development. Seeking out mentorship and leadership colleague relationships helps create a trusting and safe space for the leader to explore personal issues of leadership growth and capacity and provides a place to discuss the angst and struggles associated with personal growth as a leader (Porter-O'Grady & Malloch, 2010b).

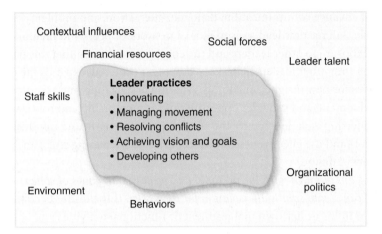

Figure 3-1 **Contextual Influences**

Personal Transparency and Openness

There is nothing more important to a community of people and their relationship to a leader than a real sense of the personal presence of the leader. Much mythology swirls around the role of the leader, who is sometimes even imbued with notions of supernatural or special characteristics. Of course, this is emphatically untrue. Leaders are people who, through growth development, role, and position, assume important roles in relationships to others. Frequently this role is formal and structured within an organizational frame of reference, but just as frequently, it is not. The expression of the role of the leader should be consistent regardless of whether the position is formal or informal. The leader's role is differentiated by the context in which it unfolds. Beyond simply being a position title, a leader must not forget her or his personal humanity; this personal aspect essentially defines the character of the leader's role, its relationship to others, and, ultimately, its impact on others. At a personal level, the leader must be able to communicate effectively with others in a way that honors their own essential humanity, supporting in others a sense of personal identity that allows colleagues to more fully engage and embrace the leader in a way that enriches their own personal work journey (Malloch & Porter-O'Grady, 2009).

In this regard, it is important that the leader represent and express a highly developed level of openness and availability to colleagues in a way that helps members of the professional community to identify with one another and with the leader. Contrary to what was believed in the past, the leader should never be identified as separate and unique from those he or she leads. In fact, more often than not, the leader should be identified as a partner in the team and should exemplify for colleagues the best human characteristics that affirm the value of each role and the integrated purpose of all team members. The leader's openness and availability should enable members of the team to become more integrated, evidenced by their connection to each other and to the leader, and through it clearly identify their purpose, value, and commitments.

CALLOUT

It is a professional obligation for all nurses to demonstrate leadership. Therefore, formal nursing leaders (e.g., nurse managers, directors, and chief nurses) are leaders of leaders. How might this change how formal leaders interact with their nursing teams?

SCENARIO

Leaders must always remember that their primary role is to create a supportive culture for the action of change in the organization. This means that the leader recognizes the forces influencing the leader's own expression of encouragement and facilitation of the change process. Understanding the issues of fit between the leader's practices and the conditions that affect them is critical to the good selection of approaches that make change successful. The leader is always aware of this need for good choices and best represents those good choices in his or her own behaviors and practices; in this way, the leader becomes a model for the staff and a signpost of how best to respond to the inevitability and engagement of continual organizational change.

Some questions related to the individual leader and his or her commitment to organizational goals follow.

Discussion Questions

1. Do you know the mission, vision, and strategic priorities of the organization, and do they influence your actions?

2. How are the organization's departmental goals incorporated into departmental priorities, actions, and measures?

3. How do you make sure that the staff's personal priorities fit tightly with the organization's goals, that their personal action is expression of their commitment to fulfilling those goals?

Connection implies support for collective wisdom. Good leaders recognize the value of the whole aggregate of individual insight, knowledge, and experience. This collective wisdom serves as a powerful force for informing deliberations, effective decision making, and advancing the critical clinical value of the discipline. As mentioned earlier, good leaders move past the need for control in relating to others and make meaningful decisions and undertake appropriate action. The difficulty, however, is that organizational control was the cornerstone of management and leadership over the course of the 20th century. As systems begin to apply newer and deeper understanding of the complexity and characteristics of organizations, a more profound understanding of how organizations work and change has emerged that reflects a new set of principles of interrelationships and interdependency. The impact of complexity thinking and quantum applications in organizations has led to a new understanding of leadership, which emphasizes the shifting understanding of relationships, interactions, and management of life mostly operating at the intersections of systems and networks. Thinkers in this arena now recognize the importance of network relationships and the synthesis of team action (Ang & Yin, 2008). In turn, traditional vertical control infrastructures and behaviors are no longer serving as the central capacity driving stability and organizational life in greater work networks. The contemporary leader recognizes the emergent skills related to addressing issues of good fit, functional linkage, relationship and interaction, and convergence and synthesis, all of which are critical elements of human dynamics in complex systems.

Contemporary leaders now recognize that building effective relationships requires constant attention and continuous reflection on the linkage to the greater intersection and interaction of all components in the system. In essence, leaders need to understand how their network of relationships can be leveraged to influence people and processes in the organization. Organizational leaders seek now to build a prevailing infrastructure that is predominantly grounded in relationships. This emphasis on the relationships between people and systems calls for leaders who understand patterns of individual behavior and their interface with the behaviors of the larger system. Such leaders can effectively manage the many

CRITICAL THOUGHT

The effective leader always prefers chaos over stability. Stability is a momentary respite in the endless movement and creativity of essential change. Although occasional stability is necessary, stability over time is the enemy of creativity and movement.

junctures of organizational networks and the human relations and behaviors that occur in response to them. They can successfully coordinate the linkages necessary to advance and sustain personal relationships and the systems with which they interact. Such leaders reassure staff that they possess the essential skill sets that are necessary to lead equitable and value-driven stakeholders collectively and congruently in fulfilling the meaning, purpose, and values of the organization as it seeks to grow and live in an ever-changing external environment.

The leader's personal attributes and skills work together to ensure that there is consonance between individual purpose and meaning and the organizational value and direction as the leader fulfills his or her role and makes a contribution to the obligations of the broader social network. The leader develops the relationships and interactions necessary to advance, through the aggregated work of individuals (teams), the purposes and values of the organization in the larger social environment. At a very personal level, the leader fully engages both self and others in the dynamic interaction that invests everyone in the high level of commitment represented in the convergence of personal talents, capacity, and skills connected to the purposes and value of the larger organization. Simply, leaders ensure that they and their teams are engaged in advancing practice, evidence, innovation, and personal fulfillment. How can this synthesis be obtained and sustained? A continuous invitation, gathering, inclusion, contribution, and demonstration of the best and most vital in everyone who participates in the concerted effort to advance the health of those they serve is necessary (Ulh-Bien & Marion, 2008). It is to this end that the activities, talents, and commitment of the leader are directed. The leader's constant and consistent focus on creating an environment of ownership, engagement, investment, and expression creates the milieu necessary for the caring network to make a sustainable difference in the health of those it serves. The personal attributes of the leader are what best represents the

REFLECTIVE QUESTION

How many times do we hear, "When this change is over, will everything be normal again?" Although there is certainly some truth to the incrementalism implied in this statement, there is no truth to its substance. Nothing is ever really done. Everything is always and forever in movement. If the movement of the universe should stop, so would everything in it. We may achieve specific objectives, but they are really a small component of a much larger journey—one that never ends. What is your best way of communicating this reality to your colleagues? What story can you tell that reflects its truth to them in a meaningful way?

character and culture of the organization. By examining the behavior patterns of leaders in any organization one can gain insights into the values, beliefs, and practices that occur in that organization. Therefore, it is important that clinical leaders reflect on how they are behaving and ensure it aligns with the professional values of the nursing profession and their own values. This will help leaders assess goodness of fit in their role and their organization. Assessing one's fit with the organization is an important action for a leader to take to support professional and personal satisfaction.

SCENARIO

Joan Black, RN, BSN, had just returned from a national conference on care redesign in healthcare reform. At the national conference, she had learned about the AAA game of ensuring patient satisfaction, consistently meeting quality metrics, and managing the price of care given the drivers of the next stage of health transformation in the United States. She also learned that the centerpiece of healthcare reform was assuring and advancing the health of those served—not just treating and curing illness and disease. Indeed, Joan was excited to learn that the focus of the future of health care was to help citizens achieve the highest level of personal health possible and thereby avoid high-cost, high-intensity illness care.

Joan realized that a good many of the elderly medical patients served on her unit could have a better health experience if the focus of care was on prevention and early engagement of these patients with many of the lifestyle and behavioral issues that often contributed to their illness.

Joan was excited to begin addressing some of these care issues with the medical unit nursing staff as a way of initiating dialogue and action that would alter the care delivery model to better serve the medical unit's patient population. While Joan was considered a clinical leader among the staff, she held no formal management leadership position. Nevertheless, she felt she could play an important role in helping drive examination and testing new approaches to delivering care. Joan realized that the medical unit staff could not transform all aspects of patient care for every patient, but she recognized that there were key groups in which change in nursing practice priorities and emphasis could alter the patient's experience of illness and even perhaps provide a higher level of health within the population. Joan knew that by taking a new approach to caring for these patients, nurses could have an impact on the triple aim of satisfaction, quality, and affordability. She knew she would need to involve and engage the nursing staff and manager on her unit to make this practice change a reality. Joan began to reflect on how she might approach making this change.

Discussion Questions

1. What do you think Joan's next first step should be as she begins to plan an approach to address this issue and engage nursing colleagues and managers in it?

2. Engaging her manager will be Joan's earliest addressed, most important issue. What do you think Joan should do to engage and excite her manager in identifying an opportunity to transform nursing practice and improve patient care?

3. Nursing staff already feel overwhelmed with the activities they are currently undertaking in rendering care. What is Joan's best approach to informing, exciting, and engaging staff colleagues in embracing this change in approaching patient care?

4. Nurses have not historically had to confront issues of financial and service value directly in their practice. How will Joan help staff move from notions of how much care they render (volume) to issues of how much difference they make (value) in the health of the patient?

5. Working with your colleagues in a team effort, consider what might be the planning stages or steps in outlining a step-by-step process for changing nursing practice from focusing on rendering illness care to focusing on population health activities that emphasize prevention, education, early engagement, patient involvement, and improving health status.

SCENARIO

Steve Kelly, RN, BSN, had just completed his critical care nursing certification and was promoted to clinical team leader on his nursing unit. Steve had never played a formal leadership role at any time in his life. He was nervous and concerned about how well he might perform his new obligations as unit clinical team leader. Steve had done well in his leadership course in the final semester of his BSN program and had worked hard to achieve

(continues)

(continued)

certification that verified his high level of clinical competence. In his role as a staff nurse, he had gained the respect and trust of both long-term and new nurse colleagues as well as members of the medical staff and clinical partners and other disciplines. However, he had always kept his focus on providing good personal clinical care and advancing the standards of practice generated by the unit's Patient Care Council. Steve had even served as a member of the Patient Care Council, making some good recommendations for improving care and demonstrating his ability to be a good team member in making decisions and applying them in the unit.

As Steve was preparing to meet with the unit manager for the first time in his new role, he overheard a couple staff members talking about him. They wondered aloud what kind of a clinical leader Steve might become. The staff members mentioned in the conversation a few previous nurses who had become "snotty" or "lorded it over staff members" in their new clinical leader position. Steve certainly did not want to be perceived in that way; he wanted to start off on the right foot so that staff colleagues would be comfortable with his approach to exercising the clinical leadership role. He was also eager to be successful in the role.

Discussion Questions

1. What do you think will be important to Steve as he begins to exercise the role of clinical team leader?

2. Do you think Steve should disclose his concerns to the unit manager? What would he say to her? What should he be able to expect from her in return?

3. What might be some things that Steve could do to both address and disclose his sense of vulnerability without "losing face" with clinical staff? How can vulnerability be identified and used as a strength for Steve as he begins to undertake this new role?

4. How might Steve begin to engage staff colleagues in a way that maintains—and even advances—their feelings of equity and value? What are some ways that Steve might affirm staff members' importance and value while maintaining his own integrity and unique contribution?

5. What do you think might be some of the first things that Steve needs to address as a new clinical team leader? What might be some of the initial concerns of the staff that need to be addressed by Steve as soon as possible? How might Steve approach addressing these issues in a way that affirms his leadership yet engages and embraces the value and role of the nursing staff?

CHAPTER TEST QUESTIONS

Licensure exam categories: Management of care: interprofessional teams, concepts of management/leadership, delegation/supervision

Nurse leader exam categories: Communication and relationship building: effective communication, relationship management, influencing behaviors, interdisciplinary relationships; Leadership: systems thinking, change management; Strategy: strategic management

1. It is better to adhere to generally accepted leadership principles than to develop an individual personal leadership plan. True or false?

2. Leadership means providing specific and clear direction to others so that they understand your intention and have a clear idea of your individual leadership vision. True or false?

3. Leadership courage indicates a specific level of self-understanding and personal knowledge about individual motivation, principles, and ethics. True or false?

4. In working with teams, it is important for the leader to let the team know about the decisions they need to make and to provide the team with the appropriate direction necessary to get to the right solution. True or false?

5. One of the differences between the management function and the leadership function is that managers are more accountable for staffing whereas leaders are more accountable for engaging. True or false?

6. The leader works hard to create trust and does everything to make sure that his or her personal principles of trust are apparent to colleagues so they can work in a trusting environment. True or false?

7. Leaders are always interested in finding answers to problems and directing colleagues to seek the most correct answers or solutions. True or false?

8. A contemporary differentiation between management and leadership is that management focuses on analysis, whereas leadership focuses on synthesis. True or false?

9. Friendship is not a critical element to leadership. Therefore, the wise leader is reserved about transparency and realizes that self-disclosure can create problems between the leader and those whom he or she leads. True or false?

10. The leader must set aside time for formal leadership reflection about personal skills and development needs and should develop a strong relationship with the leadership mentor. True or false?

References

Ang, Y., & Yin, S. (2008). *Intelligent complex adaptive systems*. Chicago, IL: IGI.

Barker, T. B. (1990). *Engineering quality by design: Interpreting the Taguchi approach*. New York, NY: ASQC Quality Press.

Bergmann, S., & Brough, J. A. (2007). *Lead me, I dare you! Managing resistance to school change*. Larchmont, NY: Eye on Education.

Bryman, A. (2011). *The Sage handbook of leadership*. Thousand Oaks, CA: Sage.

Cowen, P. S., & Moorhead, S. (2011). *Current issues in nursing*. St. Louis, MO: Mosby Elsevier.

Edwards, A., & Elwyn, G. (2009). Shared decision-making in health care: Achieving evidence-based patient choice. Retrieved from eduproxy.tc-library.org/?url=http://site.ebrary.com/lib/teacherscollege/Doc?id=10581666

Ford, L., Seers, A., & Neumann, J. (2013). Honoring complexity. *Management Research Review, 36*(7), 644–663.

Gardner, W. L., Avolio, B. J., & Walumbwa, F. O. (Eds.). (2005). *Authentic leadership theory and practice: Origins, effects and development*. St. Louis, MO: Elsevier.

Harbour, M., & Kisfalvi, V. (2014). In the eyes of the beholder: An exploration of managerial courage. *Journal of Business Ethics, 119*(4), 393–515.

Hawking, S. (1988). *A brief history of time*. London, UK: Bantam.

Kellough, R. D. (2008). *A primer for new principals: Guidelines for success*. Lanham, MD: Rowman & Littlefield Education.

Leader to Leader Institute, Hesselbein, F., & Goldsmith, M. (Eds.). (2006). *The leader of the future 2: Visions, strategies, and practices for the new era*. San Francisco, CA: Jossey-Bass.

Mackin, D. (2007). *The team building tool kit: Tips and tactics for effective workplace teams.* New York, NY: AMACOM.

Malloch, K. (2010). Creating the organizational context for innovation. In T. Porter-O'Grady & K. Malloch (Eds.), *Innovation leadership: Creating the landscape of health care* (pp. 33–56). Sudbury, MA: Jones and Bartlett Publishers.

Malloch, K., & Porter-O'Grady, T. (2009). *The quantum leader: Applications for the new world of work.* Sudbury, MA: Jones and Bartlett Publishers.

Maxwell, J. (2010). *The 21 irrefutable laws of leadership.* Nashville, TN: Thomas Nelson.

Miner, J. B. (2005). *Organizational behavior I. Essential theories of motivation and leadership.* Armonk, NY: Sharpe.

Northouse, P. G. (2015). *Leadership: Theory and practice.* Singapore: Sage publications.

O'Neill, J. A. (2013). Advancing the nursing profession begins with leadership. *Journal of Nursing Administration, 43*(4), 179–181.

Porter-O'Grady, T., & Malloch, K. (Eds.). (2010a). *Innovation leadership: Creating the landscape of health care.* Sudbury, MA: Jones and Bartlett Publishers.

Porter-O'Grady, T., & Malloch, K. (2010b). Leadership for innovation: From knowledge creation to health transformation. In T. Porter-O'Grady & K. Malloch (Eds.), *Innovation leadership: Creating the landscape of health care* (pp. 1–23). Sudbury, MA: Jones and Bartlett Publishers.

Rippin, A. (2007). Stitching up the leader: Empirically based reflections on leadership and gender. *Journal of Organizational Change Management, 20*(2), 209–226.

Rondeau, K. (2007). The adoption of high involvement work practices in Canadian nursing homes. *Leadership in Health Services, 20*(1), 16.

Simmons, S., & Sharbrough, W. (2013). An analysis of leader and subordinate perception of motivating language. *Journal of Leadership, Accountability, and Ethics, 10*(3), 11–27.

Sohmen, V. (2013). Leadership and teamwork: Two sides of the same coin. *Journal of IT and Economic Development Academic Librarianship, 4*(2), 1–18.

Tilley, D. (2008). Competency in nursing: A concept analysis. *Journal of Continuing Education in Nursing, 39*(2), 58–65.

Ulh-Bien, M., & Marion, R. (2008). *Complexity leadership: Conceptual foundations.* Charlotte, NC: Information Age.

Wager, K., Wickham, F., & Glaser, J. (2005). *Managing healthcare information systems: A practical approach for healthcare executives.* San Francisco, CA: Jossey-Bass.

Watkins, S. (2004). 21st-century corporate governance: The growing pressure on the board toward a corporate solution. In R. P. Gandossy & J. A. Sonnenfeld (Eds.), *Leadership and governance from the inside and out* (pp. 27–36). New York, NY: Wiley.

Weberg, D. R. (2013). *Complexity leadership theory and innovation: A new framework for innovation leadership* (Doctoral dissertation, Arizona State University, Tempe, Arizona).

Werhane, P. H. (2007). *Women in business: The changing face of leadership*. Westport, CT: Praeger.

Winkler, I. (2010). *Contemporary leadership theories: Enhancing the understanding of the complexity, subjectivity and dynamic of leadership*. Berlin, Germany: Physica-Verlag.

Worren, N. A. M. (2012). *Organisation design: Re-defining complex systems*. Harlow, UK: Pearson.

Zedeck, S., & American Psychological Association. (2011). *APA handbook of industrial and organizational psychology*. Washington, DC: American Psychological Association.

APPENDIX A

Old Versus New Leadership Skills

Old	New
Managing people	Managing mobility
Analyzing processes	Synthesizing systems
Setting direction	Reading the signposts of change
Using technology	Synergizing technology
Motivating others	Helping others identify their work relevance

APPENDIX B

Checking off Basic Leadership Attributes

- *Do I like people?* I will be leading many people, sometimes in directions they may prefer not to go. I must be willing to relate to many types of people and will need a positive sensitivity to the needs of others. I must like this work!

- *Can I live with a high degree of ambiguity and uncertainty?* I will be dealing with a great amount of change. I will have to be an example of excitement and engagement of this change and demonstrate a will to implement it in my own life before I ask anyone else to implement it.

- *Are my communication skills well developed?* I will be communicating with others almost constantly and will need to be informed and articulate in my expressions. Others must understand me and must respect the validity of the information I communicate.

- *Do I have the courage to handle the discipline issues that my leadership role will demand?* Can I make tough decisions and follow through with action when required without fear and uncertainty?

- *Can I stand alone on an issue when it appears that others are not embracing it?* If the position is ethical and appropriate, can I defend it with clarity and firmness, incorporating others' concerns in my own development and positions?

- *Am I a good team player?* I can make a contribution to the planning and implementing processes and then take leadership in translating decisions to others and helping them act in concert with the goals and direction others may have developed for them.

APPENDIX C

More Leader Core Behaviors

- Leaders reflect flexibility in their approach to all problem solving and in confronting all issues.
- Leaders describe the changes that will affect the staff well in advance of the staff actually experiencing them.
- Leaders translate the goals of the system into a language that others can understand and apply to their own work.
- Leaders represent in their own behavior the patterns and practices they expect to see in others.
- Leaders anticipate the changes that staff will have to make in their work and carefully design approaches to guide staff in accepting and implementing change.
- Leaders recognize the chaos embedded in all change and are not afraid of it, demonstrating engagement of it to others, mentoring acceptance and use of its energy.

APPENDIX D

What Staff Want from Their Leader

- Honesty
- Trust
- Clarity or role
- Opportunity
- Open communication
- Good problem solving
- Personal caring
- Engagement
- Respect
- Meaning in their work

APPENDIX E

Leadership

Leaders Moving Past the Age of Control

It has been said that control was the cornerstone of organizational leadership in the 20th century. As organizations seek to function in the 21st century, many of the characteristics of change are driven by a different set of principles. Recognizing the impact of complexity thinking and quantum theory, organizations are looking at an emerging significant set of relationships and intersections that require coordination and synthesis. This means that control is no longer the central issue of stability and organization in systems. The good leader recognizes that issues of fit, linkage, interaction, and relationship are the critical elements of all human dynamics.

Leaders recognize that building complex relationships requires constant attention and continual reflection on interaction of all elements in an organization, including the people who make up the organization. Building an infrastructure for relationships calls for leaders to understand linkages and intersections and to provide staff with clarity of meaning and purpose. The leader ensures those people who are led that there is value in the work and relationships necessary to advance the organization's purposes and values. In doing so, the leader fully engages the participants in an interaction that invests them in committing their work to the purposes of the organization, advancing the meaning and value of their contributions, and growing and improving their own personal skills and participation. This can be done only through invitation, gathering, inclusion, and encouraging the best and the most vital in all who participate.

Leaders can eliminate the focus on control as follows:

- Help people understand what is happening to them.
- Engage others in defining the content of their own work.
- Reduce the hierarchy to its lowest necessary levels.
- Involve stakeholders in setting their own goals.
- Eliminate secrets—disclose whatever is necessary to help others do their work.

The leader who must control others is expressing a basic insecurity that ultimately results in negative forces and behavior impeding achievement of the organization's goals.

The Leader's Commitment to Learning

The leader cannot expect to find in others what he or she is not willing to find within. When considering the role of leader, it is important to recognize the value of continuing commitment to personal change. The leader serves as a role model of the general commitment to continuing development—a pursuit that is fundamental to competence and effectiveness. Like all members of the organization, the leader cannot be competent and static at the same time. The leader must demonstrate a willingness and ability to expand the skill set necessary to exercise the leadership role and serve as a role model to others.

An endless commitment to learning is fundamental to the role of the leader. These things are critical:

- A good assessment of leadership skills and needs
- A good plan with strategies for action and implementation
- A 360-degree evaluation of the effectiveness of the application of leadership skills:
  - Reading the signs of change
  - Translating the language of change for others
  - Guiding others in adapting to change
  - Applying change in the process of work
- Entering into dialogue regarding change impact
- Evaluating the results of change
- Renewing energy for the very next change

A Leader Is Inspired and Is Inspiring

The ability to encourage others and to continue supporting their efforts through modeling, motivating, and personal commitment is critical to good leadership. The inspiring leader always recognizes that who one is, is as important as what one does. This leader always remembers the following points:

- Individuals need to know that their work has meaning and value.
- Individuals hope that their work makes a difference and has a positive effect on the lives of others.
- Everyone wants to know that they are personally valued and that they have a place and play a key role in the world.
- Everyone seeks, at some level, to make a difference and to hear that difference in the words and language of others.

- People want to know that they matter—that their lives have personal value, and that they have an opportunity to express that value in their work and actions.
- The leader always seeks what is good in others, identifies it, and makes other team members aware of the value that an individual brings to their efforts.
- The value of collective wisdom is shared between and among all team members so that their collective impact is recognized by all.
- Nothing is sustained without the concerted effort of all stakeholders committed to a common purpose.
- The leader creates the context within which others live and work in a way that encourages engagement, stimulates creativity, and builds commitment.

The leader's commitment must be such that others can sense it, and from its energy be encouraged and able to continue their own journey.

Updated Reference

Weberg, D. (2013). *Complexity leadership theory and innovation: A new framework for innovation leadership* (Doctoral dissertation, Arizona State University, Tempe, Arizona).

Let whoever is in charge keep this simple question in her head (not, how can I always do this right thing myself, but) how can I provide for this right thing to be always done? —Florence Nightingale, *Notes on Nursing: What It Is, and What It Is Not*

CHAPTER OBJECTIVES

Upon the completion of this chapter, the reader will be able to do the following:

» Understand the fundamental elements that underpin all **conflict**.

» Define normative conflict and the elements and characteristics of conflict that make it a fundamental part of all human interaction.

» Enumerate the personal characteristics affecting one's own view of conflict and individual relationship to it.

» Outline the effects of unresolved conflict and specific steps that can be taken by the individual to develop personal engagement and skills in addressing it.

» List at least five categories of major conflict, the unique characteristics of each, and key strategies for addressing them.

» State why conflict affinity and skill development are important in the role of the leader and provide the critical core functions of leadership expression.

Conflict Skills for Clinical Leaders

All conflict is normative (Smokowski & Bacallao, 2011). Conflict is simply a metaphor for difference. Without too much of a stretch, conflict is observable when one looks around at how unique and different every human being is. Although these differences add to the vitality and wide diversity of human experience, they can also lead to challenges, relational noise, and dispute. Because difference is the predominant condition of most everything in the universe, it best represents what is normative in creation—a vast and unlimited diffusion of diversity and individuality. Within the midst of that prevailing reality, the emergence of conflict is a norm of significant proportions, one that must be recognized as a primary factor influencing all human behavior and interaction. Indeed, conflict is more normal than it is exceptional and the nurse leaders must be skilled in conflict resolution to produce positive professional relationships (American Association of Colleges of Nursing, 2008).

Even so, nothing strikes more fear and anxiety in the hearts of people than the possibility of becoming involved in a conflict situation (Rodgers, 2011). Embedded in the fear of conflict are all of the issues of personal security, identity, safety, and relational integrity. The "noise" and angst associated with the acting out of conflict can range from mild incivility to blatant intent to harm (Kim et al., 2017).

The grounds of much human conflict are often ideological, identity, personality, psychodynamic, and intellectual differences that are displayed with varying degrees of passion and expression (Blackard & Gibson, 2002; Levinger, 2013). In our contemporary world, the plethora of religious, identity, sociopolitical, and cultural differences has created ideological polarization and passionate position-taking whose vitriol has moved human behavior into dangerous modes of expression. In such severely polarized circumstances, the notion of conflict has become increasingly frightening, raising the specter of a wide range of dangers associated with conflict, some of which are life threatening and destructive to the very fabric of society (Tojo & Dilpreet, 2007).

Although many significant dangers are inherent in broad-based conflict, most conflict operates at a significantly less intense level—that is, within interpersonal one-on-one and small-team differences. More than 90% of the conflict that occurs between human beings is local and completely resolvable (Avruch & Mitchell, 2013; LeBaron, 2002). Much of the fear of conflict as it arises in day-to-day relationships and exchanges is unjustified, as it simply reflects an inadequate understanding of the dynamics of conflict and a lack of competence in its management. Developing basic insights and skills related to addressing elements of interactional and relational conflict often helps take the noise off the conflict dynamic and introduces methodologies and techniques that can help people deal with their normative conflicts and move through them to resolution. The leader who recognizes the complex nature of conflict as well as its individual, interpersonal, and organizational factors can help build stronger relationships and interactions among individuals and teams.

The Early Engagement of Conflict

The most important and best first step in the management of all conflict is the early recognition of its signs and early addressing of its issues (Stahl, 2011). Health care is delivered in high-pressure, high-volume, complex environments. The critically important characteristics of caring work can accelerate the conditions and circumstances that can generate the high levels of stress, which are usually an antecedent to the emergence of conflict. The stress of clinical work provides more than sufficient opportunities for the generation of conflict, a reality that should always put the leader on the lookout for the potential emergence of conflict

CRITICAL THOUGHT

The leader listens carefully to people's conversations with or about each other, always looking for the subtext or hidden message that might indicate the presence of the seeds of conflict.

(Rodgers, 2011). Often when the individual's perceptions and needs conflict with the work and the environment as well as the activity of others, basic stressors are introduced. Many of these stressors are manifested in particular modes of communication, relationships, interactions, or expression of personal emotions. Because conflict is generally the physical manifestation of much of the expressions of individual and group stress, its potential is always present. Early engagement of conflict can help ensure that more "mild" forms of conflict (e.g., favoritism, lack of mutual trust, lack of fairness) do not escalate to more extreme forms (e.g., verbal abuse, personal attacks, bullying, physical threats) (Kim et al., 2017).

Looking for the Signs

At the personal level, a number of indicators of stress circumstances can signal the potential for conflict. When there is a sense that staff members feel overwhelmed by their work circumstances or situation and perceive that they have few choices or options to do anything about it, the seeds of conflict emerge. Often the first manifestation of early conflict is a situational clash between two individuals that reflects differences in view, opinion, role, relationship, situation, or incidents. Sources of conflict may include the following:

- Differences
- Emotions and feelings
- Opposing views
- Acting on or out
- Tension
- Interpersonal factors
- Gaps in education, experience, or generation
- Disagreeableness
- Poor communication

Sometimes the signs of conflict can be seen or are visible. For example, in an argument between two members of the staff, subsequent negative behaviors can result in exclusion, demeaning the other party, forming cliques, acting out, bad-mouthing, or rivalry.

Often a cascade of behaviors occurs over time, resulting in accelerating levels of negative behaviors and circumstances slowly and inevitably cascading out of individual control and creating a broader arc of impact among people, in teams, on units or in departments, and sometimes in the organization as a whole (Lencioni, 2002; Ramsbotham, Woodhouse, & Miall, 2011). Unless these kinds of conflicts are engaged early, they inevitably spin outward into a broader sphere of influence. Following each cascading extension of the conflict, they become increasingly more difficult to resolve. In addition, conflicts left unaddressed do not occupy the same level of intensity, are not fixed, and do not stay local. Conflict, like any other dynamic, has an accelerating pace of its own. It does not stay still; it always grows in intensity over time and becomes increasingly more complicated, difficult, and, ultimately, irresolvable (Amer & Zou, 2011). It is for this reason that the simplest and best leadership tool for conflict management is early diagnosis and intervention at the most basic stages of its expression.

Recognizing early signs of conflict requires that the leader be continuously aware of the potential for conflict. The leader's antenna should always be tuned into departmental dynamics, the character of communication and interaction, differences in individual behavioral norms, and situations and circumstances that reflect elements of controversy or disagreement (Lodge & Wegrich, 2012; Wenger & Möckli, 2003). These early signs of conflict are indicators of the potential for the next stage of conflict to emerge, which is often seen in beginning verbalizations, snide remarks, statements of discomfort, cynicism, or outright negative assessments. Each of these behaviors is an early indication of the potential for dissonance, disagreement, and deeper conflict. Addressing conflict during this symptomatic stage may help alleviate tension related to it and prevent movement into later, more intense stages of conflict expression.

Early identification of conflict helps minimize and even prevent its further development in the clinical setting. The leader should work diligently to gain insight into the origin, nature, and character of the conflict and to develop appropriate responses that fit the stage of the conflict and help address the parties involved at that time and in that place. Some common personal and systematic responses for framing the early engagement of conflict include the following:

- Develop an awareness of the norms of conflict in professional peers so they can be co-agents in the early identification of the potential for emergent conflict.
- Work with colleagues to organize a local work unit strategy for normalizing and addressing conflict that includes professional colleagues, interdisciplinary colleagues, associates, and managers.
- Develop specific protocols and processes that are automatically triggered when a particular conflict is identified and noted by any member of the staff.

- Devote a portion of the regular staff meeting to addressing a particularly challenging issue, circumstance, or event for which there is the potential for conflict or for which signs of conflict already exist.
- Regularly schedule social and relational outlets that promote socialization, friendly dialogue, celebration of key events, acknowledgment of successes or accomplishment, or recognition of important life occurrences.
- Regularly undertake feedback, evaluation, problem identification, complaints, or assessment of potential concerns with staff in an emotionally neutral, safe environment that makes such activities a regular part of the way of doing business in the unit or department.
- Establish communication, interaction, and communication norms that represent nonjudgmental, balanced, self-directed communication styles and patterns that eliminate judgment, threats, reactions, or aggression. Make these norms a part of the structure of meetings and of staff and leadership communication styles (Porter-O'Grady & Malloch, 2015).

Certain causes of conflict exist in almost every workplace. Often, individuals take these common causes for granted and ignore them as significant sources of potential conflict that can generate into increasing levels of stress and inequities at the departmental level. Professional interaction requires an awareness of the simple, usual, and ordinary issues that exist in the workplace that, if left unaddressed or are found to increase stress, create the conditions upon which conflict builds. All these elements require critical and conscious awareness, early engagement, and an organized and systematic mechanism for addressing them to prevent them from becoming drivers of conflict scenarios. Some of these usual and ordinary conflict sources that account for 90% of point-of-service conflicts are described next.

Personalities

The mix of individuals and personal characteristics in a work group is a critical determinant of the areas of concern with regard to communication and interaction in any work group. These personality differences invariably affect working relationships and may cause fallout regardless of who the people are and where the circumstances within the conflicts emerge. Recognizing the contribution that diversity makes in the team related to dialogue, decision making, problem solving, and innovation is important to developing a respect for these differences and recognizing how they can be accessed in a positive way. In addition, the challenges that differences in personality create need to be addressed. When personality challenges emerge in the course of interaction, they must be identified early so their potential to contribute to the dialogue and problem solving can

SCENARIO

Dr. Smith was particularly edgy today and appeared to be taking it out on everyone he met in the operating room. He did not act this way often, but staff could never be sure exactly when Dr. Smith would be on the emotional edge. This looming threat made it especially difficult to work in the surgical suite when people were already feeling stress about the surgery. Jane, the operating room team leader, was uncertain as to how to handle this situation. She knew that she could not let it go on unaddressed but was uncertain as to what the best approach would be.

Discussion Questions

1. When is the best moment to address Dr. Smith's behavior?

2. Where is the best place that Jane could talk with him?

3. How does Jane deal with her own uncertainty?

4. What might be the best way to open the conversation with Dr. Smith?

5. Should Jane discuss her approach with her peers before beginning?

6. Which expectations should Jane have of her conversation with Dr. Smith?

be assessed at the same time as the leader works to limit the potential negative impact or circumstances they may have on group processes.

Personal Needs, Insights, and Requisites

Everyone has a different core set of needs, drives, passions, intentions, and personal values. Each of these converge to create the unique characteristics that an individual brings to his or her profession and work. Sometimes employees may clash when their intensely felt motives rise to the surface and are expressed to other group members. Values and purpose are closely aligned with the central integrity of each individual. Giving those a voice, allowing them to be understood by each member of the team, and acknowledging the different value sets that people bring to the table can help establish a common value theme that gives the work unit a unique identity upon which the team can draw in times of challenge and difficulty. However, for this theme to emerge, these values must have a voice—and that voice must be honored, respected, and included in the mosaic of influences that informs the team's integrity and purpose in a way that represents the highest level of meaning.

Continuously Unresolvable Issues

Not every circumstance, situation, or condition can be resolved simply because people desire it. Often sociocultural, economic, technological, and regulatory requisites limit the full range of potential responses for problem resolution that people might identify as obvious or clear within their own situation or value set. Sometimes these contextual problems cannot be resolved in a short period of time or resolved in isolation in a manner that would curtail their perceived negative impact. To the fullest extent possible, problems that affect culture and relationship should be addressed and resolved early on. In those cases where regulatory influences cannot be changed, there should be opportunities to discuss them, react to them, and suggest local mechanisms for influencing their application. Participants might even develop new standards that mandate a higher level of performance or behavior than the regulations do. These can all be mechanisms that help participants to accommodate the intractable issues beyond their control or, in some ways, adapt or adjust to them.

Issues of Workload, Work Distribution, and Workload Intensity

One of the universal conditions of work is that there is always more work than there are resources to address it. Indeed, over the generations the notion has emerged that increasing resource use to meet the greater work demand is always the preferable solution. Supply chain science demonstrates, however, that such solutions are often simplistic and nonsustainable (King, 2011). Nevertheless, the perception and demands related to this notion frequently persist. Discussions and dialogue related specifically to issues of workload, work intensity, and role expectations need a forum and a regular opportunity for expression. The challenges that exist in matching demand to available resources need expression if conflict about them is to be allayed. This means having a regular opportunity in unit or department meetings to discuss issues of workload, staffing, assignments, resource management, changing demands, and the mechanisms that create balance and efficiencies among these elements. Giving these issues a voice

CRITICAL THOUGHT

Early engagement of conflict is valuable under all circumstances.

and organizational members a regular opportunity to express that voice and to respond to the issues that are raised in an equitable and efficient manner helps reduce stresses related to them. Giving a voice to these concerns allows employees to develop innovative or creative solutions for making adjustments and provides a forum for discussing modifying resources. Finally, such dialogue provides an opportunity for review and evaluation of existing workload strategies, resource issues, financial and budgetary concerns, and innovative solution seeking (Aiken, Clarke, Silber, & Sloane, 2003; Posthuma, 2012).

Personal Comfort with Conflict

Before the leader can engage in resolving conflict, the leader must be comfortable with his or her own sense of comfort in the presence of conflict. The effective leader works to create an environment where colleagues can be comfortable with their own feelings and with the ability to express them. This assumes, of course, that the individual is comfortable in the self-expression of feelings, personal insights, and challenges to prevailing views and circumstances. This leader, of course, needs an environment that is not constraining or controlling and that does not create structural barriers that make it fundamentally difficult for any individual to identify or express personal feelings. A good leader embraces his or her own feelings, regardless of their intensity, and in doing so demonstrates a level of transparency that is palpable and visible to others. As a result, the leader becomes comfortable with the expression of personal feelings and develops particular skills that frankly address and express issues of conflict through sensitive and careful consideration of the context and circumstances out of which these conflicts emerge (Shapiro, 2004).

The first thing the leader needs to be able to do is test his or her own "openness quotient":

- Am I truly comfortable with my own feelings? Is that comfort visible to others?
- Do I personally feel stress in the presence of impending or real conflict?
- Am I uncomfortable when other people express their own feelings and conflicts?
- Do I make it safe and comfortable for others to express conflicts and uncertainties to me?
- Am I able to embrace another individual in his or her moment of conflict with all the intensity and emotional expression that accompanies it?
- When there is anger or passion displayed, am I able to receive it and be available to it, or do I draw away from it?

- Am I engaging, embracing, and supportive as others express their emotional concerns related to particular conflict issues?

Each of these questions provides an opportunity for the individual to assess his or her own comfort and self-expression in the presence of conflict or conflict situations. It is difficult to ask others to be comfortable in the presence of conflict if one's own personal behavior exemplifies discomfort with the passion, emotions, noise, and expressions of conflict.

Trust: Creating a Safe Space for Positive Conflict

Everyone wants and needs trust in their lives. The ability to safely build commitment, attachment, and mutuality in relationships significantly influences just how well teams will work together, collaborate, express accountability, and have an impact. For the leader, a context of trust is the essential framework for the development of a truly safe space where conflict can be dealt with as easily and effectively as any other function, process, or relationship (Posthuma, 2012; Shani & Lau, 2005).

Trust is so important that it has a direct impact on the environment of work and the work itself. If a nontrusting environment exists, some degree of involvement and ownership will be lost; this factor will, in turn, have a direct effect on quality improvement and working methods and procedures in the clinical workplace. In addition, engagement and interaction are essential to the work. If the accuracy of communicating and reporting issues, incidents, and situations based on truth and openness is lacking, trust in the workplace begins to dwindle. Moreover, the potential for early detection of mistakes is negatively affected when the openness and honesty necessary for early detection and communication are not present; in such a scenario, the open discovery and resolution process will not work effectively. If issues of consensus, agreement, collective wisdom, common action, and other professional characteristics related to unfolding practice risks are limited or inhibited by an environment that is not characterized by openness, integrity, sincerity, mutuality, and commitment, then conflict inevitably emerges. In sum, the foundations of accountability are shaken in an environment where there is not trust or openness and there exists a lack of willingness to engage real issues, address early conflicts, resolve real problems in the workplace, and confront relational and interactional problems in a safe and trusting environment.

The Need for a Just Environment

The lack of a sense of justice and fairness in the workplace colors individual practitioners' and team members' belief in the fundamental fairness of their

BOX 4-1 ANTIDOTE FOR AN ENVIRONMENT OF INJUSTICE

- Regularly review team work processes and mechanisms for working together and problem solving.
- Use an open-ended questionnaire approach as a way of evaluating work team processes and dynamics.
- Use outside facilitation to drill down to issues of inequity or unfairness with the intent to seek equity or find solutions.

environment (Dekker, 2007). See **Box 4-1**. The sense of lack of justice stems from what is considered unfair work conditions, procedures, or relationships that are employed by the workplace and that impact the team, clinical action, individual decision making, and good leadership. Members of the clinical team begin to believe that there are inequitable opportunities to provide input and influence and make a difference. In this environment, individuals begin to experience what they perceive as biased work processes or procedures; these inequities diminish not only their own individual commitment to group action or to full participation, but also their attachment to the organization, the team, and their trust in leadership.

Fully Sharing Information

When every leader and team member shares his or her knowledge, the value that comes from experience is added to the team's decisions. Leaders and staff have many opportunities to fully cooperate in the sharing of useful and helpful information and experiences with one another. In turn, this cooperation makes it more likely that every person will fully support the group's final decision. When trust is absent in the unit or department, however, there is no commitment to the execution of the group's decisions. In fact, the staff may stall implementation efforts and sometimes actually sabotage them. Poor cooperation in fully sharing personal views, insights, or opinions is apparent in the following situations:

- You observe people nodding their heads or sitting in silence in response to a statement or question raised. This false sense of consensus signals a generalized fear or lack of consensus in sharing differing viewpoints, critical insights, or opposition in a healthy engagement and dialogue.
- People stop questioning or raising issues because they fear being labeled as not being team players and are viewed as obstructive or negative in the presence of legitimate questioning.

- Information is presented by individuals who heavily use jargon, generalized factoids, ethereal or nonspecific language, or the use of complex nonunderstandable, convoluted, or simply obtuse language.

Alienation Between Colleagues: What Happens When It Is Allowed to Flourish

Collegial attachment unfolds as team members become more familiar with one another, grow in their sense of membership on the team, and feel positive about the opportunities to work together. See **Box 4-2**. However, when alienation is allowed to flourish, individuals never arrive at that unique fellowship and strong sense of professional relationship that is a sign of a committed team. Instead, collegial relationships disappear and individuals pursue their own self-interests, often at the expense of the collective good of the team. Individuals may suffer from exhaustion and stress in a way that impedes ability to mitigate reactions to conflict (Kim et al., 2017). This predominantly individualistic behavior limits group flexibility, particularly in evaluating good choices, practice standards, and action (Bryman, 2011; Deutsch, Coleman, & Marcus, 2006).

In a professional environment, alienation is often unwittingly encouraged by permitting the reflective work of the profession to be sacrificed to unrelenting work expectations and by keeping team members busy without giving them the opportunity to think about what they are doing. Reflective work is essential for professionals to be able to determine value, importance, and priorities and to make decisions about best practices and necessary changes in patient care.

BOX 4-2 ANTIDOTES TO ALIENATION

- Ensure that performance expectations and group membership obligations are clearly and specifically enumerated and that performance evaluation includes these values.
- Establish clearly defined indicators of trust and review at least quarterly.
- Clearly delineate that team relationships, interactions, and communications are directly tied to patient care outcomes. Hold colleagues accountable for fully participating in the reflective components of practice.
- Challenge personal agendas when individual priorities predominate over team expectations and standards.

When this level of reflective interaction is sacrificed or seen as something extra by the organization or managers, the resulting lack of support for the reflective component of practice contributes to the decline of patient care and increases the security of definitive patient outcomes (Webber & Nathan, 2010). In this set of circumstances, members of the clinical team give up participating, recognize that interaction and reflection are not valued, and begin to behave in more dysfunctional employee work group patterns, ceasing to demonstrate the unique behaviors associated with professional practice.

In the midst of harried busyness and chronic addiction to action, emotional connection among colleagues never solidifies, reducing the opportunity for clinical team members to develop trust and to establish sustainable team-based patterns of work. This fragmentation emphasizes unilateral patterns of behavior, inconsistent standards of performance, and low expectations for performance and impact. The result is an uneven workload, unclear impact, competition, resentment, and challenge to the establishment of common standards of patient care practices.

Overcoming Personal Barriers to Engaging Conflict

Five personal barriers have a dramatic impact on the individual leader's ability to understand, engage, and manage conflict (**Table 4-1**). The leader must be intentional about conflict to bring it to the forefront of consciousness and to avoid simply responding to the emotional component inherent in almost every conflict situation. Often, breaking the conflict down into a logical sequence of stages helps make the conflict more objective, less personal, and more amenable to addressing and resolving it.

For the leader to be successful in managing conflict, there must be a willingness to confront conflict—that is, to overcome the barrier of fear. A survey by Mark Goulston (2015) found that 24% of people report rarely letting a colleague know when they are upset with him or her. When there is a generalized understanding in the unit or department that conflict is normative and will be incorporated into the usual and ordinary activities of managing relationships and interactions, personal reactions can be more safely confronted. Conflict management is a learned process that is developed and refined when a person has more opportunities to apply skills and test out approaches. When a safe space exists, it should be possible to objectively discuss approaches to particular kinds of conflicts and sensitivities individuals may have with regard to their relationship to that conflict. Bringing these personal issues into the open, discussing them freely, and treating the elements of conflict as a process help

Table 4-1 Overcoming Personal Barriers to Engaging Conflict

Barrier	Means to Overcome the Barrier
Fear	First, confront it. Take three deep breaths. Examine what is going on inside you. Talk to someone else about your fear. Talk yourself through the experience.
Uncertainty	Break the conflict down into parts. Identify which part has the greatest impact. Stay in touch with feelings and reactions. Identify conflict as early as possible. Validate with others your identification skills.
Negativity	Recall past experiences with conflict. Visualize yourself within a conflict. Observe family conflict dynamics. Talk with other family members. Write down and review your feelings.
No skills	Read about the conflict management process. Attend classes on conflict management. Role-play about conflict. Discuss the conflict process with others. Practice conflict scenarios.
Poor experience	Seek opportunities to practice. Begin mediating small conflicts. Have experts evaluate your progress. Build experience slowly. Evaluate your progress with peers.

diminish the fear associated with it and provide an opportunity for developing conflict-resolution experience.

The second major issue with addressing conflict is the uncertainty about the capacity to handle the conflict emotionally and personally. All conflict has a personal impact and touches individuals in a unique way. Each individual has his or her own experience with conflict and will automatically react to it in the initial stages of the conflict event. Becoming intentional helps overcome some of these issues but does not eliminate their emotional impact. If an individual can give language to the emotional experience he or she is feeling, that experience can be less obstructive and more objective. Each person will have a different alignment

CRITICAL THOUGHT

One of the most critical elements of addressing conflict is certainty regarding the feelings and insights of others. The mediator must always be sure that others' real feelings can be properly expressed.

with the conflict experience. Breaking down the emotional response into specific patterns of expression helps take from personal consciousness the sense that the whole conflict experience is necessarily rife with stress and pressure. More likely, certain stress elements or components of the conflict experience will generate 90% of the emotions that one feels in a conflict event. If the leader can grapple with the particular component that triggers his or her specific emotional response, the rest of the conflict management process reflecting that particular element of stress may be much easier to address, providing more opportunities for effectiveness.

Third, it is important to recognize that most people hold a negative attitude toward conflict. With all the discussion in the world about the positive influences and forces and normative character of conflict, personal history is generally indicative of a negative mindset or set of experiences. These experiences need to be shared among team members. When they are communicated to others and examined as a part of the dialogue together, much of the fear is diminished, resulting in a more objective assessment of the conflict experience. Sharing fears also helps others identify and personalize their own take on their conflict events. This helps defuse the negative experience, objectifies the elements of the conflict event, and makes it more manageable and useful as a tool for learning.

Conflict management reflects the fourth critical element: lack of skill. Conflict management is a learned skill—which means that the initial attempts at managing conflict are likely to be rough and unrefined. That is, the initial attempts by the staff to manage conflict are often halting, rudimentary, and not very elegant. However, with practice and opportunity, skills become refined, talent begins to grow, and effectiveness becomes a common experience. Individuals must realize that this experiential element of conflict handling is critical to personal development and a growing sense of confidence and competence with the handling of normative conflict. Through learning, application, and experiential opportunities, skills develop and become refined. During this process, the maturing conflict **mediator** becomes a role model and mentor for others who are refining their own conflict skill development (Boulle, Colatrella, & Picchioni, 2008). Some people move through this process more quickly and easily than others, which creates an obligation in them to mentor and support others whose developmental process

CRITICAL THOUGHT

The mediator does not own the problem and is not responsible for its resolution. The parties own the problem and are responsible for resolving it.

may be more challenging. In this way, skill development gets refined, common experiences get shared, and conflict becomes less dramatic as an element of shared professional relationships.

Lack of exposure and experience relates directly to the previous discussion about lack of conflict management skills. The more opportunities the leader has for actually managing conflict events, the more opportunity there is for skill development, experience, and technique refinement. The growing leader will seek opportunities first to mediate conflict in tandem with more experienced conflict managers. Later, as the leader becomes more competent and skilled, he or she can undertake conflict activities more independently and ultimately become a mentor and model for handling conflict for other colleagues. As a leader becomes more skilled in handling conflict, he or she evolves into a resource to the organization and may have the opportunity to resolve conflicts beyond the unit or department as his or her reputation for effectiveness and success grows and serves as an example of conflict effectiveness for the whole organization.

Handling Conflict

Although whole texts are devoted to the management of issues related to handling conflict, some simple rules provide the emerging leader with a basic toolset that can help guide his or her conflict skills development through the initial stages. The conflict management process is well studied, systematic, logical, and intentional. It guides parties from points of high-level conflict toward finding common ground and establishing more sustainable meaning in relationships (Partridge, 2009).

When people are given the opportunity to make choices and to manage their own lives, there is always a potential for conflict. Everyone is unique, of course. Their unique characteristics and wide variety of personalities define members of the human community as unique individuals and directly influence the roles they play and the contributions they make. At the same time, these gifts can sometimes serve as fundamental sources of potential conflict where those differences run up against the different expressions of others.

When handled creatively and effectively, these fundamental human differences can result in richer and deeper experiences and relationships among people. For this to happen, such differences must be handled with respect, through positive engagement. At the same time, the leader must handle conflicts between personalities assertively so they do not become or remain a source of constant contention and discord. If left unaddressed or ignored, important personality differences (conflict) can lay the groundwork for psychological and physiological harm. The existence of human differences creates an emotional and psychological distance between people that frequently manifests in negative feelings, aggression, oppression, antagonism, and alienation between people. In most cases (about 90% of the time) when managers call in mediators to deal with interpersonal conflicts, the conflict is found to result from a lack of understanding or misperception of personal patterns of behavior between participants (Hornickel, 2014; Kellett & Dalton, 2001). It is in anticipating these conflicts and in handling them early that the leader will spend most of his or her time in managing and mediating conflict activities.

Identifying the Problem

The leader's first task as a mediator for conflict is the ability to get the core issues at the heart of the conflict situation on the table and visible to all participants (Kritek, 2002). These core issues are identified by the involved individuals as the triggers that brought forth feelings of personal conflict. Good mediation leadership demonstrates the ability to find the central themes or issues and identify them as the drivers that most often hold people to their negative positions or feelings. Remember, these issues do not have to be right or accurate or even legitimate in the eyes of the mediator or anyone else; they simply must be felt, expressed, and clarified. Sorting through the legitimacy of issues comes later in the processes associated with resolution.

Making Sure Issues Are Expressed

The leader must be able to facilitate the individual's expression of his or her conflict in a way that is clear, frank, and understandable with regard to what is driving the individual's sense of the conflict. If the individual experiencing the conflict does not feel as though he or she has had the chance to fully express concerns and feelings, these feelings will continue—indeed, deepen—and will emerge later in the process, causing the process to slow or stop altogether. Patience and thoroughness around the issue of clarity by the mediating leader in the earliest stages of the conflict often result in fewer problems in the conflict resolution process and a quicker solution. The challenge for the mediator is to stay out of the way of expression and clarification. The mediator must always remember that he or she does not own the problem and, therefore, does not own its solution. The urge to intervene, to direct, or to control the resolution must be avoided by the mediator so the resolution that is obtained can be driven by the owners of the

CRITICAL THOUGHT

Unaddressed feelings are the most common cause of lingering conflict. These feelings smolder just below the surface, building energy, igniting fuses, and ultimately resulting in a devastating explosion that is very difficult to recover from—for all parties!

problem and they can move toward resolution in a joint effort. Remember, the mediator has no other goal than creating a safe space and helping the stakeholders resolve their own conflict.

Resolving the Five Kinds of Conflicts

Although many themes and shades of conflict occur among people, most conflicts fall into five general categories: relationship conflicts, information conflicts, interest-based conflicts, organizational conflicts, and values-based conflicts (Lansford, 2008). These five categories of conflicts have their own elements and constituents and require different insights to address and resolve them.

Relationship Conflicts

The most important ingredient for understanding relationship conflicts is being clear about how the individual feels and what he or she perceives about the conflict. The most notable kind of relational conflicts are those that build on inaccurate perceptions, especially related to what was either said or heard. Relationship conflicts are filled with emotional content. A part of the clarification process for relational conflicts is providing a safe space and time for expression for the emotional content that the individual is feeling about the relational issue. Effective mediators create a safe space that can bring individuals closer to the issues and deepen their relationship to them. To do so, they take the following steps:

- Move the parties away from each other and the place of conflict.
- Support each person in his or her feelings and emotions.
- Accept each individual's own perceptions of how he or she feels.
- Make sure each person has an opportunity to verbalize feelings.
- Do not attempt to resolve the issue before individuals express feelings.
- Be caring and supportive of each person experiencing the conflict.
- Accept whatever emotions are expressed in an appropriate place for it.

Relationships are filled with meaning and purpose, and the feelings related to the significance of this meaning must be explored sufficiently to help the parties translate their positions into language that communicates them most effectively. However, dealing with feelings and dealing with issues must be separated at the outset so they are not handled in the same way. Expressing feelings is an important part of helping individuals identify their response to their own perceptions of the conflict. As they get clear about these feelings, they can become clearer about their notion of the real issue and can be more supportive of its systematic assessment. Each party must be given sufficient time to express feelings and emotions so the full range of sensitivities related to their perception of the conflict has an opportunity to be stated and recognized. In relationship conflicts, the greatest failure in the resolution is usually found in inadequate allowances for the expression of feeling and the ability to give that feeling a language that can be understood.

There are several elements the leader will need to include in the mediation process and make the parties aware of as they explore relationship issues:

- *Mutual respect.* No matter how divided the individuals are or how attached they are to their positions, keep reminding them of their common humanity and the value each of them has. Good mediators stay keenly aware of the mutuality of weaknesses, frailties, perceptions, and positions each person brings to the table. The mediator reminds the parties of the respect they want for themselves and ensures that they offer it to each other as fully as possible in the circumstances. The mediation leader tries to direct anger to the issues, not to the person.

- *Needs versus wants.* The leader must help the participants figure out and differentiate between what they really need and what they perceive they want. The leader seeks to help the parties deepen their understanding of what they need and relate their wants to that particular need. Indeed, in this case, it is important to identify something the individual must have as a part of this self-expectation or reason to mediate. Although getting what a person needs is critical, getting what he or she wants may be less so. Helping the parties differentiate needs from wants and assisting them in achieving satisfaction of that need is a significant part of the mediation dynamic.

- *Compassion and empathy.* One of the intentions of mediation is to help the parties understand each other and to hear the other party's position clearly and with understanding. The leader creates a context for equity and value and translates that value with a sense of compassion and empathy.

- *Staying in the "I."* In relationship conflicts, there is always a temptation to blame and focus on the other party. The role of the mediator is to

SCENARIO

Rachel did not know if she could stand one more negative comment from Michael. Ever since she had arrived on the nursing unit, Michael had almost nothing positive to say to her. He seemed to track her every clinical move and knew exactly when she was overwhelmed or concerned and even when she was behind in her work. It was then that he seemed to comment about her pace, competence, and organization. Once again, this morning he had started with the comments, even suggesting that Rachel might not be able to keep up with the demands of the clinical work. His constant monitoring of her work and comments about her ability to keep up increased the stress level and made her even more tense in this new clinical situation than she would normally feel. Rachel did not know what to do. If Michael did not stop soon, she would either blow up or just throw up her hands and even consider leaving.

Discussion Questions

1. At this point in this scenario, what should Rachel's first step be?

2. Which kind of environment needs to be created to facilitate expressing conflict feelings?

3. Which kind of a relationship conflict would you define this to be?

4. Who will Rachel need to involve in her effort to resolve this conflict?

keep the parties focused on their own feelings and insights, avoiding blame, name calling, and the prolific use of "you" statements. The mediator consistently reminds the parties to begin their statements or responses with "I" statements, such as "I feel," "I think," "I need," "I want," and "I see." This keeps all parties focused on their own role, communication, interaction, and needs.

Information Conflicts

People often make judgments that reflect their own perceptions, values, and personal processing of what they know and the kind of information that supports it. Sometimes the information they access is inaccurate or inadequate to support their position. When integrated with the individual's values and perceptions, poor or inadequate information can become a potent source of conflict.

CRITICAL THOUGHT

People often think they have the right information without ever analyzing its source, the perspective it represents, the content, and the meaning it is attempting to project. A great deal of conflict could be avoided if people would really think carefully about the information influencing their actions.

Available information on its own demonstrates no bias. Bias occurs when information goes through the perceptive and values filters of the individual reviewing it. In a conflict resolution process, careful assessment of the adequacy, relevance, and accuracy of the information supporting a particular view is critical to the effectiveness of the resolution at any level of appropriate action in the mediation. Before any action can occur (including drawing conclusions or making judgments), the individuals who are involved in the conflict should deal with the following critical questions (here readers may think of a particular information-based conflict that arose because of inadequate, inappropriate, or incomplete use of information):

- What is the source of the information?
- Is the information relevant to the issue at hand?
- Does the information correlate well with other sources of related information?
- Is the source of the information credible? Is it complete?
- Is there enough information from which to draw any relevant conclusions?
- What are the prevailing views or perceptions in this mediation related to interpreting the information?
- What else needs to be done to clarify or verify information that is influencing the thinking and dialogue in the mediation?

The leader should encourage parties in the conflict to think about the following questions:

- Are judgments being made before all the information is available to support them?
- Is the meaning of the information clear to all parties before conclusions are drawn from them about which action needs to be taken?

SCENARIO

Wendy walks into the breakroom to put her lunch away prior to beginning her shift. Two other nurses are having a very vocal discussion about how no one ever involves them in decisions and how frustrating it is that the wound care supplies are being changed with no consultation from clinical nurses. Wendy values the input of the two nurses having the discussion, respects their professional opinion, and has a positive working relationship with them. Prior to hearing this discussion, Wendy's understanding of the situation was that the organization was going to trial a few new wound care products and after that make a decision regarding products.

Discussion Questions

1. At this point in this scenario, what should Wendy's first step be?

2. Which kind of environment needs to be created to facilitate expressing conflict feelings?

3. What are the perceptions of those involved with the conflict?

4. What information needs to be clarified to gain mutual understanding and insight regarding this conflict?

5. Who will Wendy need to involve in her effort to resolve this conflict?

- Are all parties' perceptions appropriately clarified so there is a mutual level of understanding and insight regarding the relevant information?

The challenge for the leader lies in managing information appropriately. Information that conflicts with an individual's fundamental beliefs or ideas about the problem is often difficult to adjust or change. People tend to hold onto their beliefs and levels of understanding whether the supporting information validates them or not. Cautiously moving through a recalibration of the personal impact of accurate information and understanding about what people know requires careful consideration of the data, the data's impact on the individuals, the potential for achieving mutual understanding about the information, and the likely usefulness of the information for subsequent dialogue and decision making.

CRITICAL THOUGHT

Most interest conflicts are characterized by the party's tremendous emotional and psychological attachment to the issue in conflict. The good mediator attempts to defuse the emotional and psychological passion and ensures the parties can get to a level of discourse that can lead to resolution.

Interest-based Conflicts

Parties to a conflict come to the table with a stake in the conflict. They have interests that need to be resolved. Much of the conflict is about differentiation of their interests. As a consequence, specifying and naming particular interests is a critical part of what the leader is attempting to accomplish in the dialogue between conflicting parties.

It is important that clarity of individuals' feelings and sensitivities related to their own concerns be established early as a part of identifying conflicting interests. Frequently, the parties are unaware that they actually may share interests; there may be common ground with regard to what they originally assumed to be conflict related to interests, or misperceptions about the interest and the conflict that generated. Indeed, the real conflict may have nothing to do with the interest that brought them to the table.

Often in the arena of interest conflict, the challenge focuses more on the different insights and perceptions each party has about how they know the issues and how they have come to understand their role in relationship to them than on the real interests. Often what occurs in these kinds of conflicts is that the legitimate interests the parties share are hidden behind an expressed interest. The mediator must work to get both parties to a place where they can recognize the underlying or real interest that is truly generating the conflict. Moving beyond the perception of interest to actual interest enhances the likelihood of conflict resolution.

Of special concern with interest-based conflict is the fact that the parties may not know what their genuine interests are: They may be actually hiding genuine interests, perceptions may be obstructing the emergence of genuine interests, or they may even be unaware of what the actual interests might be. In such a case, the mediator must bring them to sensitively, but more deeply, articulate the genuine interest issues so the real interests may be dealt with directly and effectively.

Organizational Conflicts

There are innumerable sources of organizational conflict, including the following:

- Conflicting goals
- Conflicts between groups

SCENARIO

The day shift and evening shift on a postpartum unit is experiencing conflict about the timing of patient education for families after childbirth. Each shift believes the other shift should be primarily responsible for completing the education. The day shift feels that the education would best be completed on the evening shift when other family members are present for the education. The evening shift feels that it is too chaotic when multiple family members are present and the mother cannot focus on the information. As chair of the unit's professional governance council, you have been asked to mediate the issue.

Discussion Questions

1. At this point in this scenario, what should you do?

2. Which kind of environment needs to be created to facilitate expressing conflict feelings?

3. What are the individual interests of each shift?

4. Who else can be involved to resolve this conflict?

- Intergroup competition
- Inadequate leadership
- Failure
- Compartmented departments

Although many of the sources of conflict in organizations may be obvious to all parties, most are not. Yet, organizational conflicts drive a wide range of personal conflicts because the organization essentially defines the context within which people relate and work. Organizational conflicts relate to questions of accountability, expectations, and systemic communication. In addition, questions may arise about whether a supportive environment exists that encourages the point-of-service work of the organization and provides appropriate infrastructure and resource allocation for that work to be owned and done at the point of service (Harvey & Allard, 2002; Zedeck, 2011).

The issues that drive effectiveness of the organizational culture and its facility for limiting conflict are directly related to how well people work together, how team-based activities have been constructed and sustained, how mismatches between the needs of patient care and the distribution of resources have been addressed, and how congruent the values of the organization are with the values of the people who comprise it. Conflicts in organizations can be considered as having a series of layers—the overall organizational structure, the configuration of the leadership team, the relationship and interaction between departments and services, interdisciplinary collaboration and interaction at the point of service, and the structure and relationships that operate daily at the organization's point of service. Collectively, these elements form a network that represents the character of the organization and indicates the confluence of forces in the organization and how they either constrain or facilitate effectiveness at each and every level.

The clinical leader at the point of service can have a radical impact on the roles, relationships, and effectiveness of work within the unit or department. Certainly, there should be a goodness of fit between broad organizational goals and a specific unit or departmental goals. If the general goals of the system are to be achieved, people at the point of service will need to translate those goals into action through their work effort.

Organizational conflict depends on the insight, awareness, and information level of the leader regarding organizational priorities, parameters, policies, and practices. It is important for the leader to carefully observe individuals and teams for their potential to develop and enact purposes, goals, or actions that are not directly related to the purpose, mission, and goals of the larger system. Among professional members of the system, there is a tacit agreement that a goodness of fit will exist between the purpose, mission, and goals of the system and the personal goals of the members who compose that system (Boddy, 2011). The leader is charged with making sure that there is a goodness of fit between these dynamic forces and that good alignment exists between the trajectory of the organization and that of the individual member. Some questions asked to clarify these issues might be as follows (here again, readers may identify organizational conflicts in their own experience and apply the following questions to see how those conflicts might have been better handled and resolved):

- How clear and precise are the purposes and goals of the organization, and how well does that fit with the work done at the point of service?
- Is everyone in the department or unit aware of the personal role they play in fulfilling the organization's mission and goals?
- Are there mutuality and agreements among professional colleagues, managers, and the organization regarding goals, resources, and specific actions to fulfill the effort to advance the agenda of the organization?
- Are performance measures clear and specific enough to tell the story of the staff's contribution to the organization's mission and goals?

CRITICAL THOUGHT

Organizational conflicts are best resolved when everyone in the organization is "singing off of the same song sheet." When individuals and groups play out their own agendas at the expense of others or the whole organization, they create the framework for organizational conflict. To get past this sort of fragmentation or to ensure that it does not happen, leaders must ensure that people see themselves as members of the larger organization and are committed to making it successful.

- Do leaders at every level of the organization encourage and facilitate providing the necessary resource support, goal congruence, organizational understanding for the goals, and full engagement of all stakeholders in the right response to organizational goals?
- Are financial challenges, constraints, issues of distribution, and opportunities clearly explained to all participants in a way that deepens their understanding or advances their engagement? Is financial management adjusted when performance information indicates the need for it?
- Do the clinical and management leaders in the organization participate in the system's collective effort to delineate strategy, establish priorities, define direction, construct goals, and evaluate the effectiveness of all work effort related to them?

Each of these questions alone is not sufficient to root out conflicting elements in organizational activity, but when considered together they create an integrated framework that provides a context for organizational clarity, specificity of goals and action, congruence between systems and people, effectiveness, and goal achievement. It is clear that the more the organizational framework, purpose, direction, and goals inform actions, the less likely that conflict will emerge between and among any of these characteristics. The role of every effective leader is to address those arenas, components, or elements of the organization and its goals, structures, and processes that are not congruent with the achievement of excellence in practice, process, or patient outcomes. A critical openness in organizations is the foundation for all engaged human action in systems. Varying degrees or levels of compromise in any one or more of these elements accelerates the potential for conflict in the organization and raises challenges to personal and organizational effectiveness.

Values-based Conflicts

Perhaps the most difficult conflicts to address in the workplace are those that relate to personal values. There are many sources of values conflict:

- Different cultures
- Different ethnic groups
- Different religious beliefs
- Different personal values
- Different political ideology
- Different economic and social status

Fundamental values-based conflicts may arise from almost any source significant enough to create specific identity differences between individuals and groups. Values conflicts are difficult to resolve because they generally relate to who people are, what they believe, and how they identify themselves to each other and to the world. They relate not so much to what people think as to how people feel about who they are in the world and how that is best represented in their person. It is here where the impacts of culture, ethnicity, religious beliefs, ideology, internal values, and politics are fully played out and expressed.

The quality and effectiveness of professional and work relationships over time depend, for the most part, on how well people can clarify, accommodate, and adjust to significant values differences. Here again, it is important that individuals be clear about their own personal values so that their relationship to these values can be articulated in a way that helps individuals develop a better understanding of themselves and their place in the world and that creates a foundation or premise for translating that understanding to others. Questions that need clarification at the personal level might be as follows:

- What does what you see and feel in the world mean to you at a very personal level?
- How do your culture, religion, belief system, values structure, and personal life practices inform the way in which you live your life?
- How is the answer to the previous question demonstrated in the image that you present and the way in which you show others how you live your life?
- What is it that you need others to understand about your personal values system?
- How do you demonstrate adherence to your own values and continue to respect the values differences of others as they live their lives?

- In which areas are your values significantly different from those generally expressed, and how have you accommodated them while honoring others' expression of different values?
- Are you willing to respect the diversity of values in your work culture, and are you committed to resolving conflicts between them that may affect both work and relationships?

Exploration of these questions is a critical first step for every professional and is nonnegotiable for the leader. Clarity around issues of personal value and one's relationship to the world from that values position is a foundation upon which relationships with others, the organization, and society can be developed and refined. Common responses to values conflicts often reflect a lack of clarity around these questions. These reactions may include proselytizing and position taking (lecturing, not listening); minimizing, denying, accommodating, or avoiding any issues with the potential for values conflict in an effort to keep the peace; and pretending to agree, defer, discount, or ignore values differences simply to avoid having to deal with them at all. In contrast, when participants can genuinely acknowledge particular differences, seek common ground, find a broader accommodation of multiple values positions, and develop reasonable compromise, they can build strong relationships that reflect the values incorporation as a part of mutual understanding.

Values conflicts are indeed difficult to address and resolve, but that does not make them impossible or completely intractable. For the leader, however, a unique set of approaches is needed to address constantly existing value differences among colleagues in the workplace. A number of simple, consistent, yet important contextual and role practices can generally be useful in minimizing the potential for values conflict, isolating and focusing on particular values challenges, or exploring a deeper and broader value of diversity and richness in the human experience, dialogue, and relationships. A few of those critical elements are as follows:

- Make a true and abiding commitment to finding common ground and developing win-win compromises in values adjustments between individuals and groups.
- Expand the vocabulary and language of the workplace to include broader terms, expressions, and definitions that are inclusive and respectful.
- Find the common themes and elements between and among values that can anchor relationships and demonstrate the foundation for the expressions of value.

CRITICAL THOUGHT

Values conflicts can be resolved only when common ground can be established among the parties. There must be some elements of belief and human experience with which the parties can mutually identify and through that experience find a route to building a stronger relationship upon which subsequent interaction can build.

- Articulate and define a system in your unit that includes the fundamental elements of dignity and respect, and that informs all behavioral expectations among members and colleagues.
- Explicitly state the legitimacy of individual differences, the right to have them, and the appropriate forum within which they can be legitimately expressed. At the same time, define and acknowledge environments, contexts, and situations where the expression of such differences is not legitimate or appropriate.
- Make sure a specific and well-designed ethics process or committee is in place to deal with significant values challenges or intractable values issues and to establish a common frame for behavioral expectations and expression.
- As with other differences, make values conflicts a normative expectation of the dynamics of a diverse membership group, creating a safe space for exploration, an effective process for dialogue and clarification, and *a mechanism for conflict resolution.*

Although values conflicts can create significant noise within a social system and within professional relationships, those differences need not impede or imperil the essential professional values represented in the provision of patient care. A consistent and ongoing effort to find common ground and stand on it helps create a strong set of relationships, an effective organization, and the medium for acting out of a clearly established set of common values.

The Norm of Conflict

Over time, the wise leader will come to acknowledge the universal presence of conflict and the continuing and dynamic necessity for addressing it. Conflict will not diminish, disappear, or dissipate in the human experience. It can only be well managed. In the absence of serious and effective management of conflict, it invariably accelerates, increases its intensity, and moves toward the creation of great harm.

The effective leader sees signs of conflict constantly fomenting in people and in the organization. The conflicting interests and dynamic differences between people and cultures are always a rich source for conflict escalation.

Leadership

- Poor recognition of emerging conflict
- Inadequate conflict skills
- Highly competitive
- Seeks own agenda in spite of organizational goals
- Cannot tie personal behavior to organizational expectations
- Actually likes conflict—pitting people against each other

Individuals

- Problems with work competency
- Difficulty establishing relationships
- Personal anger
- Highly competitive
- Unclear about role expectations and goal requirements
- Unable to become a team player

Groups

- Group relationship unformed or immature
- Groups aggressive or angry with other groups
- Unhealthy level of organizational competition
- Group goals incongruent with organizational goals
- Internally dysfunctional group dynamics
- Failure of the group to fulfill its obligations or achieve goals

To be effective in managing conflict, the leader first must have a defined level of comfort with the reality that conflict is a constant companion of human interaction and relationship. Out of this understanding and comfort with the presence of conflict comes the need to develop methodologies and techniques for positively addressing it. The goal is to engage conflict early enough that its positive value can be experienced and that it can ultimately make a difference in the interests of the professional community and those it serves.

SCENARIO

So much information had been swirling around the potential for patient care changes on the unit for so long that it was impossible to know what was true and what was not. The unit manager certainly tried to get clarity about which kinds of patient care changes would be coming, when the changes would be undertaken, and what the unit's staff would need to do differently in the future. There had been official notice from administration that new services and new medical staff were coming on board and that transplantation services would be added to the existing cardiac surgery services. The nurses of the cardiac unit were used to change but really needed to have clarity and specificity to deal with it with meaning and value. However, at the moment, it was difficult to sort through what was rumor and what was truth, and the confusion was creating significant unrest on the unit.

Discussion Questions

1. Is this an organizational conflict or an informational conflict (or both)?

2. Which first steps in addressing this issue does unit leadership need to take to bring some clarity to the potential for change?

3. Which format or protocol would you use to organize a change initiative and formalizing mechanism for communicating future changes in a way that reduces the potential for stress on the unit?

4. When there is legitimate uncertainty about a potential change and clarity simply cannot be obtained in the early stages, which support processes or approaches would you recommend to help the unit staff allay the potential for frustration and conflict?

SCENARIO

Cynthia Morgan, RN, was new to the mother–child unit. She was raised in a religious community that had very strong rules and restrictions on specific medical and surgical procedures related to mothers and the birth process. There were especially restrictive rules in her belief system regarding birth control and abortion. One of these restrictions related to tubal ligation (women having their "tubes tied") following childbirth. Cynthia had noticed just such a procedure on the morning schedule with one of her patients. She subsequently created a "scene" at the nurses station by clearly stating her beliefs and her refusal to have anything to do with such a procedure. She also loudly proclaimed why she felt such procedures were "immoral" and made other nursing staff uncomfortable by informing them that they, too, should not participate in such activities. This incident created quite an uproar on the nursing unit, resulting in the need for the unit manager to intercede. She changed Cynthia's patient schedule and assignment and scheduled a time for a unit conference to deliberate this issue and establish an appropriate format for dealing with it.

Discussion Questions

1. Which category of conflict does this scenario represent?

2. When would have been the earliest time to engage this potential conflict?

3. What information should inform the staff's dialogue regarding this issue and its potential for conflict?

4. Which formal process would you have created to better address conflicts associated with this issue?

5. How would you best respond to a staff member acting out in a public place in a way that creates conflict and discomfort? What should have happened in this case?

CHAPTER TEST QUESTIONS

Licensure exam categories: Management of care: concepts of management/ leadership, delegation/supervision

Nurse leader exam categories: Communication and relationship building: effective communication, relationship management, influencing behaviors; Leadership: change management

1. Discuss the essential skills to manage conflict in relation to your own personal characteristics. Which would you like to grow?

2. Discuss the best time to engage with conflict and the rationale for this timing.

3. Emotions must be controlled and separated from the conflict so that the real issues can be addressed more directly. True or false?

4. Describe the role of the conflict mediator in an interest-based conflict.

5. The conflict mediator manages all elements of the conflict and assists parties to the conflict in their personal expression and in determining who needs to get what from the experience. True or false?

6. All conflict is normative in group or team dynamics. What is the role of the leader in conflict?

7. Discuss the five personal barriers to conflict resolution and problem solving. Consider a conflict you have been involved in. Which personal factors were at play?

8. It is not the mediator's obligation to focus on the core issues of conflict; rather, it is the obligation of the parties to know their core issues and to be willing to negotiate them. True or false?

9. Identity issues are the easiest to resolve because they deal only with values and personal belief, which can be quickly identified. When they are clear, they can help move the parties to early and complete resolution. True or false?

10. All conflict is resolvable if there is a good match between commitment and effort of the parties, use of best methodology, and the clarity and effectiveness of the solutions obtained. True or false?

References

Aiken, L., Clarke, S., Silber, J., & Sloane, D. (2003). Hospital nurse staffing, education and patient mortality. *LDI Issue Brief, 2*, 1–4.

Amer, R., & Zou, K. (2011). *Conflict management and dispute settlement in East Asia.* Farnham, UK: Ashgate.

American Association of Colleges of Nursing. (2008). *The essentials of baccalaureate education for professional nursing practice.* Washington, DC: AACN. www.aacnnursing.org/Education-Resources/AACN-Essentials

Avruch, K., & Mitchell, C. R. (2013). Conflict resolution and human needs: Linking theory and practice (pp. 245–263). *Routledge studies in peace and conflict resolution, 1.* Oxford, UK: Routledge Publishers.

Blackard, K., & Gibson, J. W. (2002). *Capitalizing on conflict: Strategies and practices for turning conflict into synergy in organizations: A manager's handbook*. Palo Alto, CA: Davies-Black.

Boddy, C. (2011). *Corporate psychopaths: Organisational destroyers*. New York, NY: Palgrave Macmillan.

Boulle, L., Colatrella, M. T., & Picchioni, A. P. (2008). *Mediation: Skills and techniques*. Newark, NJ: LexisNexis Matthew Bender.

Bryman, A. (2011). *The Sage handbook of leadership*. Thousand Oaks, CA: Sage.

Dekker, S. (2007). *Just culture: Balancing safety and accountability*. Aldershot, UK: Ashgate.

Deutsch, M., Coleman, P. T., & Marcus, E. C. (Eds.). (2006). *The handbook of conflict resolution: Theory and practice* (2nd ed.). San Francisco, CA: Jossey-Bass.

Goulston, M. (2015). How people communicate during conflict. *Harvard Business Review*, *93*(6), 22.

Harvey, C. P., & Allard, M. J. (2002). *Understanding and managing diversity: Readings, cases, and exercises*. Upper Saddle River, NJ: Prentice Hall.

Hornickel, J. (2014). *Negotiating success: Tips and tools for building rapport and dissolving conflict while still getting what you want*. Hoboken, NJ: John Wiley & Sons.

Kellett, P. M., & Dalton, D. G. (2001). *Managing conflict in a negotiated world: A narrative approach to achieving dialogue and change*. Thousand Oaks, CA: Sage.

Kim, S., Bochatay, N., Relyea-Chew, A., Buttrick, E., Amdahl, C., Kim, L., . . . Lee, Y. M. (2017). Individual, interpersonal, and organisational factors of healthcare conflict: A scoping review. *Journal of Interprofessional Care*, *31*(3), 282–290. doi:10.1080/13561820.2016.1272558

King, T. F. (2011). *A companion to cultural resource management*. Chichester, UK: Wiley-Blackwell.

Kritek, P. B. (2002). *Negotiating at an uneven table: Developing moral courage in resolving our conflicts*. San Francisco, CA: Jossey-Bass.

Lansford, T. (2008). *Conflict resolution*. Detroit, MI: Greenhaven.

LeBaron, M. (2002). *Bridging troubled waters: Conflict resolution from the heart*. San Francisco, CA: Jossey-Bass.

Lencioni, P. (2002). *The five dysfunctions of a team: A leadership fable*. San Francisco, CA: Jossey-Bass.

Levinger, M. (2013). *Conflict analysis: Understanding causes, unlocking solutions*. Washington, DC: Institute of Peace Press.

Lodge, M., & Wegrich, K. (2012). *Executive politics in times of crisis*. Houndmills, UK: Palgrave Macmillan.

MacDonald, G. (2011). *Building below the waterline: Shoring up the foundations of leadership*. Peabody, MA: Hendrickson.

Partridge, M. V. B. (2009). *Alternative dispute resolution: An essential competency for lawyers.* Oxford, UK: Oxford University Press.

Porter-O'Grady, T., & Malloch, K. (2015). *Quantum leadership.* Burlington, MA: Jones & Bartlett Learning.

Posthuma, R. (2012). Conflict management and emotions. *International Journal of Conflict Management, 23*(1), 1. proxy.library.oregonstate.edu/login?url=http://OSU.eblib.com/patron/FullRecord.aspx?p=896031

Ramsbotham, O., Woodhouse, T., & Miall, H. (2011). *Contemporary conflict resolution.* Cambridge, UK: Polity Press.

Rodgers, D. T. (2011). *Age of fracture.* Cambridge, MA: Belknap.

Shani, A. B., & Lau, J. B. (2005). *Behavior in organizations: An experiential approach.* New York, NY: McGraw-Hill Irwin.

Shapiro, D. (2004). *Conflict and communication: A guide through the labyrinth of conflict management.* New York, NY: International Debate Education Association.

Smokowski, P. R., & Bacallao, M. (2011). *Becoming bicultural: Risk, resilience, and Latino youth.* New York, NY: New York University Press.

Stahl, P. M. (2011). *Conducting child custody evaluations: From basic to complex issues.* Thousand Oaks, CA: Sage.

Tojo, J., & Dilpreet, C. (2007). *Appreciative inquiry and knowledge management.* Northhampton, UK: Edward Elgar.

Webber, M., & Nathan, J. (2010). *Reflective practice in mental health: Advanced psychosocial practice with children, adolescents and adults.* London, UK: Jessica Kingsley.

Wenger, A., & Möckli, D. (2003). *Conflict prevention: The untapped potential of the business sector.* Boulder, CO: Lynne Rienner.

Zedeck, S. (2011). *APA handbook of industrial and organizational psychology.* Washington, DC: American Psychological Association.

APPENDIX A

A Brief Conflict Skills Assessment

For conflict to be properly handled, the leader must have specific skills. This is simply the basic inventory of conflict skills. For each of the points made, select the appropriate answer. The higher your score, the greater your conflict skills value. This assessment should be looked at as a developmental tool, not a test.

Scale: 1 = Almost never; 2 = Sometimes; 3 = Often; 4 = Regularly

I have a good sense of the needs of the team at any given moment.				I can anticipate important changes and alert the team before they directly experience the change.			
1	2	3	4	1	2	3	4
I work hard not to avoid conflicts.				I undertake at least one developmental opportunity per year to refine conflict skills.			
1	2	3	4	1	2	3	4
I make it safe for people to identify and express conflicts at work.				There is a staff-driven conflict resolution process in place on my work unit.			
1	2	3	4	1	2	3	4
Staff have opportunities to test their mediation and conflict resolution skills.				The environment is conducive to anyone expressing feelings of conflict.			
1	2	3	4	1	2	3	4
We have fewer conflict events on our service unit since implementing a conflict resolution process.				There is a mechanism in place for following up on conflict resolution and ensuring it was effective.			
1	2	3	4	1	2	3	4
I make it safe for people to identify and express conflicts at work.				Conflicts are identified early in the workplace so they are more easily resolved.			
1	2	3	4	1	2	3	4
The trust level on my unit is consistently high.				Staff are satisfied with the conflict process used on our unit.			
1	2	3	4	1	2	3	4
We regularly evaluate the conflict process on our unit and make changes to make it more effective.				Scoring: 1–15 Need further conflict skills development 16–30 Growing conflict management awareness 31–45 Building an effective conflict management approach 41–60 Effective conflict management leader/workplace			
1	2	3	4				

> Planning is bringing the future into the present so that you can do something about it now. —Alan Laiken[1]

CHAPTER OBJECTIVES

Upon completion of this chapter, the reader will be able to do the following:

» Develop an understanding of patient care delivery models, patient classification systems, and scheduling and staffing.

» Provide an overview of the complexities and interconnectedness of the components of workforce management systems.

» Understand the importance of evidence-driven processes, integration of research, and their impact on nurse satisfaction, patient quality, and organizational outcomes.

» Describe the current measures of staffing effectiveness.

» Gain an appreciation of the challenges in addressing inadequacies or problems of staffing and scheduling.

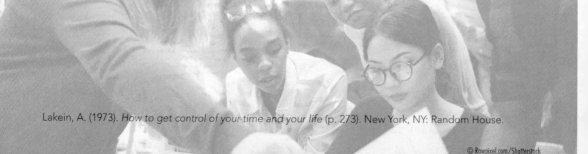

Lakein, A. (1973). *How to get control of your time and your life* (p. 273). New York, NY: Random House.

Staffing, Scheduling, and Patient Care Assignments: Models, Components, and Measures of Effectiveness

Chapter

5

Workforce management in health care requires an understanding of the nature and complexities of the dynamics involved in providing the right nurse for the right patient at the right time. Providing the right nurse for the right patient at the right time involves more than just assigning available nurses to the current list of patients on a unit. It requires an understanding of the critical elements and dynamics of workforce management processes and the translation of these elements into a staffing plan that supports the achievement of the highest quality outcomes. Staffing is not about the tools and technologies available; it is about using those tools alongside professional nursing judgment and critical thinking to achieve safety, quality, and satisfaction.

In this chapter, the importance of the patient care delivery model; basics of **staffing** and **scheduling**; regulatory, accrediting, and research standards for staffing effectiveness; evaluation of the measures of staffing effectiveness; challenges in managing variances in resources; and the role of the clinical leader in ensuring optimal staffing practices are discussed.

The nurse leader must coordinate patient workforce management to include five highly interconnected and interrelated components (**Figure 5-1**):

1. Establishment of a patient care delivery model
2. Patient needs and nurse interventions identification

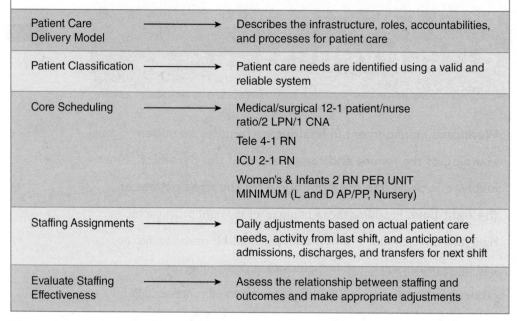

Workforce management includes distinct processes with special characteristics, processes, and goals.

Caveat: Continuing to attempt to amalgamate patient classification, scheduling, staffing, retention, and recruitment into one process serves only to decrease system validity and frustrate workers with additional unproductive tasks.

Patient Care Delivery Model	→ Describes the infrastructure, roles, accountabilities, and processes for patient care
Patient Classification	→ Patient care needs are identified using a valid and reliable system
Core Scheduling	→ Medical/surgical 12-1 patient/nurse ratio/2 LPN/1 CNA Tele 4-1 RN ICU 2-1 RN Women's & Infants 2 RN PER UNIT MINIMUM (L and D AP/PP, Nursery)
Staffing Assignments	→ Daily adjustments based on actual patient care needs, activity from last shift, and anticipation of admissions, discharges, and transfers for next shift
Evaluate Staffing Effectiveness	→ Assess the relationship between staffing and outcomes and make appropriate adjustments

Figure 5-1 Workforce Management

3. Creation of a core staffing schedule to support patient needs
   a. Knowledge of staff competencies and abilities
   b. Integration of staffing and research evidence
   c. Skill mix
   d. Registered nurse (RN) competencies
   e. Educational levels
4. Daily staffing process to match available staff with identified patient care needs
   a. Interpreting and managing the adequacy of the staffing
   b. Variance between actual staffing and patient care needs
   c. Staffing adequacy indicators/effectiveness
   d. Capacity determination

5. Evaluation of value and outcomes

   a. Qualitative and quantitative assessment of patient, caregiver, and organization outcomes

   b. Nurse retention, satisfaction, and turnover

   c. Productivity monitoring

   d. Financial performance

   e. Modification or updating of budget and performance targets for staffing effectiveness

A **workforce management** or staffing plan describes the structure and processes by which the nurse assigns responsibilities for patient care and how the work is coordinated among caregivers. In addition, it describes the mechanism for documenting and reporting staffing concerns. This integrated set of processes begins with the patient care delivery model.

The Foundation: Patient Care Delivery Model

Prior to determining how many nurses are needed for patient care, a clearly thought-out model or framework for delivering patient care is needed. A **patient care delivery model** is defined as a method or system for organizing and delivering nursing care. It includes the manner in which nursing care is organized so as to deliver care that meets the needs of the patient. The delivery system encompasses work delegation, resource utilization, communication methodologies, clinical decision-making processes, and management structure (Hall, 2005).

The patient care model emerges from the organization's mission, vision, values, and structure, which identify the desired outcomes, decision-making authority, and span of control. Thus, the model has a direct and significant impact on the number and levels of nursing staff allocated to provide nursing care. Patient care delivery models are necessarily dynamic because the healthcare environment, needs of the patients, and available technology are continually changing. The mission, vision, and values remain the stabilizing and focusing forces for the patient care delivery model. Further, the adequacy and effectiveness of the patient care delivery model are essential in supporting a positive practice environment for nurses (Drenkard & Swartwout, 2011).

An effective care delivery system is designed so that the needs of patients are matched to competent caregivers, the caregivers' roles are clearly delineated, the quality care provided contributes to the outcomes, and documentation is created to reflect the care provided and outcomes obtained. Specifically, the delivery model is designed to ensure that the right caregiver is with the right patient at the right time. This aspect of care is necessarily linked to the next phase of a workforce management system—a valid and reliable **patient classification system**, which is essential in the planning and evaluation of the patient care delivery model. The American Organization of Nurse Executives, in its document *AONE Guiding Principles for Future Patient Care Delivery* (2010), has identified the following assumptions regarding patient care delivery:

- A systems approach is needed with all disciplines, focusing on continuity of care service.
- Emerging accountable care organizations will define healthcare reform provisions and influence the delivery venues.
- Patient safety, experience improvement, and quality outcomes will remain a public, payer, and regulatory focus driving the workflow process as it responds to the demands of an increasingly informed public.
- Healthcare funding will focus on achieving the desired outcomes of improved quality, efficiency, and transparency.
- Interdisciplinary education of health professionals will become the norm, promoting shared knowledge that enables safer patient care and funding for advanced practice nurse (APN) residencies and related clinical education.

Numerous patient care delivery models have been implemented with varying levels of success. They include models based on functional nursing (work is assigned by tasks), primary nursing (a nurse is assigned as the lead caregiver to plan and coordinate care), team nursing (similar to functional nursing, in that a team provides care based on tasks and skills levels and competence), modular nursing (a two-person team provides care to groups of patients), and case management nursing (a nurse coordinates care using clinical pathways and quality criteria) (Sportsman, 2012; Sullivan & Decker, 2009). More recently, interdisciplinary models of care have emerged and include practice partnerships, patient-centered care, and primary care partnerships.

Traditionally, caregivers are assigned to work from a task perspective, a process or teamwork perspective, and/or an interdisciplinary perspective. Recently, it has become apparent that more considerations need to be incorporated into the care perspective for a delivery model to be effective. As the environment for care and clinical work becomes more specialized, additional skills are needed to blend the specialization or division of labor with the expectations for a continuum of care that integrates all disciplines involved in providing services. The importance of an effective, multidisciplinary hand-off process is now well recognized as a means to assure the desired continuity of services. Notably, facilitating knowledge work has become an important work process, as information generation and communications technology trends steadily build and form essential components of the contemporary delivery model. According to Malone, Laubacher, and Johns (2011), four areas of focus must be addressed to get work done in a complex, digital world: division of knowledge work into discrete, assignable tasks; recruitment of specialized workers based on their contributions; assurance of work quality; and integration of the work pieces. The situation is similar for healthcare workers: They face a very complex and dynamic system that requires clear delineation and **assignment** of work based on skills, licensure and competence, recruitment and retention of competent caregivers, assurance of values-based outcomes, and integration of the work of all caregivers into a whole that meets the needs of patients. Indeed, this provides a new lens for viewing the patient care delivery model expectations and reflects the expectations for continuity of care in the era of healthcare reform.

The optimal delivery model for the future is one that is driven by principles and assumptions and ensures coordination of efforts and the achievement of value-based outcomes. How that work is organized and assigned requires team focus, with each caregiver being clear about his or her work, contributions, and value to the outcome.

Identifying Patient Care Needs

After the patient care delivery model is established, the next step is to identify the needs of the patients being cared for and the required caregiver interventions to meet these needs. Time standards and levels of caregivers are then derived from the types of interventions that are performed for patients. The overall goal is to quantify the needs of the patient and family as well as the nurse interventions required to meet those needs. The needs and interventions identified in this way can then be translated into hours of work for caregiver RNs, licensed practical nurses (LPNs)/licensed vocational nurses (LVNs), technicians, and certified nurse assistants (CNAs) caregivers. In addition, the integration of hospitalists, social workers, respiratory therapists, and other professionals into the healthcare team will further increase healthcare providers' ability to determine comprehensive patient care needs.

Many healthcare organizations have considered adopting some type of work measurement technique to determine the appropriate number and type of staff for patient care units. A variety of approaches are used in health care, including historical usage, staffing grids, legislated staffing ratios, and/or patient classification systems. Many organizations use a combination of approaches. Recent technology advances have resulted in automated systems for calculation and documentation of patient care needs.

The selected technique is then customized by the facility with either a manual or a computerized patient classification system. Some organizations do not use

Table 5-1 Staffing Grid

Census	RN	Tech	Support	Clerk
24	5	2	2	1
22	5	2	2	1
20	4	2	2	1
18	4	1	2	1
16	4	1	2	1
14	3	1	1	1
10	3	1	0	0.5
8	2	1	0	0.5
< 8	2	1	0	0.5

traditional workload measurement systems but rather rely primarily on ratio or grid staffing. Historically, staffing for patient care has been based on what was actually used for staffing in the previous year rather than on an analysis of current patient care needs and projections from these data. The assumption is that patient care needs remain relatively stable over time and that the staffing levels of the previous year produced the desired quality outcomes. For many organizations, the more staff who were used in the previous year, the more staff who are budgeted for the next year. These allocations are then used to create a graduated staffing grid identifying how many nurses will be allocated based on the number of patients (**Table 5-1**).

The underlying assumption of a staffing grid or ratio-based staffing is that all patients are similar in needs and that care fluctuations can be handled within these allocations of staff hours. The grid is directly linked to the budgeted staffing. In contrast, legislated staffing ratios identify nurse-to-patient ratios based on experiences and perceptions of nurses and are not directly linked to budgeted staffing. New research continues to emerge specific to recommended nurse-to-patient ratios (Douglas, 2010; Serratt, 2013). Advantages of nurse-to-patient ratios include the following:

- Considers the historical average **patient acuity**
- Provides incentives for nurses to return to the bedside
- Uses simple-to-regulate numbers
- Increases nurse satisfaction because nurses traditionally support equal numbers of patients

- Alleviates nurse stress
- Is marginally supported by evidence
- Provides a short-term solution for a complex problem

Disadvantages of the nurse-to-patient ratio staffing methods are as follows:

- Does not fix the problems in the workplace environment
- Does not consider evidence for effective staffing
- May become maximum staffing levels rather than intended minimum staffing levels
- Does not consider the variation in patient care needs, complexity of care, unit geography, and available equipment
- Does not consider the variations in staff competence and experience
- Assumes that nurses are available to meet the legislated ratios
- Will force closure of some hospitals
- Devalues the role of nurse critical thinking and judgment
- Assumes a manufacturing model is appropriate for patient care
- Shifts staffing accountability from the organization to the government

With recent healthcare reform legislation (e.g., the Patient Protection and Affordable Care Act of 2010), the emphasis has shifted from an event-based model to a continuum accountability model that integrates all settings in which patient care is provided (Day, 2010). Patient care metrics and payment are now based on the provision of integrated care processes for each patient.

The creation and use of patient classification systems as a tool to improve the clarity and objective identification of patient care needs emerged in the 1960s along with the adoption of the **diagnosis-related group (DRG)** payment system (Malloch & Meisel, 2013). See **Box 5-1**. Multiple models for classifying and

BOX 5-1 DRG SYSTEM

The DRG system was developed by a group of researchers at Yale University in the late 1960s as a tool to help clinicians and hospitals monitor quality of care and utilization of services. It has since been used by Medicare in the United States to pay hospitals. This system categorizes the types of patients a hospital treats based on diagnoses, procedures, age, sex, and the presence of complications or comorbidities. Briefly, DRGs work by taking more than 10,000 ICD-CM codes and grouping them into a more manageable number of meaningful patient categories. Patients within each category are similar clinically in terms of resource usage.

measuring patient care needs were introduced that included the *International Classification of Diseases* (ICD), DRG, case mix index, ambulatory payment classification (APC), resource utilization groups (RUGs), Outcome and Assessment Information Set (OASIS), and home health resource groups (HHRGs) (Dunham-Taylor & Pinczuk, 2006; Shi & Singh, 2004). These models identified procedures primarily for billing purposes.

Patient classification systems for nursing care also emerged because the previously mentioned systems did not address a significant portion of nurse work—namely, patient education, family support, and interdisciplinary collaboration—that is necessary to support procedural work. Patient care needs are best identified using a framework specific to patient needs that can be translated into nursing work. The Nursing Interventions Classification (NIC), Nursing Outcomes Classification (NOC), and North American Nursing Diagnosis Association—International (NANDA-I) classification are commonly used to delineate nursing work. Examples of patient care need categories include the following (Malloch & Conovaloff, 1999):

- Cognitive needs: patient level of consciousness and decision-making capacity
- Self-care needs: support for activities of daily living—bathing, ambulating, eating, skin care, and safety
- Emotional, social, and spiritual needs: support for stress, anxiety, depression, relationships, and spiritual status
- Pain and comfort needs: support for varying levels of discomfort from acute to chronic, intractable pain levels
- Family information and support needs: intentions to assist family and support members with knowledge and information to assist the patient
- Treatments and interventions: assessments, procedures, medications, fluids, and monitoring through patient care
- Interdisciplinary collaboration needs and patient information needs: multidisciplinary communication and collaboration among team members to ensure optimal coordination of care
- Transition needs: support for the transfer of the patient from one level of care to a higher or lower level of care across multiple settings

These eight categories include the majority of nurse interventions for all clinical patient types, including acute inpatient, intensive care, women's and infants, pediatrics, rehabilitation, behavioral health, and ambulatory care. The goal of a patient classification system is to provide the most valid and reliable information specific to work that needs to be done for patients. The nature of valid and reliable

BOX 5-2 KEY CONCEPTS

Classification: The ordering of entities into groups or classes based on their similarity, minimizing within-group variance and maximizing between-group variance (Gordon, 2001).

Forecasting: Planning for operational needs through analysis of staffing data alongside organizational and operational data (American Nurses Association, n.d.-a).

Patient acuity (intensity): The level of need or dependency of an individual patient, measured in hours of care needed by skill level.

Patient classification: A process of grouping patients into homogeneous, mutually exclusive groups to determine their dependency on caregivers or to determine patient acuity (Dunn et al., 1995; Finkler, 2001).

Scheduling: The long-range plan that combines the organization's goals, legislation, regulation, and accreditation requirements and planned patient demand.

Staffing: The real-time adjustment of the schedule based on census, acuity, and the mix of available resources.

Workforce management: The comprehensive system that includes patient classification, scheduling, staffing, and budgeting systems.

systems is straightforward; however, it is difficult to achieve in a human work system. A basic understanding of the techniques and challenges in measuring human work is helpful in supporting the processes to achieve the highest degree of validity and reliability. As previously noted, this model can be used for other disciplines, such as hospitalists, respiratory therapists, social workers, etc. To be sure, there is increasing interest and documentation worldwide that seeks a means to best determine the amount of services expected and needed by patients (van Oostveen, Ubbink, Huis in het Veld, Bakker, & Vermeulen, 2014). See **Box 5-2**.

Measuring Human Work

Measuring human work, particularly in health care, to determine what is done and how long it takes is a complex process that requires a basic understanding of the techniques available to determine work quantity. See **Box 5-3**. Several techniques are available to quantify the time associated with tasks performed by workers, as well as at least 25 techniques that assist in the study and measurement of work (Myers & Stewart, 2002). These techniques are used to understand the

CRITICAL THOUGHT

Why we need a patient classification system:

- To understand the relationship among patient care needs, interventions, desired outcomes, and the skill level of caregivers as a prerequisite to determine the appropriate type and number of caregivers and support staff needed to provide safe and effective patient care
- To define the amount of staff needed for a particular situation
- To create a valid and reliable system that defines and defends the work of professionals, increases visibility of the role of professional healthcare practice, protects patients from complications, and decreases the vulnerability of professional caregiver staff to budget cuts
- To account for the constant changes in the healthcare system and subsequent adaptations that are necessary to meet patient care needs

BOX 5-3 NURSING WORKFORCE MANAGEMENT SYSTEM: VALIDITY AND RELIABILITY

Validity can be defined as the extent to which a workforce management system measures what it is designed to measure—that is, the ability to quantify and/or predict patient needs for nursing care. *Reliability* refers to the extent to which data are reproducible. Three major types of reliability are distinguished: stability, homogeneity, and equivalence. The most important for workforce management systems is equivalence. *Equivalence* refers to the extent to which different nurses use the same workforce system to measure the same individual, at the same time, to derive consistent results (Alward, 1983; Giovanetti, 1979; Hernandez & O'Brien, 1996a, 1996b).

nature and true cost of work processes and to address the ongoing challenges of reducing costs, effort, and improving the work environment.

Five of the more common techniques often used in health care are provided to better understand the strengths and limitations of each technique as they relate to measuring healthcare work. Motion and time studies, work sampling, self-reporting, standard data setting, and expert opinion are each discussed briefly.

Motion and time studies involve continuous timed observations of a single person during a typical time period or shift of work (Burke et al., 2000). An observer measures primary task occurrences and the length of time to perform the task. Motion studies are undertaken for cost reduction, and time studies are performed for cost control reasons. Motion studies focus on design, whereas time studies focus on measurement.

A motion study is designed to determine the best way to complete a repetitive job. Examples of techniques to study motion include process charts, flow diagrams, multiactivity charts, operation charts, workstation design, motion economy, and predetermined time standards systems. Workload measurement using motion and time studies has been applied to a number of military and industrial problems. Interestingly, while time and motion studies are often referred to by healthcare professionals, this technique is rarely used in health care to identify time standards.

A time study measures the length of time it takes an average worker to complete a task at a normal pace and includes predetermined time standards systems, stopwatch time studies, standard data formula time standards, work sampling time standards, expert opinions, and historical data time standards. In health care, using worked hours per patient day (HPPD) or procedures per year to budget or staff for the next year would be consistent with the standard data set approach. These techniques are problematic for healthcare work in that while many tasks are repeated (e.g., medication administration, bathing, and teaching), each task is unique for the individual patient and the context in which the care is provided.

The technique of *work sampling* is used to study work activities at systematic or random intervals. It involves the process of randomly observing people working to determine how they spend their time. The type and percentage of observations are assumed to represent the typical workload at any given point in time. Such studies do not, however, determine the duration of a particular activity.

In health care, work sampling has been the foundation for some computerized patient classification systems. The caregiver's work is examined for the entire shift or event of care for a selected number of times to achieve a representative range of services. After representative data are collected, the percentage of time spent on specific activities (e.g., taking and recording vital signs, performing assessments, administering medications, procedures, and discharge planning) is determined. These amounts then create the time standards for determining future patient acuity on a daily or shift basis.

Self-reporting is another technique used to determine the amount of time associated with activities. Generally, the individual is asked to log the work performed using a data collection tool with start and stop times of each activity recorded. Self-reporting is subjective, but it has been shown to have high face validity (Burke et al., 2000).

Standard data setting uses time standards developed from past experiences. Such a collection of time values includes a catalog of basic time standards developed from a database collected over years of motion and time study. These time standards are specific to the individual environment and not readily transferable to another environment without further validation. Standard data are typically the most accurate and least costly to determine for manufacturing settings.

Expert opinion (also known as an expert panel) is yet another technique used to determine time standards. A panel of experts or individuals with experience identify time requirements for certain work. This consensus approach uses professional judgment to determine the staff required and provides a flexible approach that focuses on a critical review of nursing practice (Dunn et al., 1995).

Patient care or service work and one-of-a-kind tasks tend to make setting time standards with the more traditional techniques cost prohibitive. Some workers never do the same thing twice, but goals are needed. An expert is needed to estimate every job and to maintain a log of estimates. The best estimation technique is a low-cost, fast, and initially acceptable way of quantifying information using estimation and self-reporting techniques. The expert opinion technique attempts to remedy the criticism levied against the work sampling technique's inability to capture professional judgment required in health care (Dunn et al., 1995). Because it can easily become biased and not always reflect current conditions, expert opinion is reliable only if the results obtained approximate the results generated by experts, and the estimates are valid and reliable.

Many of these techniques are difficult to use in health care, where both the worker and the work to be done are highly variable. Health care is very different from the manufacturing assembly-line model in which the majority of variation relates to the activities of the worker, while the machine remains stable. The time required to determine specific time standards for the range of patient care profiles and combinations of needs in health care is overwhelming and cost prohibitive to determine using motion, time, and standard data techniques.

Most recently, the expert panel approach has been used to create a comprehensive unit of service as the foundational nursing workload unit of measure for patient care (Malloch & Conovaloff, 1999). Experienced nurses develop workload standards from a comprehensive or shift perspective of the work performed, and expert nurses compile the nurse interventions provided to a patient for an entire shift or event. Collectively, they identify the time required to provide this care as a unit rather than as a summation of individual tasks. This approach is useful because it integrates the multitasking nature of caregiver work and caregiver interruptions and minimizes the risk of double-counting tasks. Typically, an expert panel consists of nurses who practice in clinical, educational, research, and administrative roles, such as experienced staff nurses, clinical nurse specialists, nurse managers, and associate nurse executives. The expert panel then collaborates using a specific nursing intervention framework to estimate the amount of time and caregiver level required to provide the total care in the comprehensive unit of service.

Patient Classification Systems: Limitations and Challenges

In addition to the challenges of measuring human work, patient classification systems are limited for other reasons. Skepticism about patient classification systems has existed since their introduction. Given the variety of patient classification systems available, and even with years of testing new and innovative ways of capturing time estimation, the nursing profession continues to struggle with the lack of a credible workforce management system (Brennan & Daly, 2014).

Five common reasons for the current mistrust of a patient classification system include low validity, misuse of the tool, difficulty in projecting future staff needs, failure to use the data generated, and lack of tool simplicity. Each is discussed briefly in this section.

Low Validity

Failing to account for the full scope of nursing practice—specifically, the relational work of nursing—is common in task-based patient classification systems. Failure to consider the relational work of professional nursing care practices, such as patient education, interdisciplinary collaboration, family support, and delegation and supervision of other caregivers, decreases the validity of the system. Because much of nursing is mind work rather than hand work, it is not surprising that the task-based methods of some systems are quickly manipulated and declared invalid.

At present, no single agreed-on patient classification system exists that adequately represents the full range of nursing interventions. Because there is no agreed-on system, few, if any, empirical data sets are available that describe nursing practice across clinical settings and client populations. In turn, this lack of standardized clinical language, which makes it difficult to know with any degree of accuracy which type of patient classification system provides the most valid and reliable data for workload management decisions, further marginalizes system validity.

One solution for improving the validity and reliability of caregiver work measurement is to attach time and skill mix standards to clinical interventions in an electronic documentation system. With documentation driving the calculations for patient needs, the issues of reliability would be decreased significantly.

Misuse of the Tool

The lack of trust between healthcare administrators and caregivers stems in part from the belief that patient classification systems are a vehicle to increase or decrease staffing levels inappropriately. This lack of trust has serious implications for the ability of hospitals and other healthcare organizations to make the fundamental changes essential to providing safer patient care (Page, 2004). Coupled with low validity, poor reputation, and expectations for the patient classification to do more than simply identify patient care needs, trust in general is minimal in many organizations. The phenomenon of acuity creep, identified by Shaha (1995), is present when the reported patient acuity increases slowly over time but the actual care does not change. In other words, with this trend acuity levels creep to higher levels to justify higher resources use. Creep represents a problem because it assumes there is an ever-increasing need for patient care resources and labor in an industry where financial resources continue to decrease (Shaha, 1995). Further, the use of a system with low validity makes it difficult to distinguish inappropriate acuity creep from real changes in patient care. Thus the validity and reliability of the patient classification used by an organization collectively constitute a critical attribute for effective use of resources.

Difficulty in Projecting Future Staff Needs

Projecting patient care needs for the next shift or time period is highly desirable for ensuring staffing adequacy. However, the amount of staff and the appropriate skill mix have proved nearly impossible to determine without an acceptable error range without using a computerized solution. Computerized applications are becoming increasingly useful in assessing current nursing work and projecting demand from a point in time; however, regardless of the sophistication and accuracy of the calculations of current work, it remains nearly impossible to accurately predict patient condition changes, new admissions, and discharges. Experts continue to work on complex mathematical **forecasting** models to project patient activities and associated caregiver support into the future. Fitzpatrick and Brooks (2010), for example, analyzed the challenges of predicting patient volumes, needs, and resources and identified the role of clinical leader as logistician. This approach integrates the science of logistics management, including systems theory, mathematical optimization modeling, and human capital planning, and results in significant improvement in outcomes. The value of reconceptualizing the planning and deployment of staff as a logistics problem is readily evident: Staff preferences are maximized, coverage is adequate, skill mix is appropriate, regulations are met, and staffing costs are minimized. Indeed, this approach presents opportunities for all staffing offices.

Patient classification system data are useful for both retrospective review of what actually occurred and for projection for next shift staffing. Attempts have been made to classify patients based on the care provided for the current shift or based on what the current caregiver believes the care needs will be for the next shift. To plan for the next shift, the nurse leader requires not only information about the patient needs but also information about the oncoming staff members' competencies; the previous, similar shift staffing (yesterday's afternoon shift compared to the upcoming afternoon shift); facility support for housekeeping, pharmacy, transportation, and teaching staff; and anticipated admissions, discharges, and transfers.

The severity of patient illness, need for specialized equipment and technology, intensity of nursing interventions required, and complexity of clinical nursing judgment needed to design, implement, and evaluate the patient's nursing plan are often not predictable. However, when nurse interventions are reframed to focus on patient care needs, the degree of accuracy increases in tandem with clear descriptions of the patient needs.

Despite its name, which implies measurement of severity of illness or patient acuity, **patient classification** is in truth more concerned with determining the time required for care; the patient acuity level is secondary information. There is some correlation between acuity and amount of care required, but this correlation is not absolute. A chronic, ventilator-dependent, paraplegic patient, for example, may score high in severity of illness yet not require many care hours because of the stability of his or her condition and the well-established plan of care.

Failure to Use the Data Generated

Too often the data generated from a patient classification system are not used in staffing allocation, particularly if the projections call for more staff hours. The lack of trust in the process and data generated is often not addressed, and the generated projections may be disregarded in favor of the staffing grid or ratio allocations. Unfortunately, when a real and valid need for additional staff hours exists, that need is often disregarded by both nurses and support leaders. The basic trustworthiness of the system may be questioned by non-nursing hospital leaders, and, in response, the system is merely tolerated or ignored.

Lack of Tool Simplicity

To address the credibility gap, and with the expectation of increasing validity, clinical experts have worked to develop all-inclusive, objective lists of interventions to create a more valid system. Some systems require the user to review and select from 100 or more intervention-related items for each patient. **Classification** systems that try to list every possible intervention become overwhelming,

CRITICAL THOUGHT

The imposition of mandatory hospital nurse staffing ratios is among the more visible public policy initiatives directed toward the nursing profession. Although this practice is intended to address problems in hospital nurse staffing and quality of patient care, such staffing ratios may lead to negative consequences for nurses involving the equity, efficiency, and costs of producing nursing care in hospitals (Buerhaus, 2009).

time consuming, and quickly abandoned. Systems that are easily misused, mismanaged, or generate inaccurate data cannot be used by managers to defend their staffing decisions.

Whenever possible, direct care or interventions specific to patient care that can be directly attributed to the patient, as well as supportive daily planning and documentation, should be included in the patient classification system. Patient care work should include work that is directly attributed to the patient, whether it takes place at the bedside, in family conferences, or in shift reports supporting the planning process. After patient needs are determined and validated, the department director can then determine the core staffing hours and skill levels necessary to meet patient care needs. The next step in workforce management is creating the core schedule.

Core Schedule

Core schedules represent an aggregated average number and skill mix required for patient care. A core schedule template for each unit includes caregivers, shift length, and calendar days. Based on the identified historical patient care needs for the unit, patient projection volume is used to create the core schedule.

Considerations in Creating the Core Schedule

The nurse leader must consider the following considerations in constructing the basic core schedule: anticipated patient needs volume, caregiver categories, shift length, licensure requirements, experience, education, regulatory minimum level requirements, contextual factors (planned and unplanned staff absences, changes in patient volume or acuity), and available research evidence for staffing effectiveness.

Anticipated Patient Needs Volume

Projected volume can be obtained from both historical trend data and budget projections and can be organized by season, day of the week, and time or hour of the day. Adjustments for fluctuations in patient care volumes resulting from vacations, seasonal variations, and time of day can be forecasted and modeled, much as Hollabaugh and Kendrick (1998) have done. These authors developed a pyramid with five differing levels of activities and seasons, a hiring plan that varied by census, a more equitable cancellation policy, and active staff involvement, all of which collectively resulted in increased continuity of care, increased job satisfaction, fewer patient and physician complaints, and cost savings.

Caregiver Categories

Caregiver categories include advanced practice nurse providers, direct care workers or knowledge workers, preceptors, technical staff, support staff, and clerical staff. Roles can also include a person who is in charge or serves as a resource person during a shift. This person provides leadership, makes assignments, and deals with unusual incidents or difficult situations. He or she supports the leadership on issues as they occur during a shift or for a specified length of time.

Staff categorization is often identified as direct, administrative, or indirect. These concepts are defined in each organization and categorize direct patient care hours, unit support hours, or hours away from the unit, such as education, vacation, or sick hours, for cost analysis and payment purposes. The core schedule focuses on identifying those caregivers available to provide care for a specified time period.

The role of the patient observer, sitter, or companion is often difficult to integrate into scheduling systems and daily staffing for several reasons; nevertheless, the hours and costs of such personnel must be accounted for. One challenge is that the level of surveillance ranges from licensed staff to support staff to family to volunteer. Allocating the hours to the patient can be further confounding if the same observer serves more than one patient. Allocating a special status and hours for observer hours requires a unique approach within existing electronic workforce management systems (Laws & Crawford, 2013). Centralized patient monitoring allows for increased surveillance of patients who are at risk for self-harm, falls, or unable to adhere to a plan of care due to confusion or disorientation. This program allows for one member of the healthcare team, often a nursing assistant, to monitor multiple patients at one time. When patient safety concerns arise, the monitor can intervene verbally with the patient and/or alert the primary caregiver, based on an established algorithm for urgency (Jeffers et al., 2013). The nurse leader may need to build the business case for the purchase, upkeep, and ongoing licensing fees for patient classification systems and centralized patient monitoring. The business case should include a return on investment financially as well as projected benefits to patients and staff.

The skill mix, or numbers of licensed and nonlicensed staff, is determined based on the work that needs to be done—specifically, the patient care needs. The specific interventions that are needed by patients are categorized based on which level of caregiver can meet those needs, such as RNs being required for work authorized by the state's nurse practice act and the organization. One anecdotal advantage noted with high RN levels is that less time is needed to communicate with less skilled workers. Determining the ideal skill mix is challenging considering the multifaceted nature of patients and caregivers.

Advanced Practice Nurse Providers and Clinical Experts

In some delivery models, a nurse practitioner or hospitalist is a member of the team. These providers write orders and provide general patient care oversight. Other practice experts include clinical nurse specialists, clinical nurse leaders, and nurse educators. These nurses provide care and assist staff in the care of patients requiring more complex care using the latest evidence in a cost-effective approach.

Direct Caregivers or Knowledge Workers: Registered Nurses

The work of the RN will continue to be the foundational and primary role in the healthcare system. Optimizing the role of the RN requires continually advancing this role to that of knowledge worker at the point of care (Marshall et al., 2014). An overview of the practice of nursing from a national perspective is provided in **Box 5-4**.

In addition to the practice of nursing from a national perspective, information specific to the evolving role of the RN as knowledge worker is identified in **Box 5-5**. Understanding and integrating these values and behaviors into the practice of nursing serve to encourage and support the full scope of RN practice.

LPN/LVN

The LPN/LVN continues to fill an important role in care delivery; however, this role is more commonly used in more stable environments, such as long-term care, than in acute care settings. The challenges of delegation and communication between the RN and the LPN have proved particularly challenging for new nurses. The LPN/LVN role is beneficial in highly functioning teams where the scope of practice of each role is clearly understood.

Unlicensed Assistive Personnel

Unlicensed assistive personnel (UAPs) assist the RN with carrying out professional activities. Healthcare organizations use these workers in a variety of roles, including some that are more focused on supporting the patient care environment than on caring for the patients themselves. The goal in using assistive personnel is to provide the highest quality patient care at the lowest cost. Thus, if support personnel can safely provide certain aspects of patient care under the supervision of an RN, then integration of these roles into the team is the prudent approach.

BOX 5-4 THE PRACTICE OF NURSING: NATIONAL COUNCIL OF STATE BOARDS OF NURSING MODEL PRACTICE ACT

Nursing is a scientific process founded on a professional body of knowledge; it is a learned profession based on an understanding of the human condition across the life span and the relationship of a client to others and to the environment; and it is an art dedicated to caring for others. The practice of nursing entails assisting clients to attain or maintain optimal health, implementing a strategy of care to accomplish defined goals within the context of a client-centered healthcare plan, and evaluating responses to nursing care and treatment. Nursing is a dynamic discipline that increasingly involves more sophisticated knowledge, technologies, and client care activities.

Practice as an RN encompasses the full scope of nursing, with or without compensation or personal profit. It incorporates caring for all clients in all settings and is guided by the scope of practice authorized in this section of the National Council of State Boards of Nursing's (NCSBN) Model Practice Act, through nursing standards established or recognized by the board of nursing.

The practice of registered nurses includes the following tasks:

1. Providing comprehensive nursing assessment of the health status of patients

2. Collaborating with the healthcare team to develop and coordinate an integrated patient-centered healthcare plan

3. Developing the comprehensive patient-centered healthcare plan, including establishing nursing diagnoses, setting goals to meet identified healthcare needs, and prescribing nursing interventions

4. Implementing nursing care through the execution of independent nursing strategies and the provision of regimens requested, ordered, or prescribed by authorized healthcare providers

5. Evaluating responses to interventions and the effectiveness of the plan of care

6. Designing and implementing teaching plans based on patient needs

7. Delegating and assigning nursing interventions to implement the plan of care

8. Providing for the maintenance of safe and effective nursing care rendered directly or indirectly

(continued)

9. Advocating for the best interest of patients

10. Communicating and collaborating with other healthcare providers in the management of health care and the implementation of the total health-care regimen within and across care settings

11. Managing, supervising, and evaluating the practice of nursing

12. Teaching the theory and practice of nursing

13. Participating in development of healthcare policies, procedures, and systems

14. Wearing identification that clearly identifies the nurse as an RN when pro-viding direct patient care, unless wearing identification creates a safety or health risk for either the nurse or the patient

15. Other acts that require education and training consistent with professional standards as prescribed by the board of nursing and commensurate with the RN's education, demonstrated competencies, and experience

Courtesy of the National Council of State Boards of Nursing.

BOX 5-5 THE KNOWLEDGE WORKER

The contemporary clinical knowledge worker focuses on a new level of accountability for moving forward to informed, evidence-based decisions. No longer does the clinical knowledge worker rely on past practices, individual experiences, and tradition. Rather, the knowledge worker em-phasizes conceptual synthesis of knowledge and experiences for practice. Such workers rely on principles and values for decision making rather than on processing policies and procedures. The focus is on the product (not the processes) of work and the value produced. Responsibility derives from how well the work is done and is based on knowledge, evidence, competence, and efficiency. It is about doing the work well and doing it right. Knowledge workers own the tools and capacities necessary to do patient care work and to be responsible and accountable for this work. Knowledge workers cannot transfer the locus of control for their patient care work accountability to institutions, organizations, or supervisors.

UAPs have been used in a variety of roles, in addition to the traditional primary support functions at the bedside. Some perform simple housekeeping or secretarial tasks, whereas others perform higher level clinical or technical tasks, such as performing electrocardiograms and phlebotomy. Because no one accrediting body certifies all types of UAPs, and because state laws vary regarding their use, hospitals have been relatively free to experiment with different care models under the guidance of their internal nursing leadership (McClung, 2000).

The nurse leader must be aware of changing legislation and regulation related to UAPs. The state of Arizona recently mandated changes that affect nursing assistants. Nursing assistants now may be either certified or licensed. While there are no differences to the training and testing requirements to be either certified or licensed, there are other implications. Unlike a certified nursing assistant (CNA), the licensed nursing assistant (LNA) must submit fingerprints for a criminal background check on initial licensure and falls under the jurisdiction of the board of nursing for any type of unprofessional conduct (Dahn, 2016). The nurse leader must carefully consider the implications of these changes and be informed as to the best option for the organization in providing safe, high-quality care.

Shift Length

Variations in shift length are much easier to manage with use of computerized scheduling and mathematical calculations of the impact of shift-length ranges from 2-hour shifts to 12-hour shifts. The selection of traditional 8-hour or 12-hour shifts must necessarily be done within the context of the type of patient care provided—specifically, care for a short time interval or a longer interval. Continuity of care and consistency in caregivers in settings where care is provided for several hours or less can accommodate more flexible shift time lengths. The hand-off process and change of shift are less complicated with short-interval patient care. In areas where care is provided over several days, the challenges of care continuity and hand-offs increase in complexity because of the nature of the patient illness. Regardless of the shift length, its selection is best made by considering first the patient care needs and second the preferences of the caregivers.

Licensure Requirements

Each state jurisdiction has established a nurse practice act that identifies the duties and responsibilities of the RN. While these standards are similar in most respects, the nurse must be aware of any differences that apply when he or she moves to a new practice setting. In general, the NCSBN's Model Practice Act clearly identifies the expectations of the role and practice of nursing.

Education

The significance of educational preparation and continuing development is well recognized in the nursing community and by researchers. Indeed, having at least a baccalaureate degree in nursing is recognized as required entry-level competence for contemporary patient care situations. Notably, Goode and colleagues (2001) described the baccalaureate-prepared RN as having greater critical thinking skills, less task orientation, more professionalism, stronger leadership skills, more focus on continuity of care and outcomes, greater focus on psychosocial components, better communication skills, and greater focus on patient teaching. Baccalaureate-prepared nurses are also better equipped to provide care to an increasingly aging and diverse population. Preparation at the baccalaureate level will better equip the nurse as a knowledge worker for leadership, systems adaptation, and health policy.

Experience/Competence

When a healthcare organization is creating its core schedule, a balance of experienced and less experienced, or learning nurses, is desirable. Such a mixture is necessary to support the highest quality care and to provide opportunities for new nurses to learn complex patient-care processes. Mentoring new nurses is a critical role of the professional nurse.

Regulatory Minimum Requirements

In several cases, minimum staffing levels are defined by state, national, and professional agencies. Such staffing requirements, which are intended to ensure safety and to support caregiver vigilance, apply to most patient care units and in particular to those areas where unstable patient conditions are the norm. The core schedule identifies the minimum regulatory requirements. In addition, regulations specific to overtime must be honored. Given that regulations change regularly at the state level, it is important for nurses to keep up to date with both state and national requirements.

Contextual Factors

Staffing effectiveness is influenced by an extensive list of contextual factors, such as facility leadership, nurse–physician relationships, available technology and supplies, and numbers of external nursing staff (Pinkerton & Rivers, 2001). In addition, Berkow and colleagues (2007) have identified wide fluctuations in patient volume, percentages of protocol-driven care, geographic locations, and teaching status of the facility as significant influences in workforce staffing.

Staffing Effectiveness Research

Significant research is emerging in which the role of the RN is correlated to patient outcomes and cost. In general, the outcomes research indicates that having

> ## BOX 5-6 AMERICAN NURSES ASSOCIATION'S PRINCIPLES FOR NURSE STAFFING
>
> The American Nurses Association supports regular and evidence-driven dialogue about staffing effectiveness (ANA, n.d.-a). In particular, this organization emphasizes the importance of recognizing the complexity of effective nurse staffing and appreciating that a simple solution is not likely to produce the desired outcomes. In addition, several other considerations must be taken into account:
>
> - The characteristics and considerations of the healthcare consumer
> - The characteristics and considerations of the registered nurses and other interprofessional team members and staff
> - The context of the entire organization in which the nursing services are delivered
> - The overall practice environment that influences delivery of care
> - The evaluation of staffing plans
>
> Reproduced from American Nurses Association. (2012). *Principles for Nurse Staffing* (2nd ed). Silver Spring, MD: Nursesbooks.org.

a higher percentage of RNs on the nursing staff results in shorter lengths of stay, fewer complications, lower mortality, lower costs, increased nurse satisfaction, and increased patient satisfaction. While a growing body of evidence supports the positive relationship and impact of the role of the nurse on patient outcomes, the results are not generalizable nationally. Also, while specific nurse–patient ratios have been identified in some research studies, these numbers are not generalizable across the United States. Instead, numerous other variables need to be considered to achieve an optimal nurse assignment. See **Box 5-6**.

Daily Staffing Process: Creating Equitable Nurse–Patient Assignments

Matching patient care needs to scheduled core staff on the day in which care is to be provided is the next step in developing the core schedule. The nurse leader evaluates the number of patient care staff, their skill mix, and the support staff needed to assist in providing the care in relation to identified patient needs. Thus daily staffing decisions are driven by informed decision makers who consider multiple factors (Cathro, 2013; Douglas & Kerfoot, 2011; Kidd, Grove, Kaiser, Swoboda, & Taylor, 2014).

BOX 5-7 WILLING TO WALK: A NEW APPROACH TO FLOATING

To address the challenges of nurse floating, the team at Aultman Hospital created a "Willing to Walk" program to minimize stress and create a positive experience for both the receiving unit and the nurse who is floating or *willing to walk*. The Aultman program is proactive in that nurses are asked to sign up for the program to be considered for floating to selected areas within their realm of competence. Nurses meet the requirements for each of the units they agree to work. In addition, nurses are asked each time there is a need for floating. The program has resulted in increased autonomy, satisfaction, and lower turnover rates over a seven-year period (Good & Bishop, 2011).

Optimized staffing processes may be achieved by using approaches that are either centralized or decentralized, or a combination of both. See **Box 5-7**. Most recently a combination, or hybrid, staffing model has emerged as the preferred means to support unit involvement, decision making, and central records management. A hybrid model also allows for consideration of both the unit and organizational needs. Situations of overstaffing and understaffing are addressed to ensure a balanced staffing plan that meets patient needs, minimizes premium labor costs, and supports staff satisfaction (Crist-Grundman & Mulrooney, 2011; Staggs & He, 2013).

Variance management is an essential component of daily staffing. One of the most often ignored processes in workforce management is the identification and management of the variance between needed staff and available staff. **Figure 5-2** presents an example of essential data for variance analysis. Managing the difference between actual hours of staff time and required hours of care requires analysis of individual caregiver variances as well as total variance hours. Figure 5-2 presents a variance analysis data form that displays the actual hours, required hours, and variances. Once a significant variance is determined, variance actions are considered, implemented, and documented. These data provide valuable trend information for nurse leaders as they continually work to create effective workload management systems.

Addressing variances is a routine activity of nurse leaders that requires an examination of the staff needed for care and the actual staff. What is not routine is the systematic documentation of the difference between required and actual hours and the interventions implemented to address and mediate the variance or gap. Both positive and negative variances need to be addressed and documented.

Variance Management: 016100 Evening Shift 02-10-2004

Actual Hours	Actual Hours	Required Hours	A-R Var Hours	%	Budget Hours	R-B Var Hours	%	A-B Var Hours	%
RN	24	29	−5	−16	24	5	19	0	0
LP/VN	16	28	−12	−43	8	20	251	8	50
Licensed Total	40	57	−17	−29	32	25	77	8	20
NA	40	16	24	155	16		−2	24	60
TECH	0	0	0		0	0		0	
Unlicensed Total	40	16	24	155	16		−2	24	60
INDIRECT	0	0	0		0	0		0	
Total Evening Shift	80	72	8	11	48	24	51	32	40

Variance Actions

NEG Called in additional help.
NEG Used staff overtime.
NEG Used resource nurse.
NEG Reassessed for over estimation.
NEG Redefined non-essential tasks.
NEG Found missing or errors in scores.
PCS Floated staff to another unit.
PCS Cancelled staff.
PCS Cancelled registry.
PCS Sent staff home early.

Figure 5-2 Variance Management

CRITICAL THOUGHT

Expecting caregivers to "do one's best" in an impossible situation continues to fuel the flames of caregiver dissatisfaction and ultimately leads to nurses' premature exit from the workforce.

Examples of both short-term and long-term interventions to address the variance or gap between needs and actual staffing include the following:

- Reevaluating patient acuity ratings
- Postponing admissions
- Calling additional staff
- Postponing nonemergent patient care
- Floating existing staff to the unit in need
- Sending staff home early
- Eliminating non-value-added work
- Hiring contract staff

In today's dynamic healthcare environment, the challenge of managing increasing workloads requires new strategies beyond working faster (Storfjell, Ohlson,

Omoike, Fitzpatrick, & Wetasin, 2009). Rather than changing the speed of work, examining work to determine which work is not adding value to the outcome and eliminating this work becomes a more realistic option and strategy to manage the variance between required work and available staff. Wasteful, non-value-added work is often subtle and difficult to identity. Decreasing the waste in required work becomes a potential pathway to increased productivity and quality care.

Evaluation of Workforce Management

Evaluation of staffing, scheduling, and patient classification systems considers the infrastructure, the processes, and the outcomes of the integrated workload management system. Assessment of these three areas includes evaluation of the presence of factors identified within each area.

Infrastructure for Excellence Assessment

1. There is a clearly defined patient care delivery system that includes support for nursing participation in decision making at the point of service, expectation for professionalism, and shared decision making.

2. A valid and reliable system to determine patient care needs drives the staffing process. Specific consideration is given to the following:
   - Number of patients
   - Acuity of patients
   - Length of stay/intensity factor
   - Unit geography
   - Skills and experience of caregivers
   - Appropriate skill mix
   - Education and training of caregivers

3. Scheduling and staffing systems are developed collaboratively by leaders, managers, and direct caregivers/knowledge workers.

4. Consideration for unit functions that support the delivery of patient care is included in staffing hours (indirect time).

5. Staff clinical competencies are identified for differing patient populations.

6. Expert resources are available to support less-experienced staff.

Process Excellence Assessment

1. Collaborative scheduling is the norm. Historical trend data, patient care needs, and staff preferences (in that order) serve as the basis for scheduling. Patient care needs are always the first priority.

2. Mandatory overtime is not used.

3. The fatigue factor is recognized; long stretches of 12-hour shifts are not considered safe practice. Nurses do not work more than three 12-hour shifts in a row. Nurses do not work more than 12 hours at a time unless there are extreme circumstances.

4. Leaders and staff work together to manage variances (staff shortages) between available staff and patient care needs.

5. Experienced clinical experts are available to assist less-experienced staff in organizing and providing patient care.

Evaluation Excellence Assessment

1. Multiple indicators are used to evaluate staffing effectiveness. Indicators include patient outcomes, staff satisfaction, and organizational cost. Performance indicators do not focus solely on hours per patient day (HPPD).

2. The analysis includes individual patient care as well as aggregate analysis. Ranges as well as averages are evaluated.

3. The analysis includes both census averages and outliers (ranges).

4. Indicators that are sensitive to nursing scheduling and staffing are examined at least monthly. These include but are not limited to the following:

   a. Patient satisfaction with response to call lights

   b. Patient increased knowledge of clinical condition

   c. Patient/family's increased ability to manage their care

   d. Absence of adverse outcomes (e.g., dermal ulcers, nosocomial pneumonia, patient falls, and medication errors)

Leading Versus Managing in Staffing and Scheduling: Concluding Thoughts

The complexity and dynamics of nurse scheduling cannot be understated. The initial work of the nurse is to understand the components of this complex system and process. The next step is for the professional RN to analyze and interpret the effectiveness of the workforce plan specific to his or her ability to provide value-based patient care. Immediate feedback to address quality concerns with proactive recommendations is critical for system success and effectiveness. Managing and adjusting current situations with a strong rationale necessarily supports improvement of patient care and the system. To be sure, it is simple to identify what is not working. It is professional and courageous to figure out what needs to be done for improvement and to build a case that is so powerful that everyone agrees with the recommendations for more effective staffing.

SCENARIO

The flaw of the averaging process for health care is that the average situation may never occur. According to Savage (2002), the averaging process distorts accounts, undermines forecasts, and dooms apparently well-thought-out projects to produce disappointing results. In healthcare staffing, average caregiver needs are often used to create monthly schedules. Although this process is efficient, it may create more challenges in the long run. Consider the situation in which the average number of staff per shift is five and the range for each day of the week is three to nine staff members, on the basis of patient activity. No shift requires five staff members, yet the core schedule calls for five personnel to be present every day.

Using the specific number within the range of relevant numbers—in this case a number between three and nine—rather than the average of five for each shift results in more accurate staffing. The wide range of time required for similar—but different—patient situations is often significant.

Discussion Questions

1. Examine two to three four-week schedules and compare the projected core schedules with the actual numbers of staff worked.

2. What are the differences between scheduled and worked hours for personnel, including percentages over and under the core scheduled numbers?

3. What is the range (from lowest to highest) of differences?

4. What are the implications of examining both averages and ranges?

5. List three strategies to decrease the differences.

SCENARIO

Eight common areas have been identified as sources of non-value-added work and result in wasted time (Jones, 2014; Storfjell et al., 2009):

- Admission, discharge, and transfer activity
- Shift report
- Supplies/equipment
- Pharmaceuticals
- Diagnostics
- Documentation
- Communication
- Staffing

Within each of these areas are opportunities to eliminate wasteful work. Examples of wasteful work include inefficient hand-offs in which information is incomplete, searching for information or reports, waiting for others to complete their work, fixing equipment, and repeating calls to fill requests. Select two areas from the previous list and brainstorm with a colleague to address the following issues and questions.

Discussion Questions

1. In examining a recent experience, which areas of waste can you identify? How much time is involved?

2. Develop a plan to share this information with members of the team and create a specific plan to decrease the wasted time for this particular event. Be sure to include a specific timeline to complete this work.

3. List the challenges in gaining support from the team and in documenting the value of this work to the team and to the patients.

4. Develop a plan to communicate the challenges in addressing basic waste at the point of patient care and the importance of continuing to address nurse work from a positive perspective.

CHAPTER TEST QUESTIONS

Licensure exam categories: Management of care: delegation/supervision, interprofessional practice

Nurse leader exam categories: Knowledge of healthcare environment: delivery models/work design; Governance: evidence-based practice and care management, patient safety

1. Staffing adequacy

   a. Is determined by multiple factors, including nurse competence and patient care needs.

   b. Does not vary by shift.

   c. Can be assured with good planning of nurses' work schedules.

   d. Requires experienced nurses and supportive managers.

2. Equitable nurse patient assignments

   a. Require experienced nurses to create nurse assignments.

   b. Are positively related to nurse satisfaction.

   c. Are nearly impossible in complex patient care settings.

   d. Are typically limited to core staff.

3. Core schedules

   a. Are based on budgeted hours.

   b. Should be adjusted at least quarterly.

   c. Are based on trended patient care needs over time.

   d. Are inconsistent with ratio staffing models.

4. Ratio staffing

    a. Is strongly correlated with positive patient outcomes.

    b. Is strongly correlated with nursing satisfaction.

    c. Requires specific state legislation to implement.

    d. Does not consider the variations in patient care needs.

5. Non-value-added work

    a. Will continue due to patient expectations.

    b. Should be identified and eliminated whenever possible.

    c. Can be identified easily during unit focus groups.

    d. Is not an area of significant concern for nurses.

6. Measuring staffing adequacy

    a. Requires knowledge of recent research evidence.

    b. Is essential for Medicare certification.

    c. Is a quarterly evaluation of evidence for nurse staffing, physician availability, and reimbursement.

    d. Is an ongoing evaluation of matching patient care needs with appropriate nurse staffing and outcomes achieved.

7. Evidence for staffing specific to nurse fatigue

    a. Is unique for each team of nurses on a particular unit.

    b. Is inconclusive for healthcare workers.

    c. Identifies work practices that can be performed safely.

    d. Includes information specific to shift hours worked, weekly hours worked, and number of days worked in a row.

8. Reliability of patient classification systems

   a. Requires the use of a standardized nursing language.

   b. Is high when the ratings by system users are identical.

   c. Requires use of the system for at least 12 months.

   d. Does not exist if the interrater reliability is less than 85%.

9. Validity of patient classification systems

   a. Is about the accuracy of the system to measure the work of patient care.

   b. Requires a minimum amount of clinical intervention categories.

   c. Does not change over time.

   d. Is only essential when the data are used for patient billing.

10. Patient care delivery models

   a. Are most commonly based on the team model.

   b. Are best used in academic medical centers.

   c. Are required for Medicare reimbursement.

   d. Form the foundation for workforce management goals.

References

Alward, R. (1983). Patient classification systems: The ideal vs. reality. *Journal of Nursing Administration, 13*(2), 14–18.

American Nurses Association. (n.d.-a). Defining staffing: Workforce management, patient classification, and acuity systems: The request for proposal process. Retrieved from nursingworld.org/WorkforceManagement-PCAS-RFP

American Organization of Nurse Executives. (2010). *AONE guiding principles for future patient care delivery.* Retrieved from www.aone.org/resources/future-patient -care.pdf

Berkow, S., Jaggi, T., Fogelson, R., Katz, S., & Hirschoff, A. (2007). Fourteen unit attributes to guide staffing. *Journal of Nursing Administration, 37*(3), 150–155.

Brennan, C. W., & Daly, B. J. (2014). Methodological challenges of validating a clinical decision-making tool in the practice environment. *Western Journal of Nursing Research.* doi: 10.1177/0193945914539738

Buerhaus, P. I. (2009). Avoiding mandatory hospital nurse staffing ratios: An economic commentary. *Nursing Outlook, 57,* 107–112.

Burke, T., McKee, J., Wilson, H., Donahue, R. M., Batenhorst, A., & Pathak, D. (2000). A comparison of time-and-motion and self reporting methods of work measurement. *Journal of Nursing Administration, 30*(3), 118–125.

Cathro, H. (2013). A practical guide to making patient assignments in acute care. *Journal of Nursing Administration, 43*(1), 6–9.

Crist-Grundman, D., & Mulrooney, G. (2011). Effective workforce management starts with leveraging technology while staffing optimization requires true collaboration. *Nursing Economic$, 29*(4), 195–200.

Dahn, J. (2016). Fingerprinting: Certified Nursing Assistant (CNA) vs. Licensed Nursing Assistant (LNA). *Arizona State Board of Nursing Regulatory Journal, 12*(1), 10–12.

Day, J. (2010). Affordable Care Act (ACA) summary and updates. Retrieved from www.wid.org/affordable-care-act-aca-summary-and-updates

Douglas, K. (2010). Ratios—If It Were Only That Easy. *Nursing Economic$, 28*(2), 119–125. Retrieved from www.nursingeconomics.net/necfiles/staffingUnleashed/su_MA10.pdf

Douglas, K., & Kerfoot, K. M. (2011). Forging the future of staffing based on evidence. *Nursing Economic$, 29*(4), 161–162.

Drenkard, K., & Swartwout, E. (2011). A commitment to optimal practice environments. *Journal of Nursing Administration, 41*(7/8), 52–53.

Dunham-Taylor, J., & Pinczuk, J. (2006). *Health care financial management for nurse managers: Applications from hospitals, long-term care, home care, and ambulatory care.* Sudbury, MA: Jones and Bartlett Publishers.

Dunn, M., Norby, R., Cournoyer, P., Hudec, S., O'Donnell, J., & Snider, M. (1995). Expert panel method for nurse staffing and resource management. *Journal of Nursing Administration, 25*(10), 61–67.

Finkler, S. (2001). *Budgeting concepts for nurse managers* (3rd ed.). Philadelphia, PA: Saunders.

Fitzpatrick, T. A., & Brooks, B. A. (2010). The nurse leader as logistician: Optimizing human capital. *Journal of Nursing Administration, 40*(2), 69–74.

Giovanetti, P. (1979). Understanding patient classification systems. *Journal of Nursing Administration, 9*(2), 4–9.

Good, E., & Bishop, P. (2011). Willing to walk: A creative strategy to minimize stress related to floating. *Journal of Nursing Administration, 41*(5), 231–234.

Goode, C., Pinderton, S., McCausland, M., Southard, P., Graham, R., & Krsek, C. (2001). Documenting chief nursing officers' preference for BSN-prepared nurses. *Journal of Nursing Administration, 31*(2), 55–59.

Gordon, M. (2001). Nursing nomenclature and classification system development. *Online Journal of Issues in Nursing.* Retrieved from http://ana.nursingworld.org /mods/archive/mod30/cec2full.htm

Hall, L. M. (2005). *Quality work environments for nurse and patient safety.* Sudbury, MA: Jones and Bartlett Publishers.

Hernandez, C., & O'Brien, P. (1996a). Validity and reliability of nursing workload measurement systems: Review of validity and reliability theory. Part 1. *Canadian Journal of Nursing Administration, 9*(3), 16–25.

Hernandez, C., & O'Brien, P. (1996b). Validity and reliability of nursing workload measurement systems: Review of validity and reliability theory. Part 2. *Canadian Journal of Nursing Administration, 10*(3), 16–23.

Hollabaugh, S., & Kendrick, S. (1998). Staffing: The five-level pyramid. *Nursing Management, 29*(2), 34–36.

Jeffers, S., Searcey, P., Boyle, K., Herring, C., Lester, K., Goetz-Smith, H., & Nelson, P. (2013). Centralized video monitoring or patient safety: A Denver Health Lean journey. *Nursing Economic$, 31*(6), 298–306.

Jones, T. (2014). Validation of the perceived implicit rationing of nursing care (PIRNCA) instrument. *Nursing Forum, 49*(2), 77–87.

Kidd, M., Grove, K., Kaiser, M., Swoboda, B., & Taylor, A. (2014). A new patient-acuity tool promotes equitable nurse–patient assignments. *American Nurse Today, 9*(3), 1–4.

Lakein, A. (1973). *How to get control of your time and your life* (p. 273). New York, NY: Random House.

Laws, D., & Crawford, C. L. (2013). Alternative strategies to constant patient observation and sitters. *Journal of Nursing Administration, 43*(10), 497–501.

Malloch, K., & Conovaloff, A. (1999). Patient classification systems, Part 1: The third generation. *Journal of Nursing Administration, 29*(7), 49–56.

Malloch, K., & Meisel, M. (2013). Patient classification systems: State of the science 2013. *Nurse Leader, 11*(6), 35–37, 40.

Malone, T. W., Laubacher, R. J., & Johns, T. (2011, July/August). The age of hyperspecialization. *Harvard Business Review, 89*(7), 56–65.

Marshall, D. R., Davis, P., Cupit, T., Hilt, T., Baer, J., & Bonificio, B. (2014). Achieving added value in a knowledge-intense organization: One hospital's journey. *Nurse Leader, 12*(3), 36–42.

McClung, T. (2000). Assessing the reported financial benefits of unlicensed assistive personnel in nursing. *Journal of Nursing Administration, 30*(11), 530–534.

Myers, F., & Stewart, J. (2002). *Motion and time study for lean manufacturing* (3rd ed.). Upper Saddle River, NJ: Prentice Hall.

Page, A. (2004). *Keeping patients safe: Transforming the work environment of nurses.* Quality Chasm series. Washington, DC: National Academies Press.

Pinkerton, S., & Rivers, R. (2001). Integrated delivery systems: Factors influencing staffing needs. *Nursing Economic$, 19*(5), 208, 236–237.

Savage, S. (2002). The flaw of averages. *Harvard Business Review, 79*(11), 20–21.

Serratt, T. (2013). California's nurse-to-patient ratios. Part 2: 8 years later, what do we know about hospital level outcomes? *Journal of Nursing Administration, 43*(10), 549–553.

Shaha, S. (1995). Acuity systems and control charting. *Quality Management in Health Care, 3*(3), 22–30.

Shi, L., & Singh, D. (2004). *Delivering health care in America: A systems approach* (3rd ed.). Sudbury, MA: Jones and Bartlett Publishers.

Sportsman, S., Poster, E., Curl, E. D., Waller, P., & Hooper, J. (2012). Differentiated essential competencies: A view from practice. *Journal of Nursing Administration, 42*(1), 58–63.

Staggs, V. S., & He, J. (2013). Recent trends in hospital nurse staffing in the United States. *Journal of Nursing Administration, 43*(7/8), 388–393.

Storfjell, J. L., Ohlson, S., Omoike, O., Fitzpatrick, T., & Wetasin, K. (2009). Non-value-added time: The million dollar nursing opportunity. *Journal of Nursing Administration, 39*(1), 38–45.

Sullivan, E. J., & Decker, P. J. (2009). *Effective leadership and management in nursing.* Upper Saddle River, NJ: Pearson Prentice Hall.

van Oostveen, C. J., Ubbink, D. T., Huis in het Veld, J. G., Bakker, P. J., & Vermeulen, H. (2014). Factors and models associated with the amount of hospital care services as demanded by hospitalized patients: A systemic review. *PLoS One, 9*(5), e98102.

APPENDIX A

Selected Staffing Effectiveness Research Evidence

Significant progress is being made in identifying the relationship between the role of the nurse and patient, provider, organization, and cost outcomes. This appendix lists the specific areas of impact and supporting references. The increasingly broad range of evidence provides support for effective staffing plans and adjustments to daily staffing assignments. Specific relationships between patient outcomes, nurse characteristics, and nurse schedules are illustrated here. Reference numbers are listed with the identified variables. In addition, the American Nurses Association (ANA, n.d.-b) maintains a Safe Staffing website with a wide range of resources (http://www.rnaction.org/site /PageServer?pagename=nstat_take_action_safe_staffing).

Patient outcomes:

- Patient mortality/failure to rescue: pneumonia, postoperative DVT/ pulmonary embolism: 1, 2, 3, 4, 8, 9, 3, 14, 16, 17, 20, 21, 22
- Patient adverse outcomes: pneumonia, postoperative infections, urinary tract infections, acute myocardial infarction, congestive heart failure, patient falls, medication errors, pressure ulcers: 1, 4, 10, 14, 15, 16, 17, 20, 21, 22
- Smoking cessation counseling rates: 13
- Pneumococcal vaccinations rates: 13
- Length of stay: 8, 18, 19
- Patient satisfaction: 7, 15
- Patient experience of care: 15
- Physician satisfaction: 15
- Readmission: 9
- Cost of care: 9, 19

Nurse characteristics:

- Clinical nurse leader role: 5, 15
- Education level: 1, 2, 19, 21
- Percentage of RN staffing: 3, 8, 10, 14, 18
- Experience at the shift level: 10
- Shift hours: 4, 9, 10, 11, 12

- Number of days worked in row: 14, 16
- Number of hours worked in a week: 14, 16
- Unit admission, discharge, and transfer activity: 12
- Nurse turnover: 15
- Nurse fatigue and sleep cycles: 13

Environment of care:

- Foundations for quality of care: 4, 6
- Nurse manager ability, leadership, and support: 4, 6
- Collegial nurse–physician relationships: 4, 6

References

1. Aiken, L., Clarke, S., Cheung, R., Sloane, D., & Silber, J. (2003). Educational levels of hospital nurses and surgical patient mortality. *Journal of the American Medical Association, 290*, 1617–1623.

2. Aiken, L. H., Clarke, S. P., Sloane, D., Lake, E. T., & Cheney, T. (2008). Effects of hospital care environment on patient mortality and nurse outcomes. *Journal of Nursing Administration, 38*(5), 223–229.

3. Aiken, L. H., Clark, S. P., Sloane, D. M., Sochalski, J., & Silber, J. H. (2002). Hospital nurse staffing and patient mortality, nurse burnout, and job dissatisfaction. *Journal of the American Medical Association, 288*(16), 1987–1993.

4. Aiken, L. H., Sloane, D., Bruyneel, L., Van den Heede, K., Griffiths P., Busse, R., . . . Sermeus, W. (2014). Nurse staffing and education and hospital mortality in nine European countries: A retrospective observational study. *Lancet, 383*(9931), 1824–1830.

5. Alward, R. (1983). Patient classification systems: The ideal vs. reality. *Journal of Nursing Administration, 13*(2), 14–26.

6. American Nurses Association. (n.d.-b). Safe staffing. Retrieved from www.rnaction .org/site/PageServer?pagename=nstat_take_action_safe_staffing

7. Finkler, S. A. (2001). Measuring the costs of quality. In A. Kovner & D. Neuhauser (Eds.), *Health services management readings and commentary* (7th ed., pp. 114–121). Chicago, IL: AUPHA Press/Health Administration Press.

8. Gabuat, J., Hilton, N., Kinnaird, L. S., & Sherman, R. O. (2008). Implementing the clinical nurse leader role in a for-profit environment. *Journal of Nursing Administration, 38*(6), 302–307.

9. Gordon, M. (1998). Nursing nomenclature and classification system development. *Online Journal of Issues in Nursing, 3*(2), 1. Retrieved from www .nursingworld.org/MainMenuCategories/ANAMarketplace/ANAPeriodicals /OJIN/TableofContents/Vol31998/No2Sept1998/NomenclatureandClassification .aspx

10. Institute of Medicine. (2004). *Keeping patients safe: Transforming the work environment of nurses.* Washington, DC: National Academies Press.

11. Kane, R. L., Shamilyan, T., Mueller, C., Duval, S., & Wilt, T. J. (2007). *Nurse staffing and quality of patient care* (Publication 07-E005). Agency for Healthcare Research and Quality.

12. Kohlbrenner, J., Whitelaw, G., & Cannaday, D. (2011). Nurses critical to quality, safety and now financial performance. *Journal of Nursing Administration, 41*(3), 122–128.

13. Kutney-Lee, A., McHugh, M. D., Sloane, D. M., Cimiotti, J. P., Flynn, L., Felber Neff, D., & Aiken, L. H. (2009). Nursing: A key to patient satisfaction. *Health Affairs, 28*(4), 669–677.

14. Needleman, J., Buerhaus, P., Pankratz, V. S., Leibson, C. L., Stevens, S. R., & Harris, M. (2011). Nurse staffing and inpatient hospital mortality. *New England Journal of Medicine, 364*(11), 1037–1045.

15. Patrician, P., Loan, L., McCarthy, M., Fridman, M., Donaldson, N., Bingham, M., & Brosch, L. The association of shift-level nurse staffing with adverse patient events. *Journal of Nursing Administration, 41*(2), 64–70.

16. Rogers, A. E., Hwany, W., Scott, L. D., Aiken, L. H., & Dinges, D. F. (2004). The working hours of hospital staff nurses and patient safety. *Health Affairs, 23*(4), 202–212.

17. Shaha, S. H. (2010). Nursing makes a significant difference: A multihospital correlational study. *Nurse Leader, 8*(3), 36–39.

18. Sochalski, J. (2004). Is more better? The relationship between hospital staffing and the quality of nursing care in hospitals. *Medical Care, 42*(suppl 2), 1167–1173.

19. Staggs, V. S., & He, J. (2013). Recent trends in hospital nurse staffing in the United States. *Journal of Nursing Administration, 43*(7/8), 388–393.

20. Stanley, J. M., Gannon, J., Gabuat, J., Hartsranfi, S., Adams, N., Mayes, C., ... Burch, D. (2008). The clinical nurse leader: A catalyst for improving quality and patient safety. *Journal of Nursing Management, 16*(5), 614–622.

21. Trinkoff, A. M., Johantgen, M., Storr, C., Gurses, A. P., Liang, V., & Han, K. (2011). Linking nursing work environment and patient outcomes. *Journal of Nursing Regulation, 2*(1), 10–16.

22. Trinkoff, A. M., Johantgen, M., Storr, C., Gurses, A. P., Liang, V., & Han, K. (2011). Nurses work schedule characteristics, nurse staffing and patient mortality. *Nursing Research, 60*(1), 1–8.

23. Unruh, L. (2003). Licensed nurse staffing and adverse events in hospitals. *Medical Care, 41*(1), 142–152.

APPENDIX B

Perfect Staffing

Perfect staffing is about having the optimal (not too much, not too little) staff resources to support the right number of qualified caregivers to do their work effectively and timely in an organizational setting that is affordable and available.

While the achievement of perfect staffing seems impossible, this must nevertheless be the goal of all caregiver teams. It is a journey that begins anew every day with the recognition that health care is complex and uncertain. It is also important to recognize that technology has increased opportunities for more efficient work and course corrections. As the caregiver team works toward perfect staffing, evidence is now our beacon for making things better, and it is readily available with the digital resources that are being introduced every day.

Perfect staffing goals include the following:

- Zero "never events"
- 100% quality compliance
- 100% patient, physician, and nurse satisfaction
- 100% working and available equipment

There are four key steps in creating a plan for perfect staffing:

1. Create the ideal story for a patient population.
2. Select data elements (focus on 15 or fewer).
3. Analyze the results.
4. Intervene at points of deficiency.

Consider the following scenario or story for a medical cardiac patient care unit and begin with one clinical condition for analysis. (Note, groups of patients can also be considered.) Outcome indicators for current performance are identified and compared to the team-developed perfect staffing metrics on the accompanying table.

In addition, nurse expectations for perfect staffing include the following:

- 12-hour patient care assignment that includes:
  - Five patients with acuity requirements for 11.5 hours of care
  - Effective hand-off from the previous shift

- An ergonomically safe environment
- Good communication/collaboration with team members
- Safe medication administration principles
- Available supplies for patient care
- Effective interactions with patients/family, including education

Given these guidelines for creating the conditions for perfect staffing, develop a plan to implement a perfect staffing plan in a selected patient care area. The plan should include the following:

1. The type of patient population
2. Current and expected performance metrics
3. A plan for analysis of data that includes the rationale for targets
4. Numbers and types of caregivers required
5. Assumptions about the patient population needs

Develop an implementation plan that includes key stakeholders, timelines, plans to address resistance, and communication of results. Include the next steps to achieve perfect staffing on a regular basis.

	Perfect Staffing	Actual Staffing	Variance
HPPD	6.0	5.9	0.1
% RN	40%	42%	2%
% New graduates	50%	30%	20%
Average years of experience	3.0	4.5	1.5
LOS	4.5	4.4	0.1
Cost/case	$4,000	$3,800	$200
Readmissions	0	0	0
Call-light response satisfaction	5.0/5.0	4.8/5.0	0.2
Pain management satisfaction	5.0/5.0	4.8/5.0	0.2
Medication errors	0	1	1

Patient falls with injury	0	0	0
Overall satisfaction	5.0/5.0	4.9/5.0	0.1
Nurse–physician satisfaction	5.0/5.0	4.7/5.0	0.3
Overall employee satisfaction	5.0/5.0	4.9/5.0	0.1
Turnover rate	< 5%	3%	2%

Enjoy the challenge of this important journey for optimal outcomes!

> Integrity without knowledge is weak and useless, and knowledge without integrity is dangerous and dreadful.
> —Samuel Johnson

CHAPTER OBJECTIVES

Upon completion of this chapter, the reader will be able to do the following:

» Describe the key concepts and related concepts of healthcare ethics.

» Identify the risks and consequences that may be experienced when nurses' personal values and their organizations' values differ.

» Identify the challenges for nurses in addressing common ethical dilemmas.

» Describe strategies to address ethical dilemmas related to patient, nurse, and organizational issues.

» Delineate strategies to develop competence in ethical decision making.

» Analyze the potential ethical risks in using technology applications specific to patient privacy and confidentiality.

» Gain an appreciation of the personal risks in taking courageous ethical actions.

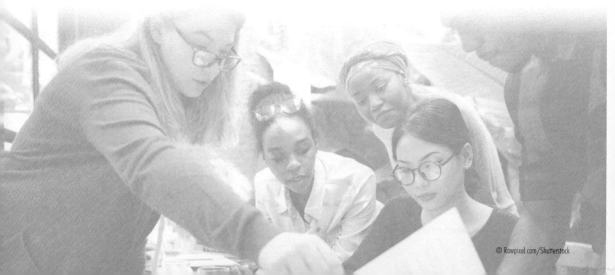

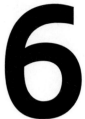
Principles of Ethical Decision Making

Doing the right thing is not always straightforward. In a complex world—and especially in today's dynamic healthcare environment—ideas, influences, motivations, principles, and individuals contribute to interactions that are far from simple. Making the best decisions in each and every situation in light of these influences is seldom straightforward, and answers to questions are rarely found in a reference book. Often, differences become evident among the patient's, nurse's, and organization's values, creating conflicts known as ethical dilemmas.

Despite the challenges involved in making quality decisions from an ethical perspective, an incredible amount of information is available to guide individuals in not only being proactive about ethical challenges, but also correcting the course when better decisions are identified. Clinical leaders must recognize and address ethical dilemmas in their sphere of influence to create better alignment of the team. Leading innovation and change can especially raise questions about ethical congruence on teams. Leaders should understand and address these incongruences early and often to support the team in changing practices. See **Box 6-1** for causes of moral distress.

In this chapter, the basic concepts of healthcare ethics are discussed, along with the challenges of making appropriate decisions and choosing appropriate strategies to support the best ethical work. The information presented in this chapter serves as an overview of ethical concepts and challenges and beginning strategies; it is intended to help nurses

BOX 6-1 THREE CAUSES OF MORAL DISTRESS

- Poor quality and futile care
- Unsuccessful advocacy
- Raising unrealistic hope

Data from Schluter, J., Winch, S., Holzhauser, K., & Henderson, A. (2008). Nurses' moral sensitivity and hospital ethical climate: A literature review. *Nursing Ethics, 15*(3), 304–321.

identify and address common ethical issues and to seek further information to better understand the complexities of such situations. In no way should this chapter be considered a comprehensive presentation of ethical issues in nursing. Every ethical situation is unique, differing based on the environment, individuals, and values involved.

The Basics

The science of ethics and ethical decision making has a language of its own. Knowledge of these basic concepts provides a foundation for nurses when exploring and discussing ethical issues in a professional manner. The following definitions, key concepts, and related concepts are described and explored to help nurses when they are providing patient care and dealing with ethical dilemmas.

Definitions, Key Concepts, and Related Concepts

Autonomy: The right to self-determination; being one's own person without constraints imposed by another's actions or psychological and physical limitations (Dahnke & Dreher, as cited in Lachman, 2006); the capacity of a rational individual to make an informed, uncoerced decision. Autonomy means that individuals are respected and allowed to make their own decisions about issues that affect them. It means we do not interfere if a person genuinely has the capacity to decide.

Beneficence: The duty to do good. This term refers to actions that promote the well-being of others. In a medical context, it means taking actions that serve the best interests of patients.

Betrayal: A person's words or actions that indicate he or she lacks good intentions toward another; the breaking or violation of a presumptive contract, trust, or confidence that produces moral and psychological conflict within a relationship between individuals, between organizations, or between individuals and organizations. Often betrayal is the act of supporting a rival group. It may also be a complete break from previously decided upon or presumed norms by one party from the others.

Bioethics: A subdiscipline of applied ethics that studies questions surrounding biology, medicine, and the health professions. Issues explored in bioethics include questions of research ethics, the use of patients in clinical drug trials, stem cell research, and human cloning, among others (Dahnke & Dreher, as cited in Lachman, 2006).

Boundary crossing: Brief excursions from an established boundary for a therapeutic purpose—for example, disclosure of bits of personal information or small gifts. The crossing is brief, with a quick return to the established limits of the professional relationship. Crossings are made based on what is best for the needs of the client (Arizona State Board of Nursing, 1997).

Boundary violation: A deviation from the established boundary in the healthcare provider–client relationship in which the healthcare provider's needs and the client's needs are confused. Boundary violations are characterized by role reversal, secrecy, and sometimes the creation of a dual relationship with the client (Arizona State Board of Nursing, 1997). Favors, self-disclosure, and/or physical contact in a professional relationship are examples of boundary violations. Performing favors such as providing lunch, transportation, or running errands are outside of the therapeutic relationship. Disclosing information about one's personal relationships, financial status, or health status are also boundary violations. Touching or hugging a patient without permission is considered an unwelcome violation of one's physical space and should be avoided.

Code of ethics: Guidelines for behavior specific to a moral framework for professional practice. Many codes look to the four basic principles of medical ethics: autonomy, beneficence, nonmaleficence, and justice.

Collective ethical wisdom: The sum total of individual and collective experience, knowledge, and good sense; know-how in which individual and collective knowledge, experience, and good sense result in sound ethical decisions and judgment everywhere and every day; the sum of experience, knowledge, and good sense, which provides subtle signals that alert us to the possibility that something is wrong and worth checking on, and which is driven more by intuition than by an assembly of facts (Gilbert, 2007).

Ethical dilemma: A problem that confronts a person, with a choice of solutions that seem or are equally unfavorable (Dahnke & Dreher, as cited in Lachman, 2006); a complex situation that often involves an apparent mental conflict of moral imperatives, in which to obey one would result in transgressing another. An ethical dilemma occurs when one value is pitted against another value. For example, one person may believe that health care should be available to everyone. Another person may believe that because of inadequate funding for health care, only those individuals between certain ages and with certain health statuses should be provided healthcare services.

Ethical erosion: The subtle, even unnoticed, slippage of ethical standards; a pervasive, subtle negative dynamic resulting from a decreased focus on values in small and often unnoticed slippages; slight deviations from the normal course of events (Gilbert, 2007).

Ethical fading: A process that obscures the ethical dimensions of a decision (Curtin, 2011).

Ethics: The philosophical study of right action and wrong action. Also known as morality, ethics delineates the highest moral standards of behavior (Dahnke & Dreher, as cited in Lachman, 2006). In this discipline, a person applies certain principles to determine the right thing to do in a given situation (Curtin, 2011).

Ethics of care: A recently developed moral theory rejects the traditional male-centered ethics that have focused on rationality, individuality, and abstract principles in favor of emotion, caring relationships, and concrete situations (Dahnke & Dreher, as cited in Lachman, 2006).

Fidelity: Duty to keep one's promise; the quality of being faithful.

Health advocacy: Actions that support and promote patients' healthcare rights and enhance community health and policy initiatives that focus on the availability, safety, and quality of care.

Justice: The elimination of arbitrary distinctions and the establishment of a structure of practice with a proper share, balance, or equilibrium among competing claims (Rawls, 2001); a concept of moral rightness based on ethics, rationality, law, natural law, religion, or equity, along with the punishment of the breach of said ethics. The act of being just and/or fair. Justice is about treating individuals fairly and equally.

Medical futility: Care at the end of life from which there is little hope of benefit (Trossman, 2011); the belief that in cases where there is no hope for improvement of an incapacitating condition, no course of treatment is called for. Withholding futile medical care does not encourage or speed the natural onset of death. One could say that it is impossible to reach a firm definition of futile medical care because this would depend on universal agreement about the point at which there is no further benefit from interventions, and different involved parties may always disagree about the amount and type of benefit under discussion.

Moral reasoning: The process in which an individual tries to determine the difference between what is right and what is wrong in a personal situation by using logic.

Morality: The conventional beliefs of a particular society (Dahnke & Dreher, as cited in Lachman, 2006); the degree of congruence between what one perceives as right and one's actual behavior (Curtin, 2011); the differentiation among intentions, decisions, and actions between those that are good (or right) and bad (or wrong). The adjective *moral* is synonymous with *good* or *right*.

Nonmaleficence: Duty to do no harm. The concept of nonmaleficence is embodied by the phrase "First, do no harm," the Latin *primum non nocere*. Many believe the primary consideration (*primum*) is that it is more important to not harm your patients than to do them good.

Organizational integrity: The means of producing stronger, sustainable performance through ethical pathways consistent with the vision, mission, and values of the organization (Gilbert, 2007).

Personal integrity: A state of wholeness and peace experienced when our goals, actions, and decisions are consistent with our most cherished values (Gilbert, 2007).

Pragmatism: An American school of philosophy that rejects the esoteric metaphysics of traditional European academic philosophy in favor of more down-to-earth, concrete questions and answers. According to Dewey, the scientific method may be used to solve moral problems from this perspective. According to Kant, a moral action is distinguished from an immoral action in that the person acts from a sense of duty, not from inclinations or feelings (Dahnke & Dreher, as cited in Lachman, 2006).

Principle: A guideline derived from philosophical perspectives (e.g., utilitarian, rights based, duty based); a law or rule that has to be followed, or usually is to be followed, or can be desirably followed, or is an inevitable consequence of something, such as the laws observed in nature or the way a system is constructed. The principles of such a system are understood by its users as representing the essential characteristics of the system or reflecting the system's designed purpose, so that the effective operation or use of the system would be impossible if any one of the principles was to be ignored.

Professional boundary: The limits of the professional relationship that allow for a safe therapeutic connection between the healthcare provider and the client. These include, at a minimum, time, location of patient care, money, exchange, favors or gifts, self-disclosure, and physical contact.

Rationalization: When a person knows what is right and does not want to do it (Curtin, 2011); a term used in sociology to refer to a process in which an increasing number of social actions become based on considerations of teleological efficiency or calculation rather than on motivations derived from morality, emotion, custom, or tradition.

Right choices: Those choices that conform to ethical norms or principles, such that others can know whether a person has made a right choice.

Trust: The degree to which one can be relied on without surveillance by the observer (Gerck, 1998). Trust has been called the ugly duckling of science, believed to be subjective, imprecise, and unreliable.

Utilitarianism: The principle of utility or the greatest happiness principle; actions are chosen that will produce the greatest amount of happiness for the greatest number of people.

Veracity: Truth telling, or the duty to tell the truth.

Whistle-blowing: Action taken by a person who goes outside the organization for the public's best interest when the organization is unresponsive after the danger is reported through the organization's proper channels (Lachman, 2008); an informant who exposes wrongdoing within an organization in the hope of stopping it (*TheFreeDictionary*, 2008).

Resources for Ethical Decision Making

In addition to key concepts and definitions, several other resources—both internal and external to organizations—are readily available. Internal resources include ethics committees, which typically focus on educating employees and providing consultative services. Each organization structures this consultative resource differently to meet the specific needs of the community and the organization. Whenever possible, nurses should consider attending ethics committee educational meetings and discussions of specific cases. Other resources—including textbooks, journals, and online information—to supplement understanding of the ethical aspects of health care are listed in the appendix titled "Selected Healthcare Ethics Resources."

REFLECTIVE QUESTION

Why is it so difficult to develop good, long-lasting relationships? Do problems in this area arise because of fear of disclosure, fear of failure, or a lack of accountability for performance? Is a lack of trust at fault—or is something completely different the culprit? Certainly, trust is a large component of healthy relationships. Healthy relationships in an environment of continual and complex change require not only that the partners have a high level of self-awareness and shared values, but also that each individual is comfortable not knowing everything and is able to trust that colleagues have the same shared values and will perform to their best ability.

On the basis of ethical principles and concepts, why is bullying unethical? When creating a course correction plan for the bullying individual, which principles would you focus on? Discuss some ethical dilemmas that might arise in a bullying situation.

Ethical Issues and Challenges

Patients and caregivers may differ in their values, perspectives, motivations, and levels of understanding. These differences often lead to various approaches to issues and conflicting perspectives on how to proceed when an ethical dilemma arises in the provision of patient care services. Discussion and resolution of these differences are essential to avoid ethical fading or ethical erosion at both the individual and organizational level. The importance of resolution should not be underestimated while the goal of reconciling personal values and organizational values is being advanced.

This section discusses several of the sources, common issues, and challenges in the provision of healthcare services that could result in ethical dilemmas. Not surprisingly, the sources of ethical dilemmas vary, with these dilemmas arising from values, communication, diversity, legislation, nurses, patients, and organizational differences. Nevertheless, ethical dilemmas seldom arise from maliciousness. Rather, an unconscious bias can arise when there is ambiguity in interpreting information, attachment to personal approval, or the expectation that an individual will support a previously approved situation (Bazerman, Loewenstein, & Moore, 2002).

The first general category to which ethical dilemmas may relate is values—which includes situations related to trust, timeliness, accountability, and personal appearance— in which individuals differ. Diversity of values and different

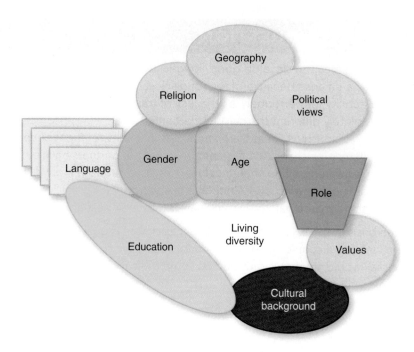

Figure 6-1 Diversity types

perspectives on age, gender, location, political views, role, education, culture, and religion are examples of the sources of differences among individuals (**Figure 6-1**). This multifaceted diversity is frequently the source of misinformation or misunderstanding that can lead to an ethical dilemma. Disrespect for differing values and behaviors among individuals is often subtle and unintentional. When these differences result in obvious conflict situations, it is helpful to use ethical concepts and principles to identify the specific issues and begin to resolve the conflict situation.

Communication style can be a source of conflict that leads to misunderstanding, divergent actions, and ethical dilemmas. Individuals have typically developed and reinforced communication styles that have worked for them, however offensive or intolerable that style may be to others. Sometimes individuals do not share complete information, or they share it in a way that is unclear, or, even worse, they remain silent and do not share information that would facilitate and enrich the discussion. Sharing partial treatment information with a patient, such as what to expect in a procedure, may be motivated by the desire to protect the patient from upsetting information; however, this decision to give only partial information disrespects the patient's right to know information that is pertinent to his or her care. Motivations for partial truth telling or withholding information vary and need to be explored when such behaviors are recognized. Ethical issues of autonomy, beneficence, betrayal, boundary crossing, justice, nonmaleficence, and personal integrity could all be involved in inappropriate communication.

Communicating in an aggressive manner can also create ethical concerns when the rights of others are violated. Consider communication behaviors between nurses that reflect horizontal violence or nurse–physician communication that is demeaning and intimidating. Bullying is another type of unhealthy communication behavior. When one person asserts physical or emotional power over another person, many ethical issues arise. Ethical issues of autonomy, beneficence, betrayal, code of ethics, justice, nonmaleficence, boundary violations, and personal integrity can all be involved in aggressive and intimidating communications.

Legislation can also be a source of ethical dilemmas when it clashes with an individual's values. Ethical issues of autonomy, boundary violations, code of ethics, pragmatism, rationalization, and personal integrity could be involved in legislative issues. For example, the right to choose an abortion, which is legally sanctioned, conflicts with the personal values of some individuals who oppose this practice. While legislation might seem like a straightforward way to resolve such conflicts in favor of the person involved, that is not always the case. Not only the values of the individual must be considered but also the context in which the individual is requesting services. If the organization's values are based on beliefs that differ from the individual's, the organization may not be willing to provide the desired services. Thus, for example, the individual who seeks an abortion may need to move to a facility that supports abortion services.

An ethical dilemma can also arise from the individual nurse's perspective. Nurses whose values are in conflict with those of the organization have several options open to them. One, of course, is to choose not to work at the organization; another is to frankly discuss the situation with managers and determine how to modify assignments so that the nurse is not involved in the areas generating the ethical dilemma. What is not appropriate is to ignore the dilemma and continue to work in a conflicted state. Unresolved ethical dilemmas can lead to toxic practice, toxic leadership, and inappropriate behavior. They can also lead to professional burnout, depression, and self-harm (Rathert, May, & Chung, 2016).

Nurse–Nurse Ethical Dilemmas

It seems natural and obvious that all nurses, given their education, would share similar values and beliefs about patient care. Given the wide range of diverse values previously discussed, however, nurse-to-nurse relationships and behaviors may demonstrate variations and give rise to ethical dilemmas. Such nurse-to-nurse ethical dilemmas may, in turn, impact perceptions and professional role behaviors.

CALLOUT

Nurses and especially nurse leaders need to recognize the symptoms of moral distress related to ethical dilemmas. Caregiver depression and suicide are becoming more prevalent. Leaders and colleagues can take an active role in addressing this trend by looking for individual and system stressors and intervening early. Resources for a healthy work environment: www.nursingworld.org/MainMenuCategories/WorkplaceSafety/Healthy -Work-Environment

An area of great concern and challenge for nurses is the nurse-to-nurse ethical dilemma in which nurses espouse different standards of practice. The American Nurses Association's *Code of Ethics for Nurses* clearly defines standards of practice, yet not all nurses follow these professional standards. Some nurses support professional standards in the strictest manner whereas other nurses tend to cut corners or ignore some professional standards, resulting in different levels of patient care. Autonomy, beneficence, betrayal, code of ethics, fidelity, nonmaleficence, rationalization, veracity, and personal integrity may all play a role in the standard practice. In some cases, these factors may even lead to substandard practice because they create moral and psychological barriers to change or challenging existing norms.

For licensure, many states require that nurses agree by law to report unprofessional and unsafe practices to the board of nursing. The requirement to report nurses who do not follow the professional standards of practice should not be taken lightly. Specific guidelines are available from the American Nurses Association and each state board of nursing. Examples include the requirement to report to the appropriate state board of nursing in the following situations:

- Information that a nurse may be mentally or physically unable to safely practice nursing
- Conduct involving practicing beyond the scope of practice of the license, such as giving a medication not authorized by a provider or an unauthorized adjustment of a dosage (boundary violation)
- Conduct that appears to be contributing to high-risk situations or harm to a patient and requiring medical intervention because of the conduct (nonmaleficence)
- Conduct involving the use of alcohol or chemical substances to the extent that nursing practice may be impaired (nonmaleficence, personal integrity)

- Actual or suspected drug diversion (nonmaleficence, personal integrity)
- A pattern of failure to account for medications or waste of control drugs (nonmaleficence, personal integrity)
- A pattern of inappropriate judgment or nursing skill (rationalization, nonmaleficence, personal integrity)
- Professional boundary violations, such as sexual conduct with a patient or patient's family member
- Conduct involving theft or exploitation of a patient (boundary violation)
- Practicing without a valid license (code of ethics)

When a nurse identifies or recognizes behaviors believed to be in violation of professional standards and regulations, the issue should be escalated to the next individual in the organizational chain of command or reporting structure to determine how and when to comply with the reporting requirements. The reporting of colleagues can be quite unsettling for the individual and can also impact team dynamics. When an issue is not addressed, however, ethical fading begins and can lead to ethical erosion. Doing the right and ethical thing requires courage and conviction of one's actions. Additionally, it is our professional obligation to the public to hold fellow nurses accountable to safe practice standards.

Substance use disorders are another area of great nurse-to-nurse conflict. Of all the professional issues among nurses, addressing impaired nurse behaviors is probably the most difficult. The number of nurses impaired by substances is of great concern to the profession and the public; such disorders represent the most common reason nurses are reported to boards of nursing (Darbro, 2011). As difficult as it is to report a colleague with probable substance abuse issues, this step is critical in getting impaired nurses into recovery.

Reentry into practice from substance use disorders often presents another dilemma for nurses. Nurses who have successfully completed initial rehabilitation and are currently in recovery from substance abuse often have difficulty reentering the practice setting. Practicing nurses are often reluctant to put forth the additional effort to monitor and mentor the returning nurse. One ethical dilemma that arises between nurses who practice safely and the returning nurse pertains to why nurses without substance abuse issues should be expected to oversee and monitor the nurse who violated professional standards. Ethical issues of autonomy, beneficence, fidelity, nonmaleficence, and rationalization are commonly encountered in these situations.

Nurse–Patient Ethical Dilemmas

Another category of ethical dilemmas is related to the nurse–patient relationship. During the course of providing patient care, numerous ethical dilemmas can emerge. Issues related to decision-making authority, pain management, the dying process, futile care, patient privacy, and communication among providers often arise; when they do, they require investigation and resolution.

Historically, physicians directed patient care treatment based on the belief that physicians possessed the best and most reliable information about medical treatments. Patient autonomy was subordinated to the expertise of the physician. More recently, this relationship has undergone a transition. Today, the patient or user of the healthcare system owns his or her decisions about healthcare treatments and has personal autonomy. For example, autonomy can come into conflict with beneficence when a patient disagrees with recommendations that healthcare professionals believe are in the patient's best interest. When the patient's wishes conflict with his or her welfare, the wishes of a mentally competent patient will prevail even if healthcare providers believe the patient's choice is not in his or her best interest. Patient knowledge, culture, religion, or other values can all be sources of disagreement with providers.

Patient restraint is another recurring challenge for nurses in ensuring a safe environment. Restraining a patient necessarily decreases patient autonomy in favor of beneficence or nonmaleficence. Similarly, when a patient or family selects palliative care rather than seeking out all possible care at the end of life in support of patient autonomy, nurses may disagree with that decision; they may believe that appropriate care is not being provided and that harm is being brought upon the patient by withholding antibiotics or tube feedings.

Another nurse–patient ethical dilemma is related to technology, specifically to monitoring alarms. The management of alarms on monitoring equipment has attracted much attention recently. As the number of monitoring devices increases, the number of associated alarms has also increased, rendering the patient care environment a cacophony of sounds. The noise and false alarms have resulted in "alarm fatigue," with nurses often turning off alarms to decrease the noise and interruptions from false alarms (Inglesby, 2011). Several concepts and principles are involved in these types of situations, including rationalization, nonmaleficence, morality, beneficence, and personal integrity.

CRITICAL THOUGHT

Trusting relationships cannot be bought or recruited from the outside; they must develop over time and through experience.

Nurse–Organization Ethical Dilemma

A third category of ethical dilemmas involves conflicts between the nurse and the organization. Interactions between an employer and an employee can lead to ethical dilemmas in several ways. Certainly, it is important to be clear how an organization addresses ethical patient care situations. When nurses' values, individual patients' needs, and the demands of the organization are not in agreement, an ethical dilemma emerges. Caregivers become disenfranchised and dissatisfied with their work. For example, if caregivers believe their primary obligation to the patient (health advocacy) is compromised, an ethical dilemma is present. Being able to work in an organization in which difficult patient care problems are discussed and decided so that the primary obligation to the patient is honored is essential for caregiver satisfaction and retention. In such an environment, caregivers are empowered, trusted, and included in the decision-making processes of ethical dilemmas. Conversely, nurse–organization ethical dilemmas may occur when disputes arise regarding error management, staffing adequacy, technology management, and other elements.

Another nurse–organization ethical dilemma between nurses and the organization is related to the management of errors. Historically, if a nurse committed an error, he or she was disciplined for poor practice. More recently, the investigation of errors and considerations of a just culture have emerged as important considerations in the management of errors (Benner, Malloch, & Sheets, 2010). Specifically, the recognition that errors are inevitable in a human system, the nature of the interconnectedness of systems, and the morality of treating individuals fairly and humanely when an error occurs have dramatically shifted the management of errors in healthcare organizations. This shift in thinking has resulted from error research and the development of systems theory, which collectively indicate that practice deficiencies can seldom be understood in isolation and that individuals are rarely responsible for anything but the most egregious errors (Goeschel, 2011). The new dilemma is to assign accountability and administer sanctions with fairness rather than to find and punish a single scapegoat.

Staffing adequacy is also associated with ethical dilemmas. When nurse staffing is less than adequate, patient care can be compromised. When a nurse does not report to work and no replacement is available, for example, the nurses on the shift must take on additional responsibilities beyond their capabilities. Nurses have accepted this situation in the belief that patient care would be worse if they refused the additional, unreasonable assignment and they were the only ones who could protect the patient. The principles of beneficence, nonmaleficence, ethical fading, fidelity, rationalization, boundaries, and rationalization are all potential explanations for this ethical dilemma.

Documentation technology is another source of ethical dilemmas. The ongoing influx of new technologies to document and monitor patient care has resulted in increased access to information and challenges in documenting care in a timely and individual manner. The wider availability of protected and private patient information in an electronic environment has sometimes resulted in inappropriate disclosure of confidential patient information. An employee who accesses patient information without a caregiver relationship to that patient may be subject to discipline and termination of employment. Principles of beneficence, betrayal, fidelity, nonmaleficence, personal integrity, rationalization, and veracity can all be involved in understanding these types of ethical dilemmas. See **Box 6-2**.

These three categories of ethical issues represent the most common situations faced by nurses. Readers can use these key concepts and common dilemmas as foundations for discussion of ethical issues that arise in their organizations. In addition, readers may use the multiple clinical scenarios in this chapter to analyze ethical situations using ethical concepts to gain skill and competence in this important area.

BOX 6-2 BEHAVIORS OF INDIVIDUALS WITH HIGH SELF-AWARENESS

Individuals with high self-awareness:

- Are aware of personal values related to culture, religion, race, gender, and other aspects of individuals.
- Articulate personal and professional boundaries specific to physical space, thoughts, sense of identity, and relationship with a higher power.
- Communicate in an open style and frequently ask questions to gain understanding.
- Communicate likes and dislikes.
- Can separate data from opinion in making decisions.
- Value multiple perspectives and diversity of ideas.
- Recognize the impact of both verbal and nonverbal communication behaviors.
- Do not talk down to others; they use language that is easily understood.
- Strive to be concise in communication and avoid rambling; do not filibuster or tolerate filibustering.
- Know the purpose for the relationship and what is expected of each person.

Strategies to Address Ethical Issues

Recognizing moral dilemmas and the associated concepts is just one step in ensuring ethical decisions and behaviors. This approach supports professional role development for nurses by encouraging them to make more thoughtful decisions when faced with ethical situations and in managing mistakes in practice (Godfrey & Crigger, 2012). Strategies to address ethical issues specific to self-knowledge, trust building, organizational team building, practice breakdown management, and managing personal risks are discussed to guide the nurse in becoming competent in this area.

Self-Knowledge

Self-knowledge specific to ethical concepts, issues, and resolutions is a necessary first step. By understanding the concepts and examples of specific applications, the nurse begins to develop his or her competence in ethical decision making. Regular discussion of ethical issues and application of the associated principles is an important practice for nurses. It is important to remember that no two situations are ever the same; however, the principles for assessing and addressing ethical dilemmas are always consistent.

Demonstrating moral courage is a competence specific to one's ability to be assertive in addressing ethical issues. When a nurse faces the situation in which he or she knows the right thing to do but does not feel able to do the right thing or live his or her professional values, moral courage is needed—courage to confront the situation in a logical, unemotional manner, focused on doing the identified right thing. To be sure, risks and consequences are present when a person asserts himself or herself to address an ethical dilemma. The reality of speaking up and risking one's position is real and often cannot be avoided. Developing moral courage begins with developing competence in concepts and scenarios specific to ethical dilemmas. In addition, working within a team setting focused on organizational integrity further assists those faced with ethical dilemmas to confront those situations with moral courage—assertiveness, clarity, timeliness, and beneficence. Managing the personal risks of ethical behaviors requires all the strategies identified in this section.

Gaining clarity regarding the nurse's professional role is another strategy for effective ethical dilemma resolution. Assisting nurses in maintaining the boundaries of the practice of nursing requires a clear understanding of the expectations of a professional, including autonomy as a professional nurse, advancement of the science and evidence for healthcare practices, and a focus on results in providing patient care (O'Rourke, 2003).

SCENARIO

Numerous healthcare situations call for courage. Examples include breaking bad news regarding a poor prognosis, challenging a colleague who appears incompetent, delivering care to an infectious patient, confronting an angry relative, and raising concerns about unethical practice. What is common to all of these situations is the fear that may be experienced as the practitioner considers the cost of the action and the consequences of a particular intervention or of getting it wrong. There may be fear of an extremely emotional reaction, violence, contamination, negative reactions from colleagues, or losing one's job. Dealing with difficult people can be addressed with principled approaches supported by the entire team (Sherman, 2014).

Discussion Questions

Ask yourself and your team members the following questions:

1. Are you willing to declare that abusive interactions will always be challenged when they occur?

2. Are you willing to no longer play it safe and speak up when an abusive situation occurs?

SCENARIO

Ample evidence exists that nurses do not always feel they can do the right thing in their everyday practice. In some instances, this may be because they lack the virtues—such as moral courage, wisdom, and integrity—that are required to speak up and bring about change. In other instances, such as when the organizational culture is defensive, unsupportive, or potentially punishing, the virtue of courage may not be adequate to change a situation.

Discussion Questions

1. In a small group, share your thoughts on this dilemma.

2. Which ethical principles are involved?

3. Which strategies should be considered to address this problem?

CRITICAL THOUGHT

Can I trust you? Can you trust me? How do I know if I can trust someone? Certain behaviors reflect trust more than others. Consider the following trust-enhancing and trust-busting behaviors as you develop your relationships.

Trust Building

Being able to communicate openly and honestly (fidelity, integrity) with colleagues, patients, and families is foundational to ethical behaviors. Caregivers know that health care is fundamentally based on personal, professional, and trusting relationships between the individuals who seek care and the professionals who care for them.

Trust implies that one individual is vulnerable to the actions of another. The greater the trust, the more positive the expectations that individuals have about others' intentions and actions based on established roles, relationships, experiences, and their interdependencies. Trust entails caregivers' willingness to be vulnerable to the patient, based on the belief that the latter party is competent, open, concerned, and reliable. See **Box 6-3**. When trust is lost, feelings of betrayal, stress, and vulnerability emerge, often resulting in ethical dilemmas. See **Box 6-4**.

Several behaviors facilitate effective ethical decision making. In particular, all members of the healthcare team should embrace the following activities:

- Support an environment in which a nurse feels comfortable speaking up to any member of the healthcare team in a respectful manner.
- Establish rules of engagement specific to ethical issues for the team. The goal is for every member of the team to know and understand key concepts, common dilemmas, and expectations, and for team members to be competent to do the right thing the first time.

BOX 6-3 BEHAVIORS THAT REFLECT TRUST

1. Share relevant information in a timely manner to support the best decisions. Sharing partial information or sharing information after the fact does not engender trust. Rather, hesitancy emerges because you never know if someone is holding back and for what reason.

2. Reveal concerns even when you are not exactly clear what the concern is. Exploring intuitions with others encourages dialogue and openness.

3. Work to understand others and their perspectives before telling others your plans and goals; allow for mutual influence to avoid a sense of personal superiority.

4. Reduce controls to engender trust in the abilities of others and decrease the need to oversee other individuals.

5. Meet expectations as promised.

6. Let others know their work is valued.

7. Recognize contributions not only by giving financial rewards but also by ensuring presence, concern, and support of effective relationships.

8. Share information regarding the rationale for changes so as to fully engage others in the change process.

9. Request input whenever possible to be sure the best decisions are made on the basis of the collective wisdom of the team.

10. Make eye contact to reflect openness and honesty (note that this does not apply to all cultures).

- Make sure that people hear the real messages that are communicated. This often requires validation of communication and reiteration of expectations.
- Make expectations clear and make sure they are understood. Communicate in several ways: verbally, in writing, and electronically.
- Develop principle-centered policies and practices. Emphasize principles for ethical behaviors and minimize specific rules. For example, the practice to provide a safe environment is a principle; a requirement to always have side rails in the up position is a rule. The principle of providing a safe environment can be met in many ways. In fact, elevating side rails may

BOX 6-4 TRUST-BUSTER BEHAVIORS

- Jumping to conclusions
- Avoiding discussion of sensitive issues
- Demonstrating insensitivity to the beliefs and values of others
- Interrupting when another person is speaking
- Expressing an opinion before a person has an opportunity to share an idea or opinion
- Being too busy for dialogue about controversial topics
- Encouraging competition—emphasizing winners and losers
- Changing a course of action depending on who is present
- Working in isolation and then presenting ideas to others as complete
- Being dishonest

decrease the safety of the environment if the patient attempts to climb over the rails to get out of the bed. Other interventions, such as lowering the bed to its lowest position or placing the mattress on the floor, may be consistent with the principle of providing a safe environment.

- Adhere to principles—do not bend them for anyone!
- Discuss areas of disagreement until common ground is found.
- Support an environment of trust and hold people to their words and promises.
- Respect every team member's contributions and build on team values.
- Work out ethical situations quickly and establish new rules as needed.

Managing Practice Breakdown Errors

As previously noted, errors in health care are now being perceived from a more humanistic perspective. Errors, recently identified as *practice breakdown*, are defined broadly as the disruption or absence of any of the aspects of good practice (Benner et al., 2002). See **Box 6-5**. This new conceptualization allows nurses to identify and examine not only the error but also the category of professional practice error, the role of the system in the error, and the opportunity to prevent other similar breakdown situations. It is important to identify the root cause of the practice breakdown—thereby identifying an area for additional

BOX 6-5 MOST COMMON PRACTICE BREAKDOWN ERRORS

- Lack of professional responsibility (77%)
- Lack of clinical reasoning (51%)
- Lack of intervention (50%)
- Documentation error (44%)
- Lack of interpretation (40%)
- Medication error (32%)
- Lack of attentiveness (25%)
- Lack of prevention (24%)

The percentages exceed 100% because some cases were classified in more than one category.

Data from Zhong, E. H., & Thomas, M. B. (2012). Association between job history and practice: An analysis of disciplinary cases. *Journal of Nursing Regulation*, *2*(4), 16–18.

education or training to improve practice and system deficiencies—not to focus on punishing an individual for an error that is believed to be his or her sole responsibility. The ethical issues of beneficence, justice, integrity, nonmaleficence, and utilitarianism are addressed with this type of approach, not with disciplining single individuals for errors that often involve team members and system flaws.

The most common sources or rationales for nurse practice breakdowns in 884 cases studied by the Taxonomy of Error Root Cause Analysis and Practice-responsibility (TERCAP) committee of the National Council of State Boards of Nursing included lack of professional responsibility, lack of clinical reasoning, and lack of intervention (Zhong & Thomas, 2012). In this study, 72% of the cases involved unintentional human errors, and 27% involved intentional misconduct or criminal behavior. More than 50% of the cases did not cause harm to the patient. When system factors were analyzed, 65% of the cases involved team members as a contributing factor, as well as communication, interdepartmental breakdown or conflict, and inadequate orientation and hand-off procedures. These data support a more humane approach to the ethical dilemma of whether to punish an individual or view the incident first as a specific type of nursing practice breakdown that can be studied and improved upon.

CRITICAL THOUGHT

- Trust is that which an observer knows about an entity and can rely upon to some extent (your spouse or coworker).
- Trust is that which can be relied upon without surveillance by the observer.
- Trust is received information that has a degree of belief that is acceptable to an observer.
- Trust depends on the observer; there is never absolute trust. Trust exists only as self-trust; trust of others will always have surprises.
- Mutual trust is a two-way street in which you trust me and I trust you.

Concluding Thoughts

Creating an ethical environment in an organization requires persistent and on-going dialogue as well as validation of appropriate behaviors. To recognize the complexities and multiple variables involved in ethical issues, nurses must develop and maintain competence so that patient values continue to drive patient care. Addressing ethical issues and dilemmas also requires logical, prompt, and principle-based actions. As noted earlier, the complexity of ethical issues cannot be understated.

Ethics Discussion Scenarios

When faced with an ethical dilemma, it is helpful to approach the situation as logically as possible. The following scenarios are intended to prompt discussion and broaden your understanding of ethical issues and potential solutions. For each scenario, consider the following seven questions:

1. What is the background of the situation? Gather and assess the relevant information, including about stakeholders.
2. What are the facts that can be verified?
3. What is the ethical dilemma? Which ethical principles or concepts are involved?
4. What are the options or possible solutions for resolution? What is the better solution? Choose and justify the better solution.
5. Which activities or resources are necessary for resolution?
6. What will be required to implement the decision?
7. What are the anticipated consequences of the decision?

Issues specific to autonomy, beneficence, betrayal, boundaries, fidelity, justice, integrity, nonmaleficence, rationalization, trust, and utilitarianism should be considered for each scenario.

Create a concept map for each scenario to illustrate the relationships involved. The concept map should identify the ethical concepts, specific to each question posed, that are involved and important in the scenario. Using lines, connect the concepts to identify their relationships. How does this analysis inform your decision making?

Additional comments are included in selected scenarios that may be considered after the ethical aspects of the scenario are discussed.

SCENARIO: NURSE–ORGANIZATION– PROFESSIONAL ROLE

The organization discourages nurses from becoming members of professional nursing organizations because of those organizations' commitment to collective bargaining. Nurses want to join professional nursing organizations because they believe those associations set the standards for nursing practice; the nurses also believe their participation on organizational committees is a professional obligation.

Comments: Nurses are hired by organizations on the basis of their nursing skill and knowledge, which is based on their profession's principles and standards. Participation in and commitment to one's profession is a hallmark of professional practice. While the bargaining arm of some organizations may be problematic to many human resources directors, it is important to recognize other purposes of the professional organization, such as standards setting, education, and mentoring. Each nurse should work to educate those in the organization who resist professional membership with information that clearly describes the essence of the American Nurses Association. Failure to resolve this issue may require the nurse to seek a more supportive employer.

SCENARIO: NURSE–ORGANIZATION– PROFESSIONAL ROLE

Several of the nurses on your unit are reluctant to participate in unit activities, discussion of patient outcome data, or nurse–physician relationships. They feel simply working their shift is enough commitment to practice. The inaction of the staff is creating ethical issues.

SCENARIO: NURSE–ORGANIZATION

The organization emphasizes the need for continuing education and excellence as core values. However, in light of the organization's limited resources and cutbacks in reimbursement, recognition and reward programs are limited to a standard annual pay rate increase for all employees, occasional movie tickets, and pizza.

SCENARIO: NURSE–NURSE

One nurse on your team continually states she is a "good nurse" because her patients love her. While observing her practice, you notice she does not practice the most evidence-based way and may put some patients' health at risk because of her antiquated practice. Is noncontemporary and nonevidenced practice considered good nursing?

SCENARIO: NURSE–PATIENT END OF LIFE

A dying patient's family is not ready for their mother to die in spite of the poor prognosis and demands that everything be done for her, including administration of antibiotics, ventilator care, and tube feedings. There is a 24-hour waiting list for intensive care unit (ICU) beds, and this patient is in an ICU bed. Therefore, the situation is blocking an admission. Several nurses reduce the ventilator settings and delay tube feedings because they believe it would be a better use of resources if the patient was allowed to die.

SCENARIO: NURSE–PATIENT PAIN MANAGEMENT

The elderly mother of a local physician in a rural setting is admitted to the hospital with pneumonia for the third time this year. The patient is somewhat confused and receiving oxygen. Her physician son orders morphine to be given every two hours around the clock to keep her comfortable. When a nursing instructor is working with students, she questions the order because the patient is not responsive and is experiencing increasing difficulty breathing. She wonders if euthanasia is being practiced.

SCENARIO: NURSE–ORGANIZATION–STAFFING ADEQUACY

The organization is experiencing declining revenues and is requesting increased efforts to control expenses. The nursing manager believes she should decrease staffing to contribute to the cost reductions, in spite of increasing patient acuity and nurse dissatisfaction. Nurses are frustrated and not able to complete the expected patient care.

SCENARIO: NURSE–NURSE TEAM

The chief nursing officer (CNO) has supported the implementation of a shared governance model and states that nurses' decisions must be respected. Nurses have become concerned because the CNO has begun to override council decisions and change council priorities.

Comments: The adage to "walk the talk" in this situation can be the ultimate challenge for leaders. Transitioning to the role of coach, mentor, and guide is difficult for even the most committed leader. The appropriate approach is a direct one, because discussing the problem without the CNO would be counterproductive. Clear identification of the overriding of council decisions by the CNO and asking for guidance on how to manage the situation are the first steps. If the CNO rationalizes that this approach is necessary, further discussion is warranted to determine what shared leadership means to the CNO and how such situations should be managed.

SCENARIO: NURSE–ORGANIZATION, NON-VALUE-ADDED WORK

All nurse managers are required to attend the safety committee in person on a monthly basis. The managers do not believe their presence is necessary because their input and opinions are never requested. They believe this meeting is a waste of their time. Nurse managers have requested to attend via conference call and/or be accountable for reviewing minutes.

Comments: Meetings that consist of only one-way communication or information giving should be eliminated in favor of memos or email.

Face-to-face meetings should be held when there is a need for dialogue and problem solving. The team should review its goals, purposes, and expected outcomes and determine the most appropriate method to get the intended work completed. With this information, the team can determine whether face-to-face communication or electronic communication, or a combination of the two, will be the most useful. Electronic communication should never replace healthy dialogue in situations where the latter type of communication is needed. Electronic and face-to-face communication both have advantages and disadvantages.

SCENARIO: NURSE–NURSE–ORGANIZATION

The manager is very concerned about overtime and has instructed nurses to clock out at the end of the shift. If more work (charting) remains to be done, the nurse is told to work on his or her personal organization and priority-setting skills and to complete the charting off the clock.

Comments: The pressure to meet budget targets should never override acceptable practices. The practice described is not acceptable for two reasons. First, it is inconsistent with federal labor laws. Second, failing to understand and manage the workload indicates a serious leadership shortcoming. This practice reflects the larger, unresolved and ever-present problem of too much work and too little time. The manager is challenged to evaluate the work that is being done to ensure that it is appropriate and positively impacts patient outcomes. New strategies to manage the variance between the required work and available staff need to be created by the healthcare team as a collective unit, not by the individual nurse at the bedside.

SCENARIO: NURSE–ORGANIZATION

The manager consistently decreases daily staffing to meet budget guidelines. Errors are increasing and patient care has been negatively impacted. The nurses are planning to file a complaint to the nursing board against the manager for failure to delegate, supervise, and protect patient safety.

Comments: The first step in this situation should be to discuss the issue with the manager and also inform him or her that you believe the manager is violating the nurse practice act. If that step does not yield the desired

(continues)

(continued)

results and patient care continues to be negatively impacted, the nurse must then follow the chain of command and communicate the concerns and the evidence of poor patient outcomes. If these efforts do not yield changes that impact patient care positively, the nurse may choose to report the situation to the board of nursing on the basis of mandatory reporting requirements for unsafe patient care.

SCENARIO: NURSE–NURSE

Most nurses on the unit refuse to precept new nurses because they do not have enough time and also believe that nurses should be better prepared by their nursing schools before they join the staff. Nurses understand their professional commitment to the development of novice nurses, but they also believe the care of their patients is compromised when they are assigned to serve as preceptors.

SCENARIO: NURSE–NURSE DIVERSITY

The nurse manager is Filipino and shows favoritism toward other Filipino nurses. She believes that if she does not honor their requests for scheduled days and lunch breaks, they will quit and there will be less diversity in the team.

SCENARIO: NURSE–NURSE DELEGATION

Critical care nurses have refused to work with nursing technicians or nursing assistants because it requires time to supervise them and delegate tasks, and the competence of the assistants is not always above average. It is believed that approximately 25% of the work in the critical care unit could be done by assistants without compromising quality. In addition, the organization would realize a significant cost savings with a decreased reliance on registered nurses for caregiving.

Comments: When there is reluctance to delegate, the root cause is often lack of knowledge of the principles of delegation and supervision and accountability principles. Basic delegation skills include being familiar with the state nurse practice act, assessing the situation, planning for the delegation, ensuring appropriate accountability, supervising performance of the task, and evaluating the delegation process. When any of these steps are omitted, nurses assume an unreasonable burden and take on overwhelming workloads that are nearly impossible to complete.

SCENARIO: NURSE–PATIENT–ORGANIZATION

An experienced nurse administered an overdose of medication that resulted in serious patient instability and the need for additional therapeutic interventions. Although this was the nurse's first medication error, she was suspended and eventually terminated for unsafe practice on the basis of hospital policy. During the subsequent investigation, it was learned that several safety checks were missed in the pharmacy department.

Comments: No nurse ever enters the profession of nursing to harm a patient. Given the inevitability of errors in a human-run system, reacting to mistakes punitively is unlikely to minimize their occurrence, even though our culture leads us to expect the assignment of blame, correction of the error, and, in most cases, punishment of those who make the mistake. Attaching blame to individuals creates a climate of shame and guilt and further decreases the likelihood of candid reporting and discussion of mistakes.

The punishment of those who make errors ultimately fails to produce the desired result—namely, the elimination of errors. The emphasis should instead be on recognizing and recovering from the error, thereby enabling the organization to learn from mistakes, to identify actions that will decrease the chance of repeating the same mistakes, and to improve performance. The goal should always be to strive for excellence, rather than to achieve perfection—the latter is an unrealistic expectation given the uncontrollable variables present in the healthcare system.

SCENARIO: ERROR TRANSPARENCY

In the situation in the previous scenario, the nurse informed the patient and family of the error. The physician and other nurses are upset and believe this step was not necessary because the patient did not experience lasting harm.

Comments: Disclosure of errors and apologies are becoming more acceptable. Errors do not necessarily constitute improper, negligent, or unethical behavior, but failure to disclose them may.

SCENARIO: NURSE–ORGANIZATION

Many states are advocating for safe staffing legislation. Some leaders believe such laws are needed because of ineffective leadership in relation to this issue in healthcare organizations. Others believe that it is the only way to address safe staffing issues.

Comments: External agencies should not be required to do the work an organization has committed to do yet failed to achieve. The strategy of enacting legislation to ensure safe staffing is representative of leadership failure to provide adequate staffing resources. Rather than work to legislate safe staffing, healthcare leaders should work to create effective systems and manage the reality of the imbalance between supply and demand.

SCENARIO: NURSE–NURSE

Peer review is a process used for evaluations. Three colleagues provide input as part of an organization's peer review program, but policy does not allow the nurse to see the specific feedback from each individual who provides such input. Nurses think it is unfair to withhold such information; the manager wishes to provide anonymity to participating staff and thereby encourage them to share information in an honest manner.

Comments: Open, honest dialogue about performance leads to better performance. Withholding or masking feedback behind an average rating within a 360-degree evaluation decreases an individual's opportunity to modify behaviors and reinforces the standard that open, direct communication is not an expectation. This policy should be modified to require open, honest sharing of feedback. Holding back information is an oppressive leadership behavior and prevents others from managing their own behavior.

CHAPTER TEST QUESTIONS

Licensure exam categories: Management of care: ethical practice, evidence-based practice, confidentiality

Nurse leader exam categories: Knowledge of the healthcare environment: clinical practice knowledge, governance, risk management; Professionalism: personal and professional accountability, ethics, advocacy

1. An ethical dilemma arises from

   a. Conscious bias.

   b. Differing values.

   c. Differing gender, generational, and educational competencies.

   d. Unsuccessful or negligent patient care.

2. Trusting relationships are essential in managing ethical dilemmas. Trust is characterized as

   a. Complete support of a colleague.

   b. An ugly duckling.

    c. A relationship in which one individual is vulnerable to another.

    d. Nearly impossible to create and sustain.

3. Ethical erosion is

    a. Subtle, even unnoticed slippage of ethical standards.

    b. A common organizational phenomenon.

    c. An increase in sensitivity to diverse values.

    d. The result of poor patient care.

4. Ethical principles are helpful in

    a. Determining the specific cause or explanation of an ethical dilemma.

    b. Assigning blame to the individual violating the principle.

    c. Forming guidelines for appropriate behavior.

    d. Resolving patient care errors.

5. Promise-keeping or fidelity is

    a. An agreement in nurse–nurse relationships.

    b. The same as nonmaleficence.

    c. A foundational ethical principle for resolution of ethical dilemmas.

    d. A difficult principle to validate.

6. Often nurses rationalize a situation because

    a. It is necessary to fully understand a situation.

    b. The right thing is not easy to do.

    c. Other, more appropriate actions might become available.

    d. The pragmatic approach is not effective.

7. Boundaries from an ethical perspective

    a. Include activities specific to nurse–patient assignments.

    b. Emphasize boundary violations as inappropriate behaviors.

    c. Require interpretations from a moral perspective.

    d. Delineate the professional limits of a therapeutic relationship.

8. Impaired nursing practice is

    a. About substance use disorders impacting safe nursing practice.

    b. Not common in the nursing profession.

    c. Readily reported by colleagues who become aware of the impaired practice.

    d. A relatively new issue in health care.

9. Practice breakdown strategies represent ethical issues

    a. In identifying the cause of errors.

    b. Specific to fair and just treatment of nurses.

    c. Requiring more stringent discipline of those making errors.

    d. Supporting rationalization of healthcare errors.

10. Conflict in ethical situations arises from

    a. Morality.

    b. Nonmaleficence.

    c. Value diversity.

    d. Financial resources.

References

Arizona State Board of Nursing. (1997). *Arizona State Board of Nursing guidelines for sexual misconduct and boundary violation cases.* Retrieved from azmemory .azlibrary.gov/cdm/ref/collection/statepubs/id/7962

Bazerman, M. H., Loewenstein, G., & Moore, D. A. (2002). Why accountants do bad audits. *Harvard Business Review, 80*(11), 97–102.

Benner, P., Malloch, K., & Sheets, V. (Eds.). (2010). *Nursing pathways for patient safety: Expert panel on practice breakdown. Overview: NCSBN practice breakdown initiative.* Philadelphia, PA: Elsevier.

Benner, P., Sheets, V., Uris, P., Malloch, K., Schwed, K., & Jamison, D. (2002). Individual, practice and system causes of error in nursing. *Journal of Nursing Administration, 32*(10), 509–523.

Curtin, L. (2011). Quantum ethics: Coming to grips with the dark side. *American Nurse Today, 6*(11), 48.

Darbro, N. (2011). Model guidelines for alternative programs and discipline monitoring programs. *Journal of Nursing Regulation, 2*(1), 42–49.

Gerck, E. (1998). Toward real-world models of trust: Reliance on received information. Retrieved from www.researchgate.net/publication/286459693_Toward_Real-World _Models_of_Trust_Reliance_on_Received_Information

Gilbert, J. A. (2007). *Strengthening ethical wisdom: Tools for transforming your health care organization.* Chicago, IL: AHA Press.

Godfrey, N., & Crigger, N. (2012). Ethics and professional conduct: Striving for a professional ideal. *Journal of Nursing Regulation, 3*(1), 32–39.

Goeschel, C. (2011). Defining and assigning accountability for quality care and patient safety. *Journal of Nursing Regulation, 2*(1), 28–35.

Inglesby, T. (2011). Being everywhere at once. *Patient Safety and Quality Healthcare, 8*(2), 44.

Lachman, V. D. (Ed.). (2006). *Applied ethics in nursing.* New York, NY: Springer.

Lachman, V. D. (2008). Whistle blowers: Troublemakers or virtuous nurses? *Medsurg Nursing, 17*(2), 126–128, 134.

O'Rourke, M. W. (2003). Rebuilding a professional practice model: The return of role-based practice accountability. *Nursing Administration Quarterly, 27*(2), 95–105.

Rawls, J. (2001). Justice as reciprocity. In S. Freeman (Ed.), *Collected papers* (pp. 190–224). Cambridge, MA: Harvard University Press.

Rathert, C., May, D. R., & Chung, H. S. (2016). Nurse moral distress: A survey identifying predictors and potential interventions. *International Journal of Nursing Studies, 53,* 39–49.

Schluter, J., Winch, S., Holzhauser, K., & Henderson, A. (2008). Nurses' moral sensitivity and hospital ethical climate: A literature review. *Nursing Ethics, 15*(3), 304–321.

Sherman, R. O. (2014). Dealing with difficult people. *American Nurse Today, 9*(5), 61.

TheFreeDictionary. (2008). Whistle-blowing. Retrieved from www.thefreedictionary .com/whistle-blowing

Trossman, S. (2011). Issues up close: The practice of ethics. *American Nurse Today, 6*(11), 3233.

Zhong, E. H., & Thomas, M. B. (2012). Association between job history and practice error: An analysis of disciplinary cases. *Journal of Nursing Regulation, 2*(4), 16–18.

Appendix A

Selected Healthcare Ethics Resources

American Medical Association. *Journal of Ethics*. journalofethics.ama-assn.org

American Nurses Association. Code of ethics for nurses. nursingworld.org/codeofethics

American Nurses Association. Center for Ethics and Human Rights. www.nursingworld .org/MainMenuCategories/ThePracticeofProfessionalNursing/EthicsStandards /CEHR.aspx

Baillie, H. M., Garrett, R. M., & McGeehan, J. F. (2012). *Health care ethics: Principles and problems* (6th ed.). Upper Saddle River, NJ: Prentice Hall.

Bioethics.net: covers information related to health care and biotechnology and includes news articles, editorials, book reviews, and a blog.

Bosek, S. D., Glenn, L. M., & Reynolds, L. (2011). Is it ethical to do dialysis but not cardiopulmonary resuscitation? *JONA's Healthcare Law, Ethics, and Regulation, 13*(2), 47–54.

EthicShare: a research and collaboration website offering reference materials, news items, group discussions, and bioethics information. www.ethicshare.org

Fremgen, B. F. (2012). *Medical law and ethics*. New York, NY: Pearson.

Hastings Center Report. www.thehastingscenter.org/publications-resources/ hastings-center-report

Health Ethics Trust. healthethicstrust.com

International Council of Nurses. *The ICN code of ethics for nurses*. www.icn.ch /images/stories/documents/about/icncode_english.pdf

Lachman, V. (2012). Doing the right thing: Pathways to moral courage. *American Nurse Today, 7*(5), 24–29.

National Institutes of Health. Bioethics resources on the web. bioethics.nih.gov /resources/index.shtml

Nursing Ethics: An International Journal for Health Care Professionals. http://journals. sagepub.com/home/nej

Pozgar, G. D. (2016). *Legal aspects of health care administration* (12th ed.). Sudbury, MA: Jones and Bartlett Publishers.

Purtilo, R. B., & Doherty, R. *Ethical dimensions in the health professions*. St. Louis, MO: Elsevier Saunders.

Santa Clara University, Markkula Center for Applied Ethics: offers online articles, end-of-life materials, case studies, and resources on medical decision making. www.scu.edu/ethics/focus-areas/bioethics

Twibell, R., & Townsend, T. (2011). Trust in the workplace: Build it, break it, mend it. *American Nurse Today, 6*(11), 12–16.

Yale Journal of Health Policy, Law, and Ethics. www.yale.edu/yjhple

Appendix B

Common Barriers to Effective Relationships

When one of these behaviors is identified, confront the issue and begin discussion to overcome and eliminate the barrier:

- Bringing up unrelated issues
- Holding a grudge—never forgive, never forget
- Insisting that the problem is entirely the other person's fault
- Being sarcastic
- Being defensive
- Being self-righteous and convinced you are right
- Using the silent treatment
- Disregarding the other person's feelings
- Pretending nothing is wrong
- Saying or doing things that are hurtful or cruel

> They must often change who would be constant in happiness or wisdom. —Confucius (551 BC–479 BC)

CHAPTER OBJECTIVES

Upon completion of this chapter, the reader will be able to do the following:

» Understand the elements and processes associated with interdisciplinary team leadership and the particular role of the team leader.

» Define the role of the professional nurse as team leader and identify the unique skills necessary to make team leadership a basic expectation of the professional role.

» Enumerate the stages of the team process and describe the leadership skill capacity necessary to facilitate, coordinate, and integrate team action.

» Outline the characteristics of team dynamics related specifically to team roles, interaction, terms of engagement, and stages of team action.

» List at least 10 team fables that often impede understanding the team process and obtaining effective team outcomes.

» State normative challenges that teams confront in undertaking their work and identify mechanisms for managing those challenges.

» Identify specific characteristics and skills of the team leader in relation to collaboration, team dynamics, team decision making, managing conflict, and achieving team outcomes.

Leadership: The Foundation of Practice Partnership

All clinical activity ultimately intersects with the activities of teams. In every work environment, regardless of the unit of service, teams are key to work effectiveness (Losoncy, 1996; Whatley & Kleiwer, 2013). This is especially true in health care, where the fundamental role of the nurse is to coordinate, integrate, and facilitate the activities of multiple players along the care continuum. As a professional nurse, it is critical to understand group dynamics; the characteristics that are essential for building caring, clinical relationships; and the management and movement of effective teams.

While the physician has traditionally been perceived as the "captain" of the clinical team, both reality and practice today demonstrate a more relevant notion of teams and leadership. Older configurations of teams, in which a single leader acted across the work spectrum and all team activities reflected an industrial model, are now considered more historical than useful (Daspit, Justice, Boyd, & McKee, 2013; Parker, 2003). This notion also often reflects a paternalistic approach to leadership of teams. In more contemporary notions that feature a deeper understanding of systems complexity and use network metaphors as a framework, teams may take a wide variety of forms. Teams are constantly in flux, shifting and changing members and processes depending on the character and emphasis of the activities that the teams pursue (Gratton & Erickson, 2007).

Because teams are social groups, they reflect the full spectrum of social life and human experience. Teams are places for interaction, learning, communication, human expression, relationship building, and the expression and use of collective wisdom. Teams represent a central element in complex systems because they incorporate and demonstrate a large number of interacting and intersecting elements that are essential to their success. These complex interactions lead to rich and important individual and group behaviors that have specific and particular impact on the healthcare experience. Within the many different roles and perspectives created through interactions among disciplines, the individual nurse, team associates, and patients, team dynamics are always at work.

The Importance of Teams in Interdisciplinary Practice

Historically, in hospitals and health systems, teamwork was perceived as a departmental and unit function. Unit teams were generally made up of partners within the discipline, including the registered nurse as team leader and associates and/or assistants as needed for the provision of clinical care (Barner, 2000). These discipline-specific teams rendered good care within the context of their own practice and functional work, but they rarely included members from other disciplines. Broader notions of team involvement often meant utilizing the skill of other discipline resources when needed in a more incremental fashion; the resulting "consulting" relationship and interaction did not incorporate team membership and contribution (Ben Saoud & Mark, 2006).

More recently, interdisciplinary, team-based development has been recognized as a critical part of clinical care delivery. In the contemporary and more complex value-driven age of network systems, evidence-based practice, and clinical integration, the notion of broad-based team construction and clinical practice has emerged as a cornerstone in developing the future of patient care (Curlee & Gordon, 2011). In fact, the Institute of Medicine (now the Health and Medicine Division) recommended that nurses lead and coordinate interprofessional teams because of the profession's position at the nexus of all aspects of care delivery (Institute of Medicine, 2011). Digital technology, mobility-based communication systems, and the need to converge the work efforts of a wide variety of clinical members have coalesced to create the demand for a much more strongly defined

CRITICAL THOUGHT

Interprofessional leadership and teamwork are now required competencies for clinical leaders. Teamwork, interprofessional communication, values/ethics, and the roles and responsibilities of other health professions must be understood and mastered to be successful in the complex healthcare environment (Interprofessional Education Collaborative Expert Panel, 2011).

foundation for interdisciplinary teamwork. Increasingly, the traditional biomedical model is giving way to a much more complex biopsychosocial model that emphasizes the need to address and sustain a health script along the continuum of care rather than simply implementing late-stage incremental interventions in a tertiary care framework.

Because of the complexities inherent in today's care model, the interdisciplinary approaches employed draw upon a wide variety of expertise and specialties. They come from separate domains but collectively focus on patient problems and issues, and they intersect in a unique way that better addresses the needs of patients. Driving much of this increased multilateral focus on patient care is the fact that much of the patient's own healing experience will occur in settings other than the hospital or healthcare system. In other words, patients will need to engage significant others in managing their response to illness and the activities associated with either maintaining health or managing some level of their health status. Also, digitalization has created a social construct where the user becomes the owner of his or her own care; the intent and direction of technological application, therefore, is to help this user better manage and direct his or her own care. This user-centric social reality shifts the accountability for impact, value, and sustainability from the provider to the individual and places full accountability for the ownership of health and the actions of the health journey on the individual rather than the health provider or the system. This shift in control from provider to user is perhaps the most significant driver of team-based, interdisciplinary collaboration.

In this increasingly complex health environment, it quickly becomes apparent that no single discipline has all the information, skills, and resources necessary to address the many intersecting needs of individual patients and patient populations. As the healthcare system continually recalibrates to focus on primary health care and early intervention, an increasingly complex array of skill sets and team players will need to converge around the health script of patients and populations and work in highly collaborative teams that seek to achieve and sustain clinical convergence and positive health outcomes (Wang, Waldman, & Zhang, 2014). These teams will not only need to include multiple professions but also patient and family care givers. Leadership of these teams will not be based on prescribed and fixed role delineations (e.g., physician-directed); rather, leadership will be determined by the particular needs of the user and the combination of skills necessary to advance particular issues and concerns along the patient's continuum of care. This more "emergent" nature of leadership reflects a more self-organizing understanding of the dynamics of the team as it unfolds around specific needs or demands. Such shifting teams may be led by a wide variety of stakeholders (including nurses), depending on the point along the continuum of health service where the intersection between the health team and the patient takes place and which particular skills are needed there.

The professional nurse must recognize that a natural attribute of the nursing role in a complex system reflects historically held role competencies related to facilitation, coordination, and integration of clinical activities around a particular patient and his or her set of needs. This role delineation does not change in a complex environment; indeed, it becomes more critical. Essentially, the fundamental role of the professional nurse within the context of team-based

SCENARIO

Mrs. Wade, a 77-year-old patient with long-term diabetes who lives alone in a high-rise apartment building, is admitted to your unit because of complications related to uncontrolled glucose blood levels that appeared to have been poorly managed for some time. She is generally immobilized by neuropathic wounds on the ankles and metatarsals of both feet and appears to have significant issues related to poor diet and malnutrition. She is alone yet alert and oriented and appears unable to continue to effectively self-manage her care.

Discussion Questions

1. As the attending nurse to Mrs. Wade, how will you decide which interdisciplinary team members need to be a part of your clinical team?

2. What role do you see for the physician on this team?

3. Which team member will take the initial leadership role on Mrs. Wade's clinical team?

4. What is the interdisciplinary team plan of care and how will you evaluate the synthesis of the efforts of all members in a way that shows how their care impacted the patient's experience?

collaborative approaches in primary patient care emphasizes the centrality of co-ordination, integration, and facilitation of the activities of the team along the continuum of care. By both disposition and definition, the unique character of the role of professional nurse places the nurse at the intersection of the continuing care journey. The nurse operates at the interface between the health system and the healthcare provider's response to the patient's needs. At this juncture between the disciplines, the nurse coordinates care to address all the patient's needs and integrates the efforts of all the providers. In a future where complex care will be the norm, this critical role will be emphasized and even expand.

Team Construction

Some elements are commonly encountered in the construction of any team. Professional nurses must be aware that while teams may often form in a dynamic fashion, effective teams need design and structure to establish their direction and evaluate their progress with regard to team role and purpose. Elements essential to viable team construction include clearly defined purpose, goals, roles, relationships, activities and functions, coordination, and leadership. The creation of the team must also account for scope of practice and regulatory environments that may limit full scope of practice. See **Box 7-1**.

Purpose

Teams are formed to fulfill a specific purpose. That is, there is a driving purpose for every team. The leader understands that the fundamental purpose for creating a team is to provide a mechanism to advance the capacity of professionals to fully engage in particular planning activities, decision making, and problem solving in a way that addresses patient care and improves team effectiveness. In other words,

---

BOX 7-1 ELEMENTS OF AN EFFECTIVE TEAM

The following elements in the construction of any team must be the focus of development at the outset:

- Purpose
- Goals
- Roles
- Relationships
- Activities and functions
- Coordination and leadership

a care team should be formed to fulfill the specific needs of the patient in the best way possible. Teams should not be formed to satisfy ego, perceived roles, tradition, or individual wants. Engaging professional partners in team-based decision making helps them better understand the decisions that are made, encourages full participation in the process of making decisions, establishes a common frame of reference for problem solving, and ultimately advances ownership and investment in the team's decisions and activities. Team leadership and facilitation help team members and stakeholders achieve clarity regarding their reasons for coming together and the end that their collective deliberation will serve.

A **statement of purpose** is usually brief and focused. Although this statement will certainly evolve over time as work progresses, it serves as an anchor for the work of the team and an indicator of the direction that is set for team activities. Some examples of purpose statements are provided here:

- The purpose of this committee is to conduct a needs assessment of the clinical education priorities that better define the foundations of safe patient care on this unit.
- The purpose of this meeting is to finalize a clear decision regarding shared governance council meeting schedules for the next year.

The simpler and more direct a statement of purpose is, the clearer the work assignment will become and the better the team members will understand the direction of team activities.

Goals

Every team has specific goals that are directed toward fulfilling that team's purpose. The goal of clinical professional teams is generally to configure the provider members in a specific or unique arrangement around patient-care processes or in specific efforts to meet the demands of advancing patient care. The identified goals outline the role and work of the team and, ultimately, the activities of each member in advancing that role. The establishment of goals is one of the more critical stages in team development. Goals give the team clear and specific direction and create a point of reference so that the team can effectively evaluate its progress and determine its movement toward achievement of those goals. Both the team as a whole and the individual members define the performance expectations for the team as part of the goals; when those expectations are broken down, they may dictate the efforts and activities of individual team members. Congruence between team goals and individual member activities is essential to fulfilling the goals of the team. See **Box 7-2** for ideas on team goal setting.

CRITICAL THOUGHT

Every team is simply the aggregation of the skills, talents, and behaviors of its participants. It is critical that the roles of all team members be clear and understood at the outset of team formation. Indeed, ambiguity around roles and contributions tends to create difficulties that hinder team effectiveness.

BOX 7-2 SETTING GOALS

1. Do the goals relate to the team's purpose?
2. Are the goals mutually supportive?
3. Are the goals clear and specific?
4. Do the goals relate to a specific action?
5. Can the goals be achieved by the work team?
6. Is there a way to measure points of progress and outcome?
7. Do the goals fit well together and aggregate in a way that fulfills the driving purpose?

When armed with clear goals, the team leader can help the team avoid frustrations related to ambiguity and lack of clarity as well as uncertainty regarding the specific activities and expectations of team members. Goals are tied to the team's purpose insofar as they become the tools for translating purpose into action and moving the team toward some level of accomplishment. Here again, the simpler and more straightforward the goal, the clearer the expectation and the more likely it can be achieved.

Using the participatory process, the team leader generally engages the team in establishing its goals. Because the goals provide the road map for the team's action, it is critical that everyone participate fully in establishing the team's direction and clarifying expectations of members' actions and goals. The leader generally establishes goals and makes them visible by writing them on a whiteboard or flip chart. During this process, the leader ensures that the following basic elements are present to help the team focus on goals development:

- The team leader asks each team member the single most important activities that must be done to address the team's purpose.

- Team members are given time to reflect on their responses and put them in writing, thereby clarifying their own positions related to the goals.
- The team identifies congruence between goals and establishes priorities with regard to goal activity and their relevance and relationship to the purpose.
- The team prioritizes the goals as they relate to the goodness of fit with the team's purpose and organizes the goals in a trajectory that will lead to fulfillment of the team's purpose.
- The team clearly identifies timelines and end dates related to specific accomplishment and fulfillment of the team's purpose.
- The team clarifies the consequences of both performance and nonperformance. Usually the purpose defines the inherent deliverable or value of the team's action and, therefore, suggests the positive consequence. However, the negative consequence also needs to be identified: "If we don't accomplish [a goal], what will happen or not happen? What will be the consequence, or what will be the impact?"
- When goals are clarified and established, and performance consequences and a timeline are determined, the team leader verifies understanding of goals, commits the team to achieving those goals, and finalizes the goals as the action steps enumerating the priorities and processes of the team's work (Curseu, 2003).

After goals have been established and clarified, the team leader should obtain affirmation of understanding of those goals from each team member. Specifically, the leader should direct each team member to indicate how he or she understands the goals, identify what personal meaning the goals have in light of his or her own role, and make a personal commitment to working with the team in achieving those goals.

Roles

The nurse team leader must sort through the participants on the team to determine which particular skills they could bring to problem solving. Clinical leaders should understand that no one individual has the capacity to possess all the skills needed for a team to function and be successful. Instead, building a team around a defined need will allow the leader to invite participants with skills that match those needs (Weberg & Weberg, 2014). A lot of teamwork can be allocated and delegated to specific individuals or groups on the team with specialized skills (Chrispeels, 2004; Eissa, Fox, Webster, & Kim, 2012). Choosing team membership carefully is a major task of the nurse team leader. Aligning skills with specified work tasks on the team is a part of the role of the leader as he or she assesses the character of the work, the distribution of that work, and the best way to break down elements of the work into meaningful components. When the objectives are clearly ascertained, some specific elements of the work generally should not be done by all team members working together. Instead, depending on the size of the team, much of the work that has been delineated through the setting of objectives can be accomplished by smaller work groups.

To meet the objectives set by the team with regard to specific work, it is important that the work is closely aligned with the skills available on the team. While members of the team must have particular responsibilities in terms of meeting goals and objectives, it is not always necessary that they meet those objectives solely through their own efforts. An effective team leader knows that additional participation in team activities may be needed and that team members who are assigned specific, additional work regarding a goal or objective may need to access additional resources that will help inform or advance these specific tasks (Belbin, 2010). Adaptability and flexibility are key behaviors for high performing team members. The more tenuous the desired outcome, the more important it is to have team members with those skills. When making specific assignments that address core objectives and goal activity regarding the team's purpose, the nurse leader needs to be sure the following elements are included in the assignment of work:

- Individuals who are charged with the responsibility for a particular goal need to be clear about what those specifics are and what the expectations are related to progress.
- The action steps associated with fulfilling the purpose of the group's work must be determined and specifically enumerated by team leadership.
- Members working on particular goal-directed activity need to be clear about the time and resources they need to undertake the work and to effectively deliberate and act in a way that fits their assigned responsibility.
- A specific timetable and clear expectations regarding the completion of the action related to a goal must be established early and coordinated with the time parameters within which the goal must be achieved.
- Measures and markers related to the specific goal must be incorporated into team members' work so that appropriate progress toward success or real challenges in meeting the work group's performance expectations can be identified.

TEAM TIP

Leaders always need to prepare for the team's work before the team ever meets. To ensure team effectiveness, the leader must establish the following foundational elements:

- Rules of behavior
- Purposeful information
- Requisite financial data
- Good deliberation processes
- Clear sense of the role of members
- Information
- Terms of engagement

Relationships and the Terms of Engagement

The overall success and effectiveness of a team depends largely on the relationships and interactions through which the team does its work (Dunin-Keplicz & Verbrugge, 2010). Maintaining positive team dynamics and healthy interactions form the foundation for successful communication and progress with regard to team efforts and accomplishments. A major part of successfully moving the team toward achieving its purpose is making sure that all members understand the rules of engagement and communication, thereby ensuring that the team remains positive and constructive in both its relationship and its work.

Terms of engagement are the general rules that govern relationships and interactions within the team and serve to maintain a positive communication and interaction environment within the context of the team as it completes its work. All teams are driven by human dynamics, which means they are inevitably subject to the foibles and challenges of making these dynamics effective and productive. In turn, the nurse team leader needs to be aware of his or her role in firmly enumerating the rules of communication and interaction that are critical to maintaining balance, equity, and fairness in team processes. Those terms of engagement might include the following elements:

- Members should be required to stay within the context of the issues and deliberations currently on the table (keep to the purpose). Reaching far afield in dialogue and making extraneous points rather than sticking specifically to the points under discussion wastes time. It causes anxiety with regard to maintaining focus on the specific work of the team. The leader works to maintain focus on the issues at hand and limit the tendency toward digression and off-topic discussions.

- The nurse team leader works diligently to make sure that judgment-laced language is not a part of the team's interaction or deliberation. Avoiding judgments about others' views or statements is important in keeping the group on an even keel and advancing positive contributions.

- Team leaders encourage all participants to contribute fully to the dialogue and processes associated with the team's work. Team members should recognize that presence on the team does not simply mean being a warm body sitting at the table. Instead, team member presence means full engagement in, investment in, and pursuit of the team's objectives, as demonstrated by full participation in the dialogue and interactions necessary for good teamwork.

- Team members avoid judgment words that reflect other people's thoughts or contributions to ensure that everyone's participation is honored. The nurse leader should help team members avoid moderating and judging language that negatively impacts individual contributions. Phrases such as "I agree," "I disagree," "You are right," and "You are wrong" (almost any "you" statements are judgment statements) should be carefully identified as unacceptable and eliminated from the dialogue among team members.

- Interaction parameters for communication should be established early in the team process and incorporated into a team communication charter as the foundation for established team communication behavior. Enumerating these elements and carefully affirming them as a part of the foundations of team processes is important to the effective work of the team. These elements may need to be reviewed on a regular basis, as they tend to be forgotten over time.

CRITICAL THOUGHT

Team leadership and working well with others is always a learned skill. No matter how well we know other team members, working in the context of a team requires a higher level of managing relationships and building team effectiveness. This work will consume much of the energy of the leader.

Challenges, problems, or emergent concerns should be addressed as part of effective deliberation in teams. The nurse team leader should be aware that such issues are likely to arise routinely during the functioning of a team. In his or her moderating role, the team leader must not just be aware of these potential realities, but also revisit the terms of engagement periodically. This review serves as a reminder of the methods of communication that have been agreed to by members as their way of doing business, and it is critical to pursue when individual members either flaunt or ignore the terms of engagement (Salas, Goodwin, & Burke, 2009). In such a case, the team leader must have specific and focused conversations with the individual who is violating these ground rules. The individual should be challenged and reminded of the obligations of team membership or encouraged to alter aberrant behavior so as to facilitate the work of the team. Consistent failure on the part of a team member to adhere to the terms of engagement, despite counseling, should be regarded a disciplinary issue; such behavior needs management intervention and involvement as a final stage of resolution.

SCENARIO

You have been a member of the nursing unit for the past 12 months. The staff members get along very well, and there is a clear team commitment to patient care. However, there has been a great deal of difficulty with appropriate shift staffing coverage, and staff members' commitment to their schedules appears to be passive, almost lackadaisical. The nurse manager works diligently to develop the schedules but appears to have a great deal of difficulty getting staff acceptance of schedules and making sure the staff follow their schedules. The problem with this variable response to the schedule is evident in misunderstanding of work times scheduled.

To rectify this situation, the unit is considering adopting a self-scheduling process. It is agreed that a team of staff members will work together to develop a self-scheduling methodology, and you have been appointed the team leader. Explore the following questions as they relate to your role as team leader of this work group.

Discussion Questions

1. What will be the purpose statement for your team's action?

2. How will you select the team's members?

3. How large should the team be?

4. What information do you need to have available prior to the first team meeting?

5. Which decisions will you make about personal characteristics of participants, and how will those decisions influence your effort to create sufficient diversity on the team?

6. Who would you select as your advisor/mentor to assist in your own team leadership development and assessment?

Team Fables

As a team leader, you will need to confront much of the mythology around the process of building effective teams—and there is a lot of this kind of mythology. While much literature focuses on creating effective teams, there is also a need to be aware of what can impede good team effectiveness. The following fables are 10 key moderators of effectiveness that should be addressed and kept in mind by the team leader.

Fable One: Team Members Always Feel Committed to Implementing a Good Team Process

This myth can be really quite dangerous for the leader. Most people on health-related teams come from a clinical frame of reference. While they may have worked with one another, they may not have necessarily related to one another in a formalized team process. Working in the same place, within the same department, and even with the same patient population does not guarantee that the people work together well in a structured team format. Constructing a team-based frame for understanding the collective work of the service is very different from simply doing clinical work with other people. Also, the team leader should be careful not to assume that people really want to work well in teams. Often, while members may have good intentions, they are really not clear about what teamwork entails. Most people have not learned how to work within the context of formalized teams. Just like leading a team is a learned skill, being a member of a team is a learned capacity. However, given appropriate time and use of the developmental and implementation tools available, carefully constructing a realistic approach to building team effectiveness will help staff come on board quickly. Understanding that team construction includes development of team members will be an important insight that can help build an effective team.

REFLECTIVE QUESTION

Is it possible to influence and change team behavior through preplanning and building good structures and processes within which the team will work? In other words, can good structure determine good team behavior?

Fable Two: All Team Members Are Created Equal

Perhaps one of the most dangerous considerations in building teams is the belief that all team members will have something of value to contribute to the team just by virtue of their presence. In reality, the team members come to their roles on the team with different beliefs about their own person, contribution, interactional skills, and relationship to others on the team. The leader should address some early concerns related to creating the foundation of equity, balance, and involvement of members on the team. Notably, a physician comes to the team with a certain sense of self and role perception that is entirely different from the professional nurse's, the respiratory therapist's, or the physical therapist's. The nurse also comes to the team with a certain understanding of his or her unique role. The nurse needs to be able to participate from a strongly facilitative perspective.

Thus each member will approach the team process within individualized insights, precepts, and levels of self-confidence regarding the expression of member roles that will need to be understood and clarified at the outset of the team formation. Many of the early developmental processes associated with growing an effective team require the team leader to work through issues of participant equity in an effort to build effective and truly collaborative team deliberation.

Fable Three: People Really Want to Reach Agreement and Move Past Their Issues of Concern

One of the most difficult elements of the team process that the leader will confront relates to effective decision making and the ability to build consensus around meaningful decisions. Unfortunately, most people who come to a team do not know how to make good decisions. Members often do not understand the process of consensus building, nor do they recognize that consensus can be obtained through a number of decision-making and problem-solving techniques that, once learned, are very effective in moving the group to make good decisions.

Clearly, for the team leader, knowing these techniques will be critical to team effectiveness and advancing decision making. For the team leader, this is an early learning requirement that will require some concerted and intentional effort to master. The new team leader must engage in early learning activities around the techniques and modalities of good team decision making and must build personal and collective skill, develop insight with regard to progress, and accelerate the capacity for leading effectively.

Fable Four: Team Members Generally Use Good Critical Thinking to Resolve Their Questions and Issues

Initially, one of the more disheartening realities of team management is the leader's eventual recognition that team members do not necessarily exhibit the capacity for problem solving or the skill set for structured thinking that the leader might have hoped for early in the team construction process. Often, analytical, objective, deductive, or reductive processes are not used by team members in the process of doing this new and more disciplined, collective work. Much of the skill that team members use in their own patient care activities tends to be intuitive and responsive, reflecting talents and skills honed over time that are second nature to their practice work. In team-based activities, however, the discipline necessary to engage in critical thinking and problem-solving applications becomes more visible and is more essential in effective team deliberation and organized problem solving. While this may not be exciting work, refining deliberative and critical thinking skills as part of the team's activities will be important to effective skill development. The nurse leader must ensure that time is spent in verifying and advancing the team's problem-solving skills during the team's early days. Where the efforts of reflection, discernment, and discourse articulate well with the functions, activities, and priorities of good teamwork, good results can be achieved. Good techniques that incorporate evidentiary dynamics, the utility of accurate and timely information, good analysis and rationale development, and decision-making synthesis will be important to enhance the effectiveness and sustainability of the team's work.

Fable Five: Team Members Will Set Aside Their Emotional Issues in the Interest of Effective Team Decision Making

Ideally, team members will balance their emotional sensitivities with the requirements of the team and the elements of good team decision making. While this kind of balance can ultimately emerge and contribute to team effectiveness, the

CRITICAL THOUGHT

Each of us develops our own patterns of behavior over the years of our lives. It is a false expectation that we always know why we do what we do. Careful and caring attention to addressing the habits and rituals of others is important to building team effectiveness. Good leadership and facilitation techniques and methods can make the process work of teams operate effectively and create an open and responsive framework for accommodating the delicate personal issues that are always a part of good team function.

team leader should not expect emotional maturity to be generally present at the outset. Achieving such balance is a learned skill; thus its development requires some specific focus and even some developmental activities undertaken by the team as a whole. Early in the team's formation, the leader should initiate a careful dialogue around the role that emotion plays and the impact of feeling, expression, and the obligations of healthy communication in team dynamics. The team leader must remember that "people work" never ends within teams, and that individual circumstances and behaviors will always be a part of the team management process. However, making space for dialogue around the impact and implications of member feelings, emotions, interactions, and ownership is always part of the dynamics of team interaction and should be expected—even encouraged—as well as effectively managed by the team leader.

Fable Six: All Team Members Fully Understand Why They Act as They Do

One of the mysteries of human relationships is the recognition that people bring different meanings, values, behaviors, and insights to their activities and to team interactions. While much of this behavior is unconscious activity, such individual behavior affects collective behavior. Surprisingly, many people do not fully understand the impact of their individual expressions on others. Human beings behave in ways that may make sense to themselves but do not necessarily positively impact their relationship with others. In team interaction, however, the unconscious must be made conscious. Whether consciously or unconsciously, the team leader attempts to identify and advance normative interactions and to minimize aberrant behavior that in any way fails to support good communication and effective deliberation. Certainly, the terms of engagement help establish effective rules of communication and interaction. The team leader must depend on these interactive principles as a way of guiding appropriate dialogue and discussion and minimizing communication that is either negative or poorly expressed.

Fable Seven: People Always Want to Work with Others

While we often idealize the notion of team-based behavior, the truth is that people do not necessarily want to, or know how to, work well with others. In clinical environments, much of the work that is done is driven by individual action. Team-related interaction is often a secondary consideration in such individual work.

Teamwork, however, is significantly different from unilateral action. Recognizing the unique character of a team and the characteristics of work in team relationships is very different from working in loose work groups. Team participants may not be always precisely clear about the dynamics of teamwork and the steps necessary to create and sustain an effective team. Becoming a functional, well integrated, fluid, effective, and synergistic team can require significant personal effort to tame unhealthy unilateral characteristics.

The working synergy of a good team has a major influence on the team's ability to achieve positive outcomes. This synergy is not achieved quickly, nor is it easily affected by the team leader. Instead, synergy develops over time and through a focus on good team interaction, deliberation, and decision making. To achieve this goal, the team leader must develop the facility to build team congruence, effective interaction, good deliberation, strong decisions, and critical outcomes.

Fable Eight: Effective Teams Grow Naturally

Teams do not grow accidentally or naturally. Rather, teams are deliberately constructed groups that undergo disciplined development before they can contribute to the fulfillment of the purposes for which they have gathered. Teams, much like other aspects of life, grow intermittently and incrementally; they do not grow in a straight line. Teams experience pushes and pulls, ups and downs, flurries of positive and meaningful activity, and periods of dormancy and nonproductivity. Incremental, intermittent processes and energy associated with teamwork represent highly variable elements of human relationship and interaction. Therefore, the team leader should not expect good team processes and effective deliberation to flow in a seamless continuum of good deliberation but rather should anticipate the many challenges inherent to the collection of a wide variety of competing human behaviors.

Fable Nine: Building Trust Is an Important Role of the Team Leader

Trust cannot be built; rather, it represents or demonstrates something that is already in place. Trust is actually a visible representation of the work and

CRITICAL THOUGHT

Trust is not something that can be created. Trust is evidence of what is already present between people. In a safe, effective, rewarding, and well-functioning team with confidence in its values and positive continuing relationships, those characteristics serve as the evidence that trust is present.

methodology already under way, the effectiveness and success of which indicate the presence of trust. Trust, then, is a reflection of all the elements that give evidence of its presence.

The only thing the team leader can do to build trust is to undertake positive and productive activities that result in a sense of inclusion, engagement, openness, confidence, and good feeling among members of the team. For the team leader, it is important to recognize that building the elements of team effectiveness and constructing a framework for positive relationships and safe dialogue create the conditions that support trust; such an environment supports team members' belief that the team is a safe and positive place where one can contribute, be valued, and make a difference. Just as trust can reflect what is good in team dynamics, however, so it can be broken through major breaches in process, or relationships, or through a series of minor breaks in the interactions among team members at any point along the continuum of team processes.

The effort of the team is directed not so much toward building trust but more toward generating relationships, processes, and methodologies that address the circumstances and conditions supportive of the presence of trust. The role of the leader in this scenario is to advance the integrity and strength of the relationships of team members, enhance their ability to problem solve and seek solutions, build the team's skill in dealing with performance issues and challenges, and bolster the team's ability to consistently obtain expectations and outcomes. Progress in each of these arenas will be critical to maintaining and strengthening the conditions that ultimately demonstrate the presence of trust.

Fable Ten: Team Members Will Always Focus on the Outcomes to Which Their Effort Is Directed

Team members do not always focus on their work or their outcomes. Indeed, group members often become unclear about their team's purpose and its related activities; they may even forget the outcomes to which their efforts are directed.

Part of the functional work of the team leader is to help the team continuously renew its understanding of its purpose, the value of its processes, the direction of its work, and the proximity of the team to its outcomes. Building in a continuous mechanism for evaluating place and progress is a good way for the team leader to check in with regard to where the team is in its work and what progress is being made toward the team's expectations and purpose. Achieving short-term or small outcomes may signal to the team leader that the team should move on to the next phase, step, or goal of its effort to fulfill its purpose. Furthermore, team leaders remind their teams of specific conditions or circumstances impacting the team's purpose and goal in a way that helps the team continually evaluate its processes and outcomes. Teams often find themselves so enmeshed in their processes and activities that they forget the ends to which their work should lead. In such a case, the work may become an end in itself, and purpose and meaning may get lost inside activity and function. Reacquainting team members with the questions related to purpose and value helps the team reaffirm its work and firmly establishes a goodness of fit between what the team is doing and the values it is seeking to advance.

Team Progress

Progress in teamwork does not always follow a straight line from initiation to success. Most human teams experience varying degrees of progress, with increments of high achievement intertwined with times of minimal progress (Chau & eLibrary, 2008; Pinar, Zehir, Kitapci, & Tanriverdi, 2014). The leader must expect that these differences will operate in the course of any level of effective teamwork and must plan for them accordingly. Teams often reflect working relationships or a set of interactions that do not unfold in the same way as individual work. Teams are essentially artificial constructions that are not permanent and do not represent the usual or traditional relationships and interactions in the workplace. Often members of a team may not work with one another regularly and may have interactions with one another only during the course of the team process. While this particular dynamic can yield both strengths and weaknesses, it is important for the leader to recognize these forces are at work during team activities. Even as the teamwork progresses constructively with some measure of success, these more negative dynamics may continue to operate just below the surface and should be anticipated, so people are not surprised when they erupt. Accordingly, because these forces may make team progress difficult or slow, or even nonexistent, recognizing them as a normative part of team dynamics helps create a more positive frame for the issues (O'Neil & Allen, 2014; Parker, 2008). Team members can then envision the possibility of getting past them or even resolving the issues they may engender. In the ensuing positive framework, team relationships can compensate for the negative behaviors or interactions that can represent people's level of frustration, lack of progress, and difficulty in working through apparently intractable problems with each other.

The nurse team leader is called upon to both monitor and moderate the effect of progress and challenges to the work of an effective team. To do so, the team leader must not be overwhelmed by the team's seesawing between small successes as they intertwine with moments of challenge. This unevenness is normal and usual as teamwork is directed toward specific goals. In fact, the team leader should anticipate these swings and affirm to members that these elements will be a part of the team dynamics at a number of points in the team process. What is important is for the team leader to anticipate these events and to plan for them in advance of their occurrence (Hartigh, Gernigon, Van Yperen, Marin, & Van Geert, 2014; Mash et al., 2008).

Team members need to celebrate the team's small successes as they occur. Recognition of success should not be saved only for the major accomplishments. Instead, the team leader should provide opportunities for the team to take time out by identifying and positioning small successes as critical steps along the trajectory of major progress, and by celebrating them as indicators of positive movement toward goal completion.

Surprisingly, the same approaches are just as effective for dealing with momentary challenges. The leader needs to point out to the team members that these challenges are also signposts of significant moments and signs of progress. This progress simply needs further refinement, deliberation, clarification, and renewal of effort to better direct the team's work toward the goals or as a part of the effort to clarify the strategies necessary to keep the team moving (McAlvey & Nikolovska, 2010; Rondeau, 2007). Through these actions, the leader recalibrates the team's action steps toward particular efforts and achievements. In these moments of challenge or team delay, the team leader needs to take on the relevant issues with transparence and specificity. Some immediate response strategies the team leader could initiate within the team process are as follows:

- Reaffirm specific goals and activities that were identified as essential to the team's progress toward fulfillment of its purpose. Reaffirming the goals and stages of the team's work helps reestablish their relevance and upholds the direction of the team in relationship to its purpose.
- Recognize the context of the problem, barrier, or challenge and identify the relevant stages or elements of change management; this can help prevent the generalization of the problem and impeding the progress of the team.
- When the context of the issue has been clarified, break the problem down into smaller issues so it can be better understood and more

specifically dealt with in the context of the stage, gap, or elements of the goal affected by the problem. Here again, the team leader attempts to see the problem in context and to suggest that no one problem can derail the purpose or goals of the team. Instead, a problem may actually help the team refine and hone its focus. These smaller issues can assist the team in moving forward more effectively, while addressing concerns that affect progress and/or affirm direction.

- When team goals and efforts have been reaffirmed by the team and articulated by the team leader, identifying particular responses and solutions helps keep the team's effort focused, enables clear delineation of team-derived responses and opportunities, and removes the issue as a barrier.

- The team leader may bring in experts and skilled problem solvers who can help broaden the team's insight, present new information, or help the team recalibrate its efforts and strategies to overcome problems or barriers in a more creative and unique manner. New insights and understanding of the problem can reenergize the team and refocus on new solutions that will further the process and move the team forward.

The nurse team leader must be aware of the various strategies that can help the team advance toward fulfilling its purpose and achieving its goals. It is important that the team leader recognize that he or she must be flexible and fluid in terms of

TEAM TIP

In an effort to be thorough, team leaders and members often set more priorities for the team than they can ever address. Team leaders should create an agenda with no more than three to five items on which work activities are focused. This helps ensure that the goals for the meeting can be addressed in the time available.

CRITICAL THOUGHT

Occasionally, the team may need to access external consultation to obtain information or serve as an impetus regarding a particular deliberation. The team leader should always seek whatever resources and support are necessary to help inform or advance the team's thinking and work.

anticipating challenges and changes within the team process. This leader must be consistent with and faithful to the team's purpose and goals, and must be willing to adjust the team's approach as necessary to advance the members' interests and competence, maintain a high level of commitment to the work and keep up the team's energy, and help the team implement new strategies that can ensure successful movement toward goals and the fulfillment of the team purpose.

When the Problem Is a Team Member

The nurse team leader will often encounter challenges related to specific members of the team by virtue of individual patterns of behavior, problems in relationships among team members, or varying levels of commitment or contribution of team members to the purposes and efforts of the team. This is not an uncommon set of circumstances; indeed, it should be seen as a normative expectation in the course of any interactive, relationship-based process. However, even though such dynamics are normative, the team leader should develop strategies for addressing these challenges early. The leader's efforts must support ongoing team interactions over the course of the team's work. When the problem is an individual team member's behavior, early engagement and intervention are critical to protecting the progress of the team and to ensuring that the anomalous team member's negative behavior does not have lingering effects on the integrity and effectiveness of the team's work.

There will always be challenging elements of human behavior that the team leader must be prepared to address. Professionals need to be aware of the reality that even the best-intended members will present challenges to team leader activity and team member progress. These challenges reflect the dynamics inherent in human interaction and simply demonstrate the need for continuing good facilitation, problem solving, and competence building. When aberrant behavior arises, none of these circumstances should be seen as a terminal event for the leader and team effectiveness; rather, they are simply human characteristics that are part of the collective work of deliberation and teamwork. Their occurrence also reflects the need for the team leader to have good facilitation skills that can address the noise created by human dynamics and team interaction (Raes, Decuyper, & Lismont, 2013; Rouse, 2007). Development of such skills is the most critical component of successfully addressing team relationship and interaction problems. These skills evolve over time with maturation, experience, and personal experimentation. Ideally, the team leader will seek out mentorship and guidance in his or her process of learning and exercising the leadership role. The openness of the team leader to accessing expertise and guidance from mentors and leaders in the organization can ensure that the leader capitalizes on these valuable resources while building skill competence in team facilitation. The team leader's ability to deal with personal conflicts and anomalous team member behaviors can be enhanced by good technique, opportunity, patience, and continuous and faithful application of honed skills, all of which can make a difference in facilitating team interaction and performance effectiveness.

Collaboration

Information on the development and use of teams for decision making and work processes could fill many textbooks; indeed, it already has. While this chapter merely introduces this topic as a concern for the professional nurse leader, team-based dynamics are sure to be prevalent throughout the nurse's professional life. Historically, leader education has not emphasized the critical understanding that team-based frameworks are the primary way in which professionals advance decision making and work processes. Collaboration is the essential, central methodology through which the diverse team stakeholders work to both define the team's response to patient needs and advance the team's competence in serving its population well.

Collaboration implies the capacity to have team members work well together, deliberate purposefully, and decide and act in ways that are in the best interests of both the patient and the team (Lorinkova, Pearsall, & Sims, 2013; Peterson & King, 2007). The team leader is responsible for ensuring that the structure and framework of the team's actions represent what is necessary to advance the collaborative care process.

TEAM TIP

To minimize misunderstandings and problems with individual team member behavior, the team leader should clearly review and affirm the operating expectations of team members, including each of the following:

- Functions
- Activities
- Relationships
- Interaction
- Processes
- Expectations
- Outcomes

BOX 7-3 COMMON MYTHS ABOUT TEAMS

- Good teams do not need strong leaders.
- Teams can always be self-directed.
- Failure is a sign of an ineffective team.
- Good teams do not experience conflict.
- Teams should never experiment.
- Individuals, not teams, are important.
- You cannot really evaluate teams.
- When left alone, teams get into trouble.
- Teams are always well supervised.
- Individuals perform better than teams.
- Team players are compliant and quiet.
- Teams who err are failures.

Teams in the healthcare setting should ideally operate very much like a well-designed and -structured symphony. Much like the symphony's conductor, the team leader within a collaborative work model is responsible for carefully and judiciously planning the character and content of the team's work (its "music") and anticipating how the team members (the "orchestra members") will accomplish that work. The discipline of good planning for collaboration requires that the team leader use whatever skills are necessary to facilitate good team collaboration—that is, to help the group make "beautiful music." Leaders should also be aware of myths that might impede team development. See **Box 7-3**.

Decisions

The most important aspect of team leadership is the team leader's clarity regarding the decisions around which the team will gather. One of the great errors of teamwork is the idealization that teams gather to undertake processes that will result in the achievement of some goal or outcome. The true foundation of team effectiveness is bound up in whether that team is dealing with the right questions and whether those questions are clear enough for members to find the right answers. Therefore, the team leader must make sure that everyone is certain of the purpose around which the team is gathered and the questions that are driving that work. See **Box 7-4**. Questions addressed by teams can range from organizational objectives to clinical behaviors to personal fulfillment of standards,

BOX 7-4 TEAM LEADER'S CHECKLIST

- Make sure all the elements of the team and team performance are acting congruently.
- Maintain a consistent leadership style that best fits the character and content of the teamwork.
- Make sure that the team adheres to all the terms of engagement and that corrective action is undertaken early when those rules are violated.
- Manage team errors and conflicts early and well, establishing processes that address these issues calmly as a normal part of team processes.
- Watch for individual behavior that acts in opposition to the synthesis and effectiveness of team performance.
- Meet frequently with individuals and the full team to assess progress, confront issues, undertake learning, and measure goal achievement.

practices, or activities. When the team is forming and questions arise about which kind of decision making will be used, the selection of an approach should be clear and precise. The sooner the leader learns that his or her focus is on a question specific to each stage of the deliberative process, the more effectively the group will be able to focus on doing its work (Porter-O'Grady, 2009).

Creating Equity: Overcoming the Uneven Table

When the questions around which the team will gather are clear to the facilitator, it becomes important to make decisions about how those questions can be best constructed to address the diversity at the table. The team leader's interest lies in ensuring that the questions driving the team's work are broadly enough informed and served by the breadth of membership at the team table. **Setting the table** means knowing how all the decisions need to be served, which talent or expertise needs to be gathered, how the size of the team will affect the issues the team is addressing, and which particular gifts and skills will be available to the team members as they deliberate the questions before them.

Breadth of representation on the team is important and must be reflected in the kind of people selected to deal with the issues at hand. One of the greatest difficulties in team management is focusing the team on its work while providing for an adequate array of resources at the table. Often teams are formed because of the relationship of members to particular disciplines or to a geographical

CRITICAL THOUGHT

All teams experience conflict; all conflict has value. The good team leader looks at conflict as a normal part of team effectiveness and engages it early and often.

location or even some affinity to the issue itself. These are not the best reasons for gathering people together in a team process. If the team is to perform its work effectively, team members need to have the right mix of skills, talents, and capacities to address the issues before them. A careful selection process based on the members' personal alignment and commitment to the team goals helps establish the strength of the team before it even begins to tackle the work and provides a healthy foundation for the collaborative process. Ultimately, aligning team membership with team goals and work is one of the most critical elements in ensuring team effectiveness.

Diversity is not only essential to the decision-making process and team collaboration, it is also vital in terms of the kinds of team members sitting around the table and the particular behaviors that they bring. Nothing is worse than having a team's behavior patterns limit progress and rule out good relationships, thereby making it difficult for the facilitator to coordinate and integrate the decision-making process with the collaborative team. Behavior patterns are critical to the success of deliberation and team processing. Achieving behavioral balance while capitalizing on members' different skills and personal dynamics will be important to good team functioning even before the team has formed (Larson, 2011).

People bring as much diversity in their patterns of behavior as they bring in terms of their personality characteristics. Setting the table by embracing the diversity of personality characteristics that need to be present in the deliberation of an issue requires that the nurse leader carefully reflect on the dynamic that needs to be expressed to make the deliberation process effective and move the team in a valid direction. Loading a team with highly articulate but dramatic and aggressive operators will create a lot of action on the team but may not yield much consensus. Conversely, loading the team with highly reflective, thoughtful, and nonexpressive people means the team will deliberate a great deal but not necessarily move to decision making and action in a timely fashion. The goal is to mix actors and reflectors so that the team's diversity is balanced between members who can effectively drive the team toward decision making and action and members who can thoughtfully and carefully reflect on the meaning of the discussion and its implications for people and for organizations.

In addition to care and caution with table setting for personality and behavioral characteristics, the attitude of team members toward the team and the issues it will address is an element of team facilitation that is frequently underaddressed. The team leader needs to be aware that in every deliberation process, some negative elements inevitably operate. This negative undercurrent can slow the team's progress or, at worst, it can cripple the team's deliberative dynamics. Negative behaviors and responses can create a milieu within the team that discourages member participation, diminishes the energy necessary to address critical issues, and often delays or derails the team's deliberation and decision-making process. Here again, the team leader must be prepared to handle the negative dynamics that inevitably arise in the course of almost any kind of teamwork. Ideally, before the team comes into being, the leader will develop the techniques and skills necessary for dealing with negative behaviors and for establishing terms of engagement for team processes. These terms of engagement are critical to the collaborative dynamic because they provide the framework for dialogue and establish a rule set within which team members can operate, and the application allows team members to build a sense of personal safety and trust in the course of the team's work. These terms of engagement create a sense of discipline among the team members and serve as a framework for the team leader to access when team behaviors do not match the standards established by team members at the outset.

SCENARIO

Sam is the leader of a relatively new team. The team is finishing the first stage of development and is creating rules of engagement, performance expectations, and common goals. The team has been making good progress with its formation activities; however, it is having difficulty dealing with conflict emerging between two strong team members. Sam sees this conflict coming fairly early in the process, but he is a little concerned about how he can properly address it. Two other team members are becoming aware of the conflict between the strong personalities, and both have come to Sam with their concerns that this problem may be growing and is beginning to affect team cohesiveness and team processes.

Sam wants to take care of this problem as quickly as possible. In the past, he has always managed these issues through a one-to-one exchange, by exerting his personal leadership. He realizes, however, that this conflict is

(continues)

(continued)

a team issue and should be addressed within the context of the team. He knows that the team must own its relationships between team members and work to resolve this conflict as soon as possible. Furthermore, Sam knows that, as team leader, he must facilitate the processes that will lead to confronting this issue, ultimately creating a framework for the team's ability to work together and achieve outcomes. Sam feels stuck and needs some insight and assistance. He has come to you for guidance.

Discussion Questions

1. What are the elements of the conflict resolution process that Sam must be aware of as he walks through the stages of addressing the conflict between these two individuals?

2. How does Sam engage the team in owning and investing in this conflict resolution process?

3. How does Sam keep the environment safe, push for resolution among team members, and ensure a successful conflict resolution process?

4. How does Sam evaluate the effectiveness of the process and determine whether it made any difference?

Terms of engagement may contain the following elements:

- Each member of the team has an opportunity to speak. A procedural caveat: The discussion facilitator challenges any person who has spoken to not raise his or her position again or otherwise respond until at least one or two other team members have responded.

- Team members avoid the use of judgment terms, such as "I agree" or "I disagree." These statements are not relevant to the deliberation, and they do not contribute content to the discussion. They are merely fragments of personal judgment that do not add value to the common good at the table. Members should be encouraged to simply share their views rather than react by reflecting others' views.

- Team members communicate with ownership of their notions. They are encouraged to use "I" statements as a way of contributing their thoughts to group deliberation in a responsible way.

- The use of appreciative strategies in conversation (techniques that add value to conversation rather than reactions to prevailing negatives in a conversation) are encouraged and stimulated. Participants must continually see themselves contributing to further deliberation and refinements of decision making in a way that moves them forward rather than reacting to or acting on negative statements regarding the process or the deliberation. Keeping this appreciative frame recalibrates the discussion within the context of the possible and the relevant in a way that positively supports the team's efforts to advance meaningful change.
- The leader encourages the team to take timeouts to evaluate their sense of progress and their operating dynamic. This process of checking in helps them re-anchor their deliberations and make some judgments about progress and challenges in their work.

Interdisciplinary Alignment

Clinical teams in health care have some unique issues that need to be addressed prior to the team undertaking work. Historically in health care, hierarchy has been a significant impediment to the collateral, horizontal nature of collaborative relationships. That is, specific healthcare professionals have had different status levels and relationships within the system, creating issues of equity, value, and integration of decision making in the system. For example, physicians have historically not been classified as employees in hospitals and healthcare systems. The majority of physicians have been self-employed and have a different relationship to the hospital or healthcare community than any of the other players on the deliberative team. This consideration becomes important when one includes physicians in the deliberative work group because the implicit characterization of the physician's role is that of leader or director of healthcare decision making. While questions arise about whether that notion is still valid, it remains a commonly perceived characterization within the healthcare system. This role identity places at the center of the team's deliberation a mental model contributed to by both the physician and other team members; in turn, this model may create some difficulty in establishing common ground, equity, and respect for all contributors on the team. Furthermore, its impact on team dynamics becomes clear when the physician is not happy with the team's work. Because of preset notions about the physician's role and position in health care, the team often assumes that the physician's nonapproval serves as a veto of the team's direction, decisions, or progress. Characterizations and behaviors of "subordinate" team members may then make it difficult to get equivalent value from all team contributors—the table is uneven.

The team leader must recognize these historical influences on expectations, performance, and behaviors and address them at the outset of the team's deliberative process. Simple rules need to be established. For example, clear, upfront rules about how people on the team will be addressed (e.g., use of first names for everyone) ensures a common understanding of how they will be recognized, the roles they will play with one another, and the expectation of equal contributions from and value assigned to all members (Finkelman, 2011). Teams often fail because this step has not been carefully deliberated and decisions related to the team's processes are not thoroughly articulated in a way that sets the team up for sound collaborative processes and good decision making. Such efforts directed toward creating an even table are among the most critical steps undertaken by the team leader in forming an effective framework for team dynamics (Kritek, 2002; Tost, Gino, & Larrick, 2013).

Focus on the Team Leader

The team leader has huge influence over the team—influence that can drive the team toward effective and responsive processes and ensure good alignment among reflection, group energy, engagement, coordination, and communication (Yukl, 2009). Early commitment by the team leader is vital to ensuring that the team is structured appropriately and has the information it needs to do its work and access to the resources, processes, and creativity it needs to obtain the best outcome. All these factors reflect the talent of the leader in structuring teamwork in a way that can ensure effective processing and meaningful outcomes.

The team leader essentially creates the facilitative context, conditions, and circumstances that lead to effective team performance (Plsek, 2010). Construction, structure, purpose, and team dynamics all converge to create the conditions that positively predict effectiveness. In addition, the team leader is aware of the need to maintain membership stability and thereby enable the team to work effectively. High turnover usually reflects a failure to address many of these forces, leading team members to perceive that their membership and contributions to the team's work have little value and relevance. See **Box 7-5**.

The long-term effectiveness of the team reflects the leader's ability to encourage and develop members' blossoming as participants in processes of interaction, relationship, and collective deliberation (Wolfe & Sparkman, 2010). The team leader must see his or her role as providing an opportunity to help team members develop higher levels of contribution, thereby more strongly influencing the team's long-term effectiveness and the individual member's own skills and capacities.

Team leaders should consider seeking mentors as they develop their team leadership skills. Personal team leadership coaching helps construct a frame for both

BOX 7-5 RESOLVING TEAM PROBLEMS

- *Identifying the problem:* All teams have the potential for experiencing difficulties and challenges. In the context of human relationships, the potential for conflict always exists. The leader knows this, anticipates it, and is constantly prepared to deal with it. The leader, therefore, always keeps an eye out for problems and helps the team maintain awareness of that potential and identify such problems as soon as possible. Problems left too long or dealt with too late have the potential to become greater impediments to accomplishing the work than problems addressed early.

- *Creating individual awareness and ownership of problems:* After the leader identifies a problem or concern, it is vital that this information be shared with individuals or a collective body of team members. The leader must always remember that team members own their own problems. The team leader never makes the problem his or her own; when this occurs, the locus of control for the problem's resolution is also transferred from its rightful owners (the team members) to the leader. In reality, the solution is always operating within the context of the team members and in the process of their work. The leader facilitates dialogue, discernment, and problem solving with the appropriate owners of the problem.

- *Moving the group to resolution:* Resolution is more a journey than a destination. The leader helps the team assess the most appropriate responses to problems or concerns and identify the best strategy for addressing the problem in a particular time frame or within the context of a particular circumstance or process. In doing so, the team leader focuses on techniques and methodologies that might be applied to problem solving, offering them as tools for the team members to use in creating objective formats for problem solving. The team leader draws from these objective processes to help the team apply these techniques, to address an issue, find a solution, and move the team toward its goal.

evaluating the behavior of the leader and assessing the effectiveness within a particular team format. The mentor should be encouraged to assess the utility and effectiveness of the leader's work by examining capacity, approach, and affect, assessing these aspects of leadership within the context of the team's progress toward fulfilling its purpose and goals. In addition, a mentor can enhance the team leader's skill development by emphasizing more effective interaction between team leader capacity and the overall effectiveness of team dynamics and goal achievement.

When you anticipate yourself filling the role of team leader, which personal developmental and role skills do you think you will need help in honing?

A mentor can also help the team leader assess and translate his or her own personal effectiveness into measures of team effectiveness in achieving the team's purpose and the desired product of its work. The three major factors that are critical to the effectiveness of the team leader's role relate to adequate structuring of the team, use of good process, and progress of the team toward its goals or in fulfillment of its purpose. A mentor can be helpful in assessing these strengths and challenges experienced by the team leader and can address specific talent development to guide the team leader to higher levels of competence.

The motivation, energy, and commitment of the team leader establish an emotional framework for the team and reflect the kind of personal energy that demonstrates commitment, enthusiasm, and a strong desire for the team to be effective in its work (Northouse, 2007; Taylor, 2013). These personal attributes of team leaders help establish a positive, energetic, and safe context for team members that can then be translated into a culture of collective value, where the real potential for contribution comes from each team member. The confidence and trust of team members can be assured if the team shares the broad perspective that each member is valued, that the work of the team is purposeful, and that the team is a safe space for collective interaction and engagement, and if the team actually achieves its intended ends.

Virtuality and Team Performance

Digital technology has created significant shifts in the way in which teams are constructed and the processes through which they do their work. Although many of the dynamics of good team construction and management are similar between geographical and virtual teams, some obvious differences arise. Application of technology can create an environment that is structurally and emotionally neutral; moreover, in the digital team environment, the human-intensive patterns of visceral responses may be hidden to some extent (Gibson & Cohen, 2003; Jawadi, Daassi, Favier, & Kalika, 2013). Although the relational challenges are more obvious in this milieu, it is also clear that digital team processes and dynamics have the potential for moving quicker, deliberating more succinctly, and performing specific tasks faster. At the same time, depth of understanding, uncertainty, and

CRITICAL THOUGHT

The team leader is always sensitive to including team members in decisions that affect what they do. The wise leader never acts unilaterally or in any way that does not demonstrate team ownership and team value.

challenges that are normally visible through critical assessment of body language and interactive emotional cues are less available to the team leader. To compensate for the more two-dimensional team interaction, team leaders in such settings must check in more frequently to ask team members about their sense of the team process and their evaluation of its progress (Chhay & Kleiner, 2013; Singh & Waddell, 2004).

Spatial and temporal differences in team interaction will cause the team leader in the digital team environment to be more purposeful in articulating the progress of the team. The leader must check in to validate the general consensus of the team's sense of effectiveness or progress. Thinking through the structural elements of team dynamics and creating a rubric for monitoring and evaluating team interaction and task progress will give team leaders an objective tool for more accurately determining team members' sense of engagement and progress with the team effort.

In the 21st-century, digital environment for teamwork, team leaders must recognize that unilateral team direction that was once successful in more vertical and geographical team processes may not be as effective in the digital infrastructure. Teamwork must often be broken down into smaller components, and leaders and small groups of team members must become more focused on particular goals and tasks associated with the team's progress. Breaking down task function and leadership engagement spreads the expectations for performance and progress among team members and suggests that leadership itself is more collective and engaging. Such smaller work groups with more narrowly designated team leaders become able to focus intently on particular dialogue, tasks, and goals. They can take ownership of components of the process, achieving success more quickly, and team member contributions can be more easily enumerated in the context of this dynamic. In the digital team environment, team leaders must develop more effectiveness in coordinating and integrating the work of these smaller work teams. Such leaders must ensure that each smaller work group produces outcomes that fit well with the broader objectives of the team and are well integrated into the full team's effort. Effective smaller teams demonstrate subsequent positive contribution, quickly moving the whole team more strategically toward accomplishing its collective goals.

Concluding Thoughts

Teams are the basic unit of much contemporary work, especially in knowledge-driven work settings. Certain broad and intensive elements and characteristics of teamwork and effectiveness are elemental to the role of the nurse leader. The professional nurse will respond to a lifetime of opportunity and challenge by leading many team efforts that advance the interests of healthcare organizations and meet the obligations of the profession for addressing all areas of patient care. Every professional nurse must expect that he or she will play a major role in team processes as both leader and participant. The critical factors related to the nurse's role on teams and as a team leader are reflected in the leader's capacity and skill in constructing the team effort around clear purpose, goals, and processes. Building on functional clarity for the team, the leader demonstrates the value of constructing a well-functioning team by aligning its members with the specific breadth, capacity, and range of skills necessary to address the team's work focus in an effective way (Porter-O'Grady & Malloch, 2015).

The team leader sets the table for effective team functioning by achieving clarity around equity and membership, terms of engagement, team process dynamics, relationship building, and management of the interaction of team members. Developing effective personal leadership skills requires the nurse team leader to be aware of his or her personal attributes and identify and work with a mentor to build facilitation, integration, and coordination skills.

Today's healthcare environment includes a growing emphasis on digital team activities, which means that the team leader must develop a range of approaches that best reflect this kind of team and its unique characteristics. As teams become a more common medium for deliberative work processes, and as the nurse's role in coordinating interdisciplinary team dynamics becomes a more central aspect of the clinical work environment, the professional nurse will need to develop a wide array of team leader skills.

SCENARIO

Jane Rosen, RN, BSN, has recently been promoted to clinical team coordinator in the medical geriatric diabetic unit. While she has been a nurse for only 18 months, Jane has demonstrated strong leadership potential and an enthusiasm for problem solving and innovation. Jane's manager soon approaches her with the first opportunity to exercise her new leadership role in a major change initiative.

Nursing leadership has been considering how clinical practice could be altered for at-risk populations in a way that would engage them earlier and manage their chronic conditions by addressing the continuum of care and reducing the incidence of late-stage, late-engagement, high-intensity hospital care. The geriatric, diabetic patient population has been one of those patient groups selected for testing out new models of care. The proposed model would emphasize earlier engagement in patient care management and the longer-term continuum of care service structure for delivering care to this population of patients.

Jane has been asked by her manager to put together a small team of nursing colleagues to plan ways in which care could be designed and delivered differently for the geriatric diabetic population so as to directly effect a reduction in hospital inpatient admissions, a higher level of quality of service, and a stronger positive impact on the lives of geriatric diabetic patients. This is a new challenge for Jane and her colleagues, but Jane is excited by the opportunities provided and looks forward to the work of the team.

Discussion Questions

1. Before pulling her team together, which kinds of strategic planning activities should Jane consider doing with her manager?

2. What would be a simple and definitive purpose statement that would guide Jane in structuring the team's work?

3. How should Jane "set the table" with the right diversity of team members to address the issues the team will need to confront?

4. After selecting members of the team, what are the first activities Jane should lead the team members in addressing before beginning the team's work?

5. Which goals should the team set out for itself? Which measures should the team use to evaluate the achievement of those goals?

SCENARIO

Kevin James, RN, BSN, has been leading the quality improvement team for the past six months. The team has done some significant work in establishing quality metrics for a number of clinical indicators on the medical-surgical unit where Kevin is a clinical leader. Most of the team members have worked well together and cooperated to do important work and to achieve some small successes.

One of the team members, however, is not making good progress with the team. As a nurse who has been on the unit for more than 20 years, she constantly expresses negative comments about Kevin's leadership and the work of the team. When she is present at the team meetings, she is often negative, even to the point of lack of kindness to specific team members. Kevin has tried to engage her on a number of occasions, only to have her either negatively respond or inform Kevin that the issue addressed is his problem, not hers.

Kevin has not directly addressed his concerns with this nurse's behavior in the past. However, he recently set up a meeting with this nurse with the intent of raising his concerns with her negative communication pattern. The meeting is planned for tomorrow. Kevin is anxiously reflecting on how he will structure and manage that meeting.

Discussion Questions

1. As Kevin is planning for this meeting, which kinds of things should he be thinking about?

2. Should Kevin have any "terms of engagement" to address issues of communication with this individual?

3. Which ideas might Kevin give to help this individual become a more focused and positive contributor to the team's deliberation and work?

4. What expectations should Kevin address and clarify prior to closing his meeting with this individual?

5. Should Kevin define a specific communication mode or any relational expectations for this individual? What expectations might you recommend to him?

CHAPTER TEST QUESTIONS

Licensure exam categories: Management of care: interprofessional practice, concepts of management, delegation/supervision

Nurse leader exam categories: Communication and relationship building: relationship management, influencing behaviors, interdisciplinary relationships; Knowledge of healthcare environments; Professionalism: personal and professional accountability

1. Teams are the central component of the delivery of healthcare services. True or false?

2. Healthcare reform and transformation have made teams less important by advancing the value of individual clinical functions over team activities. True or false?

3. The professional nurse is a critical and key leader of clinical and health delivery teams. True or false?

4. Purpose, goals, roles, and relationships are the four central elements upon which team effectiveness depends. True or false?

5. It is the obligation of the team leader to establish the goals for team members and make clear to them their obligation to meet these goals. True or false?

6. Conflict is always a barrier to team effectiveness and success, so it is the role of the team leader to eliminate conflict between team members so the team can proceed to successfully complete its purpose. True or false?

7. Team members need a clear understanding of their individual roles so they know what they are committing to and what is expected for their participation in team activities. True or false?

8. Measures of team success are identified only after the team has made progress with its goals, thereby establishing a foundation for measuring the team's degree of success. True or false?

9. The team leader must reaffirm the team's purpose and check its progress frequently to help its members understand where they are in the team process, the progress they have made toward their goals, and the need for adjustments and accommodations to changes affecting the team's action. True or false?

10. All team leaders should have external mentoring, guidance, or advisement to help advance personal insights and skills for team leadership. True or false?

References

Barner, R. (2000). *Team troubleshooter: How to find and fix team problems.* Palo Alto, CA: Davies-Black.

Belbin, R. M. (2010). *Team roles at work.* Oxford, UK/Burlington, MA: Butterworth-Heinemann.

Ben Saoud, N., & Mark, G. (2006). Complexity theory and collaboration: An agent-based simulator for a space mission design team. *Computational and Mathematical Organization Theory, 13*(2), 113–147.

Chau, V. S., & eLibrary. (2008). Relationship of strategic performance management to team strategy, company performance and organizational effectiveness. *Team Performance Management, 14*(3–4), 111–191. West Yorkshire, UK: Emerald.

Chhay, R., & Kleiner, B. (2013). Effective communication and virtual teams. *Industrial Management, 55*(4), 28–30.

Chrispeels, J. H. (2004). *Learning to lead together: The promise and challenge of sharing leadership.* Thousand Oaks, CA: Sage.

Curlee, W., & Gordon, R. L. (2011). *Complexity theory and project management.* Hoboken, NJ: Wiley.

Curseu, P. (2003). *Formal group decision-making: A social-cognitive approach.* Cluj-Napoca, Romania: ASCR Press.

Daspit, J., Justice, T., Boyd, N., & McKee, V. (2013). Cross functional team effectiveness: An examination of internal team environment, shared leadership, and cohesion influences. *Team Performance Management, 19*(1/2), 34–56.

Dunin-Keplicz, B., & Verbrugge, R. (2010). *Teamwork in multi-agent systems: A formal approach.* Hoboken, NJ: Wiley.

Eissa, G., Fox, C., Webster, B., & Kim, J. (2012). A framework for leader effectiveness in virtual teams. *Journal of Leadership, Accountability and Epics, and Ethics, 9*(2), 11–22.

Finkelman, A. W. (2011). *Case management for nurses.* Boston, MA: Pearson.

Gibson, C. B., & Cohen, S. G. (2003). *Virtual teams that work creating conditions for virtual team effectiveness.* San Francisco, CA: Jossey-Bass.

Gratton, L., & Erickson, T. (2007). Eight ways to build collaborative teams. *Harvard Business Review, 85*(11), 100–111.

Hartigh, J., Gernigon, C., Van Yperen, N., Marin, L., & Van Geert, P. (2014). How psychological and behavioral team states change during positive and negative momentum. *PLoS One, 9*(5), 5–9.

Institute of Medicine (US). (2011). Committee on the Robert Wood Johnson Foundation Initiative on the Future of Nursing. *The future of nursing: Leading change, advancing health.* Washington, DC: National Academies Press.

Interprofessional Education Collaborative Expert Panel. (2011). *Core competencies for interprofessional collaborative practice: Report of an expert panel.* Retrieved from www.aamc.org/download/186750/data/core_competencies.pdf

Jawadi, N., Daassi, M., Favier, M., & Kalika, M. (2013). Relationship building and virtual teams: A leadership behavioral complexity perspective. *Human Systems Management, 32*(3), 199–211.

Kritek, P. B. (2002). *Negotiating at an uneven table: Developing moral courage in resolving our conflicts.* San Francisco, CA: Jossey-Bass.

Larson, W. J. (2011). *Team member characteristics contributing to high reliability in emergency response teams managing critical incidents.* Tucson, AZ: University of Arizona.

Lorinkova, N., Pearsall, M., & Sims, H. (2013). Examining the differential longitudinal performance of directive versus empowering leadership in teams. *Academy of Management Journal, 56*(2), 573–596.

Losoncy, L. (1996). *Best team skills.* Boca Raton, FL: St. Lucie Press.

Mash, B. J., Mayers, P., Conradie, H., Orayn, A., Kuiper, M., & Marais, J. (2008). How to manage organisational change and create practice teams: Experiences of a South African primary care health centre. *Health Education (Abingdon), 21*(2), 132.

McAlvey, J., & Nikolovska, I. (2010). Team collectivist culture: A remedy for creating team effectiveness. *Human Resources Development Quarterly, 21*(3), 307–316.

Northouse, P. G. (2007). *Leadership: Theory and practice.* Thousand Oaks, CA: Sage.

O'Neil, T., & Allen, N. (2014). Team task conflict resolution: An examination of its linkages to team personality composition and team effectiveness outcomes. *Group Dynamics: Theory, Research, and Practice, 18*(2), 159–173.

Parker, G. M. (2003). *Cross-functional teams: Working with allies, enemies, and other strangers.* San Francisco, CA: Jossey-Bass.

Parker, G. M. (2008). *Team players and teamwork: New strategies for developing successful collaboration.* San Francisco, CA: Jossey-Bass.

Peterson, L., & King, S. (2007). How effective leaders achieve success in critical change initiatives part 4: Emergent leadership—an example with doctors. *Healthcare Quarterly, 10*(4), 52, 59–63.

Pinar, T., Zehir, C., Kitapci, H., & Tanriverdi, H. (2014). The relationships between leadership behaviors team learning and performance among virtual teams. *International Business Research, 7*(5), 68–79.

Plsek, P. (2010). Directed creativity: How to generate new ideas for transforming health care. In T. Porter-O'Grady & K. Malloch (Eds.), *Innovation leadership: Creating the landscape of health care* (pp. 87–106). Sudbury, MA: Jones and Bartlett Publishers.

Porter-O'Grady, T. (2009). *Interdisciplinary shared governance: Integrating practice, transforming health care.* Sudbury, MA: Jones and Bartlett Publishers.

Porter-O'Grady, T., & Malloch, K. (2015). *Quantum leadership: Advancing innovation, transforming health care.* Burlington, MA: Jones & Bartlett Learning.

Raes, E., Decuyper, S., & Lismont, B. (2013). Facilitating team learning through transformational leadership. *Instructional Science: International Journal of the Learning Sciences, 41*(2), 287–305.

Rondeau, K. (2007). The adoption of high involvement work practices and Canadian nursing homes. *Leadership in Health Services, 20*(1), 16.

Rouse, W. (2007). *People and organizations: Explorations of human-centered design.* New York, NY: Wiley.

Salas, E., Goodwin, G. F., & Burke, C. S. (2009). *Team effectiveness in complex organizations: Cross-disciplinary perspectives and approaches.* The organizational frontiers series (pp. xxxiv, 589). Hove, UK: Society for Industrial and Organizational Pyschology.

Singh, M., & Waddell, D. (2004). *E-business innovation and change management.* Hershey, PA: Idea Group.

Taylor, G. (2013). Implementing and maintaining a knowledge sharing culture via knowledge management teams: A shared leadership approach. *Journal of Organizational Culture, Communication & Conflict, 17*(1), 69–91.

Tost, L., Gino, F., & Larrick, R. (2013). When power makes others speechless: The negative impact of leader power on team performance. *Academy of Management Journal, 56*(5), 1465–1486.

Wang, D., Waldman, D. A., & Zhang, Z. (2014). A meta-analysis of shared leadership and team effectiveness. *Journal of Applied Psychology, 99*(2), 181–198.

Weberg, D., & Weberg, K. (2014). Seven behaviors to advance teamwork: Findings from a study of innovation leadership in a simulation center. *Nursing Administration Quarterly, 38*(3), 230–237.

Whatley, L., & Kleiwer, H. (2013). Contextual influences on team effectiveness and consultant identity: Implications for consulting and consultation. *Journal of Leadership, Accountability, and Ethics, 10*(1), 92–108.

Wolfe, B. D., & Sparkman, C. P. (2010). *Team-building activities for the digital age: Using technology to develop effective groups.* Champaign, IL: Human Kinetics.

Yukl, G. (2009). *Leadership in organizations.* New York, NY: Prentice Hall.

Appendix A

Sample Techniques for Team Decision Making

There is a whole range of approaches to disciplined decision making and incorporating the team within the decision-making process. Processes such as flowcharts, workflow diagrams, Pareto charts, cause-and-effect diagrams, matrices and stratification instruments, checklists, scatter diagrams, brainstorming, and multivoting are just a few of the tools that teams can use in making good decisions. The team leader carefully makes choices with regard to which decisions need to be made in the processes that support decision efforts. Some decision-making techniques are as follows:

Nominal group technique:

- Is useful when time is a concern.
- Provides controls for issues of power.
- Helps establish priorities.
- Can aggregate ideas.
- Builds group acceptance.
- Is transparent.

Affinity groups:

- Build consensus and acceptance.
- Use a smaller group for process.
- Let participants know how broadly the idea is supported.
- Offset power.
- Make effective use of time.
- Value and support individual and group ideas.
- Take more time than nominal group technique.
- Allow one idea to help spark others.

Delphi technique:

- Can be used to gather information from outside the team.
- Is good for brainstorming.
- Allows key ideas to be identified and related ideas to be drawn.
- Is good for gathering much information from a broad group.
- Allows participants to feel safe to share controversial ideas.

Appendix B

Team-Based Decision-Making Process

Team decision making is always a structured process and, therefore, is a learned skill exercised by all members of the team.

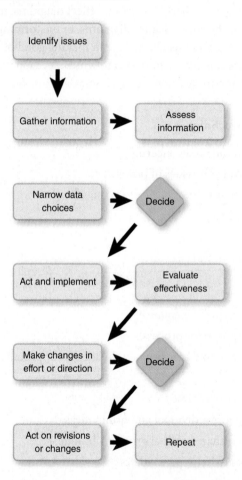

Appendix C

Keeping the Team Focused

- Make sure the team is always aware of its mission.
- Know who has accountability for which decisions.

- Make sure planning is thorough and done ahead of the work.
- Ensure that each team member is aware of his or her role and individual contribution to the team's work.
- Do frequent consensus testing to make sure that every individual's understanding of the work matches the understanding of the team as a whole.
- Clarify misunderstandings, misperceptions, or conflicts in roles and performance early to minimize their impact on the team's work.
- Evaluate the team's process, relationships, and progress frequently.
- Integrate the efforts of the team and evaluate their interface to ensure that each team member's effort is synthesized with the work of the team as a whole.

Appendix D

Some Dos and Don'ts of Team Leadership

Dos	Don'ts
Give the team the information it needs to work well.	Oversupervise the team and control the team processes.
Help the team with skill building in relationship to its work.	Criticize or punish team members in the presence of others.
Build effective communication mechanisms among team members.	Personally own the work of team members as though it belongs to you.
Undertake corrective action potentially impeding teamwork as early as possible.	Ignore internal or external dynamics with the potential to impact team effectiveness.
Evaluate the effectiveness of the team as you go—do not wait.	Let the team get tangled up in peripheral and nonessential issues that impede their work progress.
Confront conflict early and assess often.	
Review goals and progress toward them with team members regularly.	Let team members forget that their work serves a purpose and has value.
Reward and encourage team members' successes frequently and well.	Take credit for the team's work and identify them as "my people."
Assess external and internal impediments to team effectiveness and remove them as soon as possible.	Overwork the team without providing ample time for relationship building, social interaction, and celebrating successes.
Celebrate team successes frequently.	Limit information or access to resources that might affect team goal achievement.

Appendix E

Creating Team Infrastructure

- For teams to be successful, they must be the way of doing business and a part of the continuous dynamic of the organization from the inside out.
- Teams are a strategic imperative.
- Senior management supports the team approach.
- All leaders operate within the context of team processes and are skilled in team management.
- Staff operating in teams is the expectation of the organization and is supported through continual team learning.
- Team processes are used for all decision making and problem solving and are evaluated for effectiveness.

Appendix F

Considerations for Team Effectiveness

As teams move through their specific stages of development, the team leader, working on the periphery, is constantly monitoring and measuring the effectiveness of team members' interactions, relationships, problem solving, and work processing. The team leader recognizes that resolving issues in any of these arenas early creates a framework for team effectiveness and success that can operate over the long term. Creating a culture of openness to issues of concern with regard to problem solving, work processes, and relationship building establishes a frame of reference for the team that is positive, disclosing, and safe. Through this early engagement of issues, the leader sets up a foundation upon which subsequent problem solving can build and team success can be ensured.

- *Forming*: The initial stage of team development in which rules are uncertain and team expectations, rules, and roles are unclear.
- *Storming*: The formative stage of the group process, which is filled with conflict as the group begins to establish roles, relationships, and rules around purposes and the work of the team.
- *Norming*: Work processes are established, rules are agreed to, systems are set up, and creative work patterns emerge in ways that more clearly define the team.

- *Performing*: The team now begins to work well together, undertake processes, work through difficulties, achieve objectives, and measure results.
- *Evaluating and retooling*: The team assesses internal and external dynamics, makes decisions about more effective processes, and refines the team work rules, roles, and relationships.

> It's not enough to be busy, so are the ants. The question is, what are we busy about? —Henry David Thoreau

CHAPTER OBJECTIVES

Upon completion of this chapter, the reader will be able to do the following:

» Understand the six basic categories of resources associated with the provision of healthcare services.

» Describe the interactions among the economic concepts of demand, supply, and price from a healthcare perspective.

» Compare and contrast the purposes, utility, and importance of value and volume measurements in health care.

» Understand basic data measurement concepts, analysis, and interrelationships in determining healthcare value.

» Explain the importance of variance management and the role of the clinical nurse leader in responding to variances in financial, productivity, and performance data.

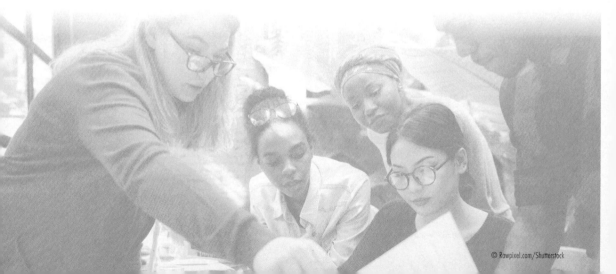

Resources for Healthcare Excellence

For the healthcare system or any healthcare organization to function effectively, resources for personnel, fiscal support, physical settings, supplies, technology, and time to do the expected work are needed. These six major resource categories are incredibly complex and intertwined. While it is important to understand current practices, it is far more important to be thinking about how we can dramatically change the management of those resources in the future. Current practices and policies related to how we finance, organize, deliver, and evaluate health care serve only as an informational baseline. Working to sustain most of these practices will result in reinforcing the existing, less than effective healthcare system; thus there is an urgent need to rethink how we select, manage, and evaluate our resources. Current practices must change dramatically if we are to improve system quality, cost, and value.

This chapter examines the foundations of current practices for managing resources and presents new ideas to consider for the future. Topics covered include basic economic principles specific to price, supply, and demand; major resource categories in health care; differences in value and volume measurements; and the basics of budgeting, data analysis to inform decisions, and managing variances.

Basic Economics Are Not So Basic: Price, Demand, and Supply Complexities

A basic understanding of **healthcare economics** is helpful for clinical nurse leaders to advance their understanding of the complex nature of the workings of health care. Multiple resources are available for studying healthcare macroeconomics and microeconomics in greater depth if the reader is interested. The accompanying box includes a list of some of these resources. To be sure, healthcare economics is a fascinating field that provides vital insights in managing resources and advancing change in the marketplace.

Healthcare economics is the branch of economics that focuses on efficiency, effectiveness, and behavior in the production and consumption of healthcare goods and services (Shi & Singh, 2014). See **Box 8-1**. It is the study and science of how human needs are perceived in relationship to the available supply of health care. Price is always a factor and changes based on the dynamics of supply and demand. In the early 1960s, Arrow (1963) pointed out differences between healthcare economics and other types of economics. The involvement of the government, the intractable uncertainty in many healthcare areas, the barriers to accessing services, and the role of third-party agents in brokering and managing funds are all unique characteristics of healthcare economics versus general economics. These distinctions further reinforce the complexities of healthcare economics. Nevertheless, this branch of economics shares some basic concepts with other types of economics—namely, price, demand, and supply.

In general, prices for healthcare resources, such as supplies, people, and physical settings, are based on what one has to give up to buy a good or service. They

BOX 8-1 SELECTED HEALTHCARE ECONOMICS RESOURCES

- Feldstein (2012)
- Foland, Goodman, and Stano (2012)
- Getzen (2010)
- Shi and Singh (2014)
- Public Health Economics and Methods (www.cdc.gov/stltpublichealth/pheconomics)

are also based on available dollars and the need for a good or service. Prices are considered from multiple perspectives: the actual cost of the service, the actual charge determined by the seller of the goods, and the overall expenditure of dollars. Several factors affect the price of healthcare services and are intertwined in complex ways. Most notably, changes in the need for people (human) resources, materials, equipment, and technology will result in a price change.

The supply of goods or services is the amount that is available at a specific price. The supply of healthcare goods and services includes people, supplies, technology, and time, as well as the funds to pay for these services. Overall, supply includes all healthcare workers, the physical facilities for patient care, materials, equipment, technology, financial assets, and the time resources required to provide health services.

Each type of supply reacts differently in the environment. For example, the supply situation for healthcare workers has ranged from undersupply to oversupply and tends to follow cyclical trends based on changing conditions in price and demand. The supply of nurses is a continual area of analysis and requires ongoing discussion and strategizing to ensure the right nurse is with the right patient at the right time. Both short-term and long-term nursing supply processes are important for allocating the appropriate numbers of nurses. Most recently, the demand for and supply of nurses have been influenced by emerging evidence focusing on safe staffing and staffing effectiveness. Lessons from these staffing effectiveness studies, however, must be customized to the individual facility, geographic location, and available technology for the purpose of making appropriate supply and demand projections.

Of interest is the traditional estimation of the demand for nurses. Currently, the average number of nurses per population unit is used to estimate the demand for and supply of registered nurses. This approach is limited in that it is specific to the quantity of available nurses and does not take into account the types, education, skill levels, and clinical areas of need (StateHealthFacts.org, n.d.). **Figure 8-1** depicts the current nurse supply for each state in the United States.

To determine the adequacy of the Arizona nurse population and develop a plan to change the number of Arizona nurses, more information is needed. Specifically, data about the patient population being served, the skills and competencies of the Arizona nurse population, and the geographic location of the nurses are needed to adequately inform the forecasting of nursing demand. It would be futile to increase the supply of surgical nurses if that supply was already in excess and surgical nurses were looking for jobs. An additional analysis of the supply numbers is needed to best determine the characteristics and geographic locations of nursing demand (Malloch, Davenport, Hatler, & Milton, 2003).

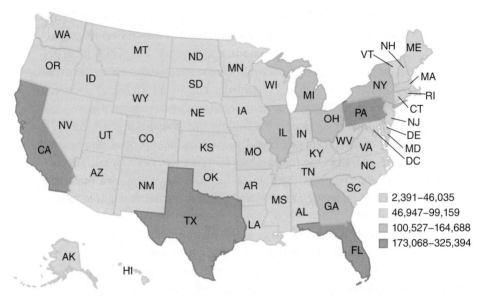

Figure 8-1 Registered nurses in each state

Data from Kaiser Family Foundation. (2017). State health facts: Total number of professionally active nurses. Retrieved from https://www.kff.org/other/state-indicator/total-registered-nurses
/?currentTimeframe=0&selectedDistributions=registered-nurse-rn&sortModel=%7B%22colId%22:%22Location%22,%22sort%22:%22asc%22%7D

The supply category also includes physical facilities in which patient services are delivered—that is, the number, location, type, and quality of locations for health-care services across the country. The numbers and locations of healthcare facilities are affected by demand for services, geographic location, and available funding for services provided. Likewise, physical facilities are impacted by changes related to technology, such as development of telemedicine and the model of care delivery. In recent years, one of the most notable trends related to physical facilities has been the shift from medical centers to community centers and services.

Material supplies include those items that are typically used only once and then discarded. Examples include dressings, medications, and food needed for patient care services. Material supply levels are affected by the types of services provided, the access to supplies, and the cost of supplies. Healthcare organizations and systems are requiring standardization of material supplies in order to streamline the supply chain processes and costs.

The equipment supply is influenced by several factors, such as the ability to use items more than once. Patient beds, wheelchairs, lift equipment, computers, and monitoring equipment are examples. The availability of equipment, the effectiveness of the equipment in advancing patient care, and the cost all affect the type and quantities of equipment supplies that are available in the healthcare system.

The availability of financial resources is similarly complicated and is highly interrelated with the supply and demand factors. Financial resources are available from government and private sources. Federal healthcare spending reflects the types of programs approved for funding by Congress and each of the 50 states, as well as funding provided by employers to insure their employees. Time is also a significant supply resource. Put simply, the time required to analyze, plan, and facilitate effective healthcare programs is significant and often overwhelming. The available supply of time is often not analyzed or categorized as an essential economic resource, yet an understanding of the time available to address supply and demand needs is critical for effective dialogue and evaluation of ongoing activities. Although it is difficult to accurately estimate the time required or needed, discussions and reflections specific to estimation of the capacity of individuals need to occur, and the supply of time for each one is finite.

Demand for goods or services is generated by the number of consumers (patients in the healthcare model) who desire the available goods at a certain price.

SCENARIO

Your state's supply of nurses is 10% below the national average. Your team has been asked to create a plan that will result in an optimal number of nurses and lead to patient quality outcomes at the 99 percentile.

Discussion Questions

Create a plan that includes the following:

1. Rationale, metrics, and quality indicators, including target registered nurses per 100,000 population

2. Assessment of clinical specialties (adult, critical care, pediatric, behavioral health, rehabilitation, surgical, ambulatory, and community health) available to the state, specific to geographic regions

3. Areas of clinical need

4. Areas of geographic need

5. Timeline to achieve goals

6. Facilitators to this work

7. Barriers to this work

8. Plans to support facilitators and address barriers

BOX 8-2 COMPONENTS OF THE CURRENT U.S. HEALTHCARE SYSTEM

- Financing: The payment of premiums to provide coverage for insured individuals
- Insurance: The vehicle to manage risk across populations
- Delivery: Provision of healthcare services by providers, hospitals, diagnostic clinics, and suppliers
- Payment: The process of reimbursement to providers for services rendered

Data from Shi, L., & Singh, D. A. (2014). *Delivering health care in America: A systems approach* (6th ed.). Burlington, MA: Jones & Bartlett Learning.

Demand is about the desire to own a good or service, the ability to pay for it, and the willingness to pay the asking price at a given point in time. It is influenced by the available resources, the prices of related goods, the number of interested buyers, and consumers' preferences. Thus, multiple dynamic influences affect the demand for healthcare goods and services. See **Box 8-2**.

In general, as the price increases, the demand for a good or service decreases; as the price decreases, the demand increases; and as the quantity of goods or supply increases, the price decreases. These relationships are studied extensively to better understand future prices, supplies, and demands from the healthcare economics perspective. **Figure 8-2** illustrates these basic relationships in the economic model.

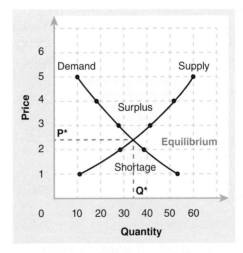

Figure 8-2 Supply and demand

SCENARIO

Change Healthcare is an organization dedicated to transparency in healthcare charges and costs. In a recent news release, the organization reported a wide range of prices within one town, from $230 to $1,800, for a pelvic computed tomography (CT) scan.

Discussion Questions

1. List at least five supply and five demand factors that might have created this situation.

2. Is it possible to standardize these prices?

3. What would be the facilitators and obstacles to standardization?

Data from Change Healthcare. (n.d.). The actionable cost transparency solution. Retrieved from www.changehealthcare.com; Kennedy, K. (2011). Health care costs vary widely, study shows. *USA Today.* Retrieved from web.archive.org/web/20160927191831 /http://usatoday30.usatoday.com/money/industries/health/2011-06-30-health-costs -wide-differences-locally_n.htm

Resource Categories: Human, Fiscal, Material, Technology, and Time

Five resource categories within the healthcare marketplace are continually influenced by the price, supply, and demand concepts in healthcare economics.

The first category, known as human resources or people resources, includes individuals who provide direct patient care as well as those who support patient care processes (i.e., who provide indirect care). The comprehensive management of human resources includes the recruitment, management, and retention of these people. Recruitment of individuals is based on the defined or anticipated needs for services. Advertising, interviewing, selecting, and hiring are all part of the recruitment process. The demand, supply, or availability of individuals for healthcare work varies by geographic region, type of worker, and wage and benefit levels.

The more effective the recruitment process is in identifying and selecting individuals who closely match the needs of the unit and organization, the stronger the team will be and the higher the quality of patient outcomes will be. An ineffective recruitment process negatively affects the supply and demand cycle, resulting in increased work effort and unnecessary expenses.

Management of human resources demand can be enhanced by a strong, evidence-based retention program. Nurse retention is a basic consideration for all healthcare organizations and groups of nursing. Ensuring that competent nurses are satisfied and continue to thrive in their environment requires proactive planning and programming.

SCENARIO

Nurse retention involves more than just handing out pizza and movie tickets to nurses. Recent research identified focused and structured processes with clearly defined evaluation criteria for effective nurse retention. Specifically, the following five practices have been identified as important in decreasing turnover:

- Onboarding: "An ongoing process of building engagement from an individual's first contact with the organization until the individual has fully assumed his/her role and responsibilities within the organization" (Harper & Maloney, 2016).

- Employee rounding: Regular rounding in work areas to identify employees' most critical needs, safety issues, and clinical concerns.

- Social networking: Specific social activities to support team building, seasonal challenges, and common needs.

- Employee recognition: Acknowledgment of outstanding behaviors, communication, accountability, valuing diversity, delivering excellence, and teamwork.

- Developmental stretch assignments: Assignments to improve employee satisfaction and engagement through autonomy and leadership practices.

Discussion Questions

1. In a team setting, make a list of activities specific to each of the five practices that are occurring in your organization.

2. Make a list of activities that should occur in the next year for each of the five categories.

3. What are the facilitators and barriers to improving retention?

Data from Hinson, T. D., & Spatz, D. L. (2011). Improving nurse retention in a large tertiary acute-care hospital. *Journal of Nursing Administration, 41*(3), 103–108.

The costs associated with turnover of experienced nurses are better spent in retaining competent nurse experts who are acclimated and socialized to the setting (Li & Jones, 2013). Focusing on retention is especially important when resources are limited. According to Hinson and Spatz (2011), focused initiatives on retention can be quite successful in retaining nurses. In their study, the implementation of five retention concepts—**onboarding**, **employee rounding**, **social networking**, **employee recognition**, and **developmental stretch assignments**—reduced voluntary nurse turnover by 91%, led to 100% retention of 43 newly hired nurses, and produced a savings of $655,949.

The second resource category is financial resources. Fiscal or financial resources include the dollars required to purchase and pay for human, material, and technology resources. The current U.S. financial system for health care includes financing, insurance, payment, and delivery (Shi & Singh, 2014). This system has evolved over many years and is quite complex and costly. Some of the characteristics of the U.S. system are as follows:

- Public and private funding resources: Federal and state government and private insurance companies are the major financiers of health care.
- Insured and uninsured individuals: Insured individuals include those with employer-sponsored health plans and selected populations for government programs (senior citizens, military, veterans, disabled citizens, and impoverished groups); uninsured individuals include those that do not fit into insured groups.
- Varying costs to individuals: Costs to individuals vary across plans (e.g., copayments and deductibles).
- Financing models: A variety of models of financing, insurance, and/or payment exist that are not integrated across the healthcare continuum (e.g., managed care organizations and integrated networks by large employers and self-insurance by private insurance plans).
- State versus federal systems: Some states assume accountability for federal programs, such as Medicaid.
- Varying coverage: Coverage or payment varies across government and private insurance plans for selected conditions and procedures.
- Inconsistency: Charges are inconsistent for services and quality control mechanisms.

It is these widely varying characteristics in the financing of health care in the United States that recently spurred the passage of national healthcare reform. This national legislation, known as the Patient Protection and Affordable Care Act of 2010 (ACA), is intended to provide healthcare coverage to every citizen and eliminate many of the challenges associated with the existing system, such as disqualifications for preexisting conditions, portability of benefits, and lack of quality and cost control. Specifically, reform is intended to create an integrated network of interrelated components that work together coherently and effectively. See **Box 8-3**.

Interestingly, the management of fiscal resources continues to challenge the best healthcare leaders for several reasons. In addition to the perceived limited availability of resources, the wide variation in charges for similar healthcare services is especially problematic. These charges for healthcare services differ from the actual costs of specific healthcare products and services. The actual costs of products and services are difficult to determine given the need to include administrative and delivery costs into the total amount paid for each product and service. The specific charge for a product or service, therefore, includes its cost plus any administrative fees. Furthermore, costs and charges vary by provider,

---

BOX 8-3 GOALS OF THE AFFORDABLE CARE ACT OF 2010

- Rein in the worst excesses and abuses of the insurance industry with some of the toughest consumer protections the United States has ever implemented.

- Hold insurance companies accountable for keeping premiums down and prevent denials of care and coverage, including for preexisting conditions.

- Make health insurance affordable for middle-class families and small businesses with one of the largest tax cuts for health care in history, reducing premiums and out-of-pocket costs.

- Provide the security of knowing that if you lose your job, change your job, or start a new business, you will always be able to purchase quality, affordable care in a new competitive health insurance market that keeps costs down.

- Strengthen Medicare benefits by providing for lower prescription drug costs for individuals in the "doughnut hole," chronic care, free preventive care, and nearly a decade more of solvency for Medicare.

- Improve the United States' fiscal health by reducing the country's deficit by more than $100 billion over the next decade, and more than $1 trillion in the decade after that.

Data from HealthReform.gov. (n.d.). About HealthReform.gov. Retrieved from healthreform.gov/about/index.html

geographic region, and type of organization providing the service. For example, patients may pay as much as 683% more for the same medical procedure, such as magnetic resonance imaging or a CT scan, in the same town depending on which provider they select (Kennedy, 2011).

The third category of healthcare resources is material resources. Material resources for physical setting, supplies, and equipment include items needed for the environment and supplies and equipment to provide the required patient care. See **Box 8-4**. Similar to human and financial resources, there is significant variation in material resources and continuing demand for new and improved material resources. For example, as evidence emerges specific to the relationship between attributes of the physical setting and patient outcomes, redesign of facilities is being demanded.

The fourth resource category is technology. Technology resources include those resources required for the electronic or virtual management of information, such as hardware and software applications for clinical documentation, data analysis, clinical monitoring systems, communication devices, and robotics. While most of the emerging technology provides improvements in selected patient care processes and supporting information processes, not every new technology is appropriate for every organization, especially if that organization has limited financial and other resources. The addition of technology must necessarily be

BOX 8-4 PHYSICAL SETTING: CHANGES IN DEMAND

- Private rooms
- Patient rooms with views of nature
- Enclosed medication administration rooms
- Decentralized and centralized workstations
- Multiple hand washing dispensers located based on human factors research
- Multipurpose interventional suites for surgery, catheterization labs, endoscopy, and interventional radiology
- Admission units for all patients except critical care
- Family space in all patient rooms
- Healing modalities of music, water features, and gardens
- Attractive space for staff lounges
- Separated greeter and unit clerk space

evaluated for the fit with current technologies and manual practices, the anticipated value to patient quality and safety outcomes, employee safety and performance, physical setting safety and effectiveness, and affordability. The potential
for saving time, reducing errors, and increasing the reliability of information
management is an important consideration when the demand for new technology
is being considered.

The fifth resource category in healthcare economics is time. Time resources
include the available time to provide the care and support services for healthcare
work. Very few individuals believe they ever have enough time to do the things
that need to be done. Thus, time emerges as an important resource to manage.
Learning to identify what needs to be done, what the priority level of that work is,
who needs to do the work, and how to create boundaries between work and personal time is an underdeveloped competence for most healthcare workers.

The following strategies are helpful in assessing and managing one's time. First,
self-assessment is essential. Determine what your personal abilities are in managing your work across a span of time. Take into consideration your own personal
assessment and feedback from others on your team. Such personal reflection
may address meeting deadlines; feeling less stressed or overwhelmed; managing
interruptions; prioritizing; avoiding time wasters, idle chatter, and complaining; focusing on perfection; and reducing procrastination. Develop a personal
plan to optimize your time management. Select one or two strategies to address
the areas of concern. Do not overwhelm yourself by setting unreasonable goals
and timelines; they will soon be forgotten and pushed aside. Consider planning
at the beginning of a work period, by allowing a short time for reflection on the
work to be done, prioritization of work, and estimates of the time required for
small blocks of work. Estimating time often provides invaluable insight into time

CRITICAL THOUGHT

- Recognize that everyone has the capacity for improving their use of
  time.
- Focus on the importance of balancing energy rather than efficiency.
- Share the spirit of the reality that there will always be a shortage of time
  and an excess of desires—and therefore a never-ending struggle to
  close the gap!
- Stay focused and aware of personal performance.
- Support others who are less successful in time balancing, knowing there
  are opportunities to improve for all.

requirements and helps to identify sources of overuse and underuse of time. The third activity is to review the results at the end of the work period and recognize what went well and what could be improved.

Numerous techniques to improve time management exist; some will work for you and some will not. Being open to new ideas will provide insights into other successful approaches.

SCENARIO

Your team has a reputation for poor time management on some days and excellent time management on other days. Patient call lights are not always answered in a timely manner, pain medications are late, documentation is usually done after the shift, and overtime is greater than 5% of the budget.

For a clinical ladder project, you and two other nurses have decided to learn from individuals who have excellent time management skills and those who are struggling. You believe you can learn something about work habits and systems issues if you work with both groups.

Discussion Questions

Using the following categories, brainstorm with team members to create a plan to share ideas and improve management of time. Include both positive and negative behaviors. Ask each individual to create a personal plan for time management. Feel free to add other categories that you believe are involved.

1. Prioritizing

2. Planning

3. Procrastination

4. Interruptions

5. Perfectionism

6. Complaining

7. Communication

8. Feeling overwhelmed

Value Measurement: Productivity, Quality, and Volume

Productivity measurement is a long-standing, quantitative measurement of the efficiency of the use of specific resources. Productivity is a ratio comparing what is produced to what is required to produce it. Usually this ratio takes the form of an average, expressing the output divided by the total. Productivity is also a measure of output from a production process, per unit of input (Shi & Singh, 2014). Aggregate productivity ratios are helpful in determining the overall efficiency of processes and individuals at a macro level.

Productivity values generally increase as volumes of work increase. This implies that few obstacles or deviations from that standard process occur and that less time for a process will result in the desired quality outcome with higher volumes. Historically, higher productivity levels have been associated with higher profits.

Examples of productivity metrics include the following:

- Registered nurse hours per patient-day (HPPD)
- Registered nurse hours/treatment or procedure
- Admissions, discharges, and transfers/shift
- Direct care hours/total care hours
- Overtime hours/total worked hours
- New staff orientation hours/total worked hours
- Total salary cost/diagnosis-related group (DRG)

While emphasis is often placed on productivity targets, it is only one part of the picture. In reality, more information about processes and outcomes is needed before it can be stated that the productivity level is either positive or negative. An out-of-range productivity result may, in fact, be more than acceptable if the patient care conditions (demand) exceeded the standards expressed in the productivity target calculations.

Historically, many healthcare workers have confused high work volumes or high productivity with high quality and value. Also, some have considered completion of process requirements, such as completion of a checklist, to be a sign of high levels of quality and value. Completing checklists 100% of the time or distributing healthcare information to all patients with a certain disease does not guarantee that value outcomes were achieved. Instead, we need to know what value was produced from completing the checklist or from distributing the healthcare information. The value outcome requires specific use of the data from the checklist to better plan patient care or improvement in patient knowledge and healthy behaviors. Specifically, it is essential to know if patient care was positively impacted in such a way that it produced an outcome that was significant and valued by the patient.

Another challenge in measurement arises with the use of single versus multiple re-lated measures. Single metrics are limiting and measure only one aspect of the overall performance of the organization. Not only are single metrics limiting in the informa-tion that can be produced, but the type of analysis is also limiting. Traditionally, a return on investment or cost–benefit analysis is performed to determine the worth or value derived from expending resources; that is, spending resources is expected to result in increased financial value. However, there is more to analyze in this scenario. Consider expending resources for a women's wellness service. The financial outcome may be positive, yet the desired changes in women's level of wellness may not be achieved. Thus, determining the value and achievement of the goals of a program in addition to the financial benefit is essential to support effective allocation of resources.

Five types of value analyses should be considered when expending resources (Buerhaus, 1998):

1. Cost-minimization analysis (CMA)
   - The emphasis is on keeping costs as low as possible.
   - Only costs are evaluated.
   - Clinical outcomes are assumed to be the same.
   - Example: Practice guidelines for thrombolytic therapy; streptokinase via tissue plasminogen activator.
2. Cost–consequences analysis (CCA)
   - Consequences of two or more alternatives are measured, as well as the costs, but costs/consequences are listed separately.
   - Example: Comparison of early discharge of low-birth-weight infants whose care was managed by advanced practice nurses compared to traditional physician care.
3. Cost-effectiveness analysis (CEA)
   - Outcomes are measured in the same units between alternatives, such as dollars per life-year gained or cases avoided.
   - Example: Evaluation of pain management interventions for patients with chronic arthritis.
4. Cost–utility analysis (CUA)
   - This special type of cost-effectiveness analysis includes measures of both quantity and quality of life.
   - Individual preferences for different health outcomes are sought and included.
   - CUA is a difficult comparison; the goal is to compare expenditures to quality adjusted life-years.

5. Cost–benefit analysis (CBA)

- Outcomes are measured according to a monetary unit.
- A single dollar figure, representing cost minus benefits, is calculated.
- Example: Is the cost of a pain management clinic covered by the amount of revenue generated? For example, if the cost of service is $500.00 and the reimbursement from an insurance company is $750.00, the profit is $250.00 or 50% (250/500) return on investment.

Use of additional measures that identify the quality of the processes and the outcomes of providing patient care is gaining favor, particularly in light of the goals of healthcare reform. The specific positive impact on functionality, reduction of pain, and time expended for care, for example, must be included in the determination of value along with costs, reimbursement, processes, and completion of procedures. For example, while the charges and reimbursement amounts are readily available for a surgical procedure, such a procedure may not yield any value to an elderly individual who is in hospice care. In such a case, the surgical procedure meets all the quality parameters for a safe procedure, yet the patient experiences no value or change in functionality or pain level.

Table 8-1 is an example of a multilevel measurement evaluation for macro patient, employee, organization, and payer categories. Using the same framework,

Table 8-1 Value Evaluation: Multiple Measures for Consideration

	Quality	Productivity	Cost
Patient	Clinical outcome Functionality Comfort status Satisfaction	Length of stay Length of procedure Time to treatment	Cost of service Charge per case Out-of-pocket expenses
Employee	Competence, credentials, certifications, experience Level of education Satisfaction with work	Hours per unit of service Skill mix percentages Turnover Registry staff percentage Overtime percentage	Wages and benefits
Organization	Reputation in the community Licensure status Accreditations	Full-time equivalent/ adjusted occupied bed	Net income margin Departmental margins Available capital
Payer	Reputation with providers and organizations	Claims processed per 24-hour period	Cost of claims

Dashboards and Measures

Dashboards and scorecards have become useful to leaders in managing the plethora of data in the healthcare environment in a strategic manner. Typically, **dashboards** combine graphics and numbers so as to quickly display important data elements. Basic information, technology considerations for accessibility to data, and meaningful measures over which users have some control are important considerations when constructing a dashboard (Serb, 2011). According to Mick (2011), administrators and stakeholders want to know if financial investments in programs are achieving the desired outcomes as well as compliance with regulatory requirements. Dashboards with a combination of financial, performance, and productivity measures reported in real time become critical resources for clinicians. Continually monitoring progress and data allows providers to make course corrections or change strategies in a timely manner. If quality of care is to be improved, however, the data displayed in the dashboard must be of high quality (Ko, 2012). Dashboard users should regularly assure the quality of data being extracted to the dashboard.

Effective dashboards include data that individuals can react to and have control over. For example, a unit clinical dashboard would include the number and type of caregivers present; a summary of the caregivers' levels of education, experience, and expertise; and comparisons to target hours of care and cost projections. Another dashboard would be specific to patient feedback and satisfaction with specific areas of care, such as caregiver responsiveness, information provided, and level of pain relief achieved. Using a focused method that attempts to select those most critical variables is an important first step. **Figure 8-3** provides an example of a dashboard focusing on critical measures for the nursing staff on an oncology unit.

The greatest challenge in using dashboards is to identify and measure what really matters—that is, which metrics are the critical variables that indicate value, service, and cost outcomes accurately and comprehensively. As previously noted, multiple related metrics are required to explain the causality of relationships; seldom does one variable completely explain one outcome. By its very essence, the complex and dynamic nature of health care renders it resistant to simple linear, cause-and-effect metrics. For example, no single intervention is accountable for a patient's recovery from pneumonia; diet, fluids, medications, and activity all contribute to the resolution of chest congestion. Similarly, the HPPD metric cannot be linked simply and traced to the activities of a single unit leader; the competence of staff, the level of illness of the patients, the number of interventions required, and the availability of equipment and supplies all impact the level of HPPD.

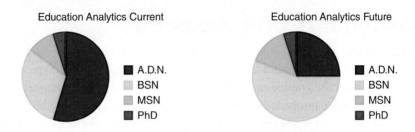

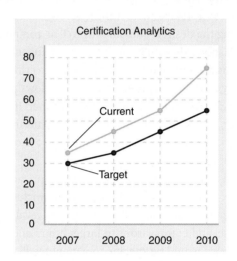

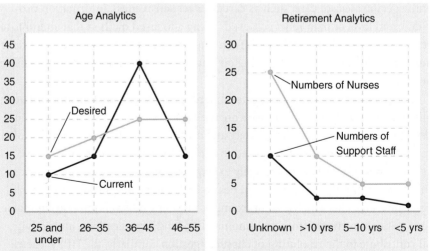

Figure 8-3 Dashboard: Oncology unit retention

It is seldom readily apparent which combinations of metrics provide the desired information. Further, as the work of health care continues to evolve, the evidence changes; thus the metrics will also need to change.

Comparing multiple metrics often provides new insight into performance. For example, safe medication administration is a major challenge for all healthcare workers in the United States. Multiple structure and process variables interact to produce safe medication administration. Attempts to decrease preventable adverse drug events (PADE) without making additional changes to structures and/or process variables could be futile. For example, increasing nursing hours of care without adding electronic processes to support patient identification and ensure legibility of orders could result in no change in the number of PADEs. To effect change, combinations of variables known to impact the structure and processes are needed. In **Table 8-3**, Scenario One reflects the optimal conditions for medication administration and patient care excellence based on the structure and processes available. See also **Box 8-5**.

Another important issue is the fact that focusing on combinations of metrics or aggregate metrics has advantages and disadvantages, as well as supporters

Table 8-3 Preventable Adverse Drug Effects: Multiple Inputs, Processes, and Metrics

Structure	Processes	Metrics	Expected level of performance
Scenario One			
Electronic health record Enclosed medication-preparation rooms Bright task lighting at least 1,400 lux Single-bed rooms Decentralized pharmacists Positive patient identification	Computerized physician order entry with standard order sets Computerized medication administration documentation Bedside documentation Patient/medication barcoding	Number of **Preventable Adverse Drug Effects** (PADEs) Nursing care hours per patient-day (HPPD) Pharmacist HPPD Total cost of care/patient-day Number of verbal orders Turnaround time from order to dispensing for first dose, nonstat medications	Fewer than 4 PADEs/month or 0.001 error/100,000 doses Nursing hours < 6.0 HPPD Pharmacist hours < 0.2 HPPD Cost of patient-day < $240/day < 2% verbal orders Turnaround time (TAT) < 60 min for first dose, nonstat medications

(continues)

Table 8-3 Preventable Adverse Drug Effects: Multiple Inputs, Processes, and Metrics (*continued*)

Structure	Processes	Metrics	Expected level of performance
Scenario Two			
Manual documentation system 75% single-bed rooms Centralized pharmacy services Overhead lighting less than 1,400 lux	Manual documentation at central station Handwritten physician orders Manual order transcription Visual patient name identification	Number of PADEs Nursing hours of care per patient Pharmacist HPPD Total cost of care/ HPPD Number of verbal orders	Fewer than 20 PADEs/month or 0.005 error/100,000 doses Nursing hours < 6.2 HPPD Pharmacist hours < 0.25 HPPD Cost of patient-day < $300 < 10% verbal orders TAT < 3 hours for first dose, nonstat medications
Scenario Three			
Electronic medication administration record 75% single-bed rooms Centralized pharmacy services Overhead lighting less than 1,400 lux	Manual documentation at central station Handwritten physician orders Manual order transcription Electronic documentation/ reconciliation of medications Visual patient name identification	Number of PADEs Nursing care HPPD Pharmacist HPPD Total cost of care/ HPPD Number of verbal orders	Fewer than 15 PADEs/month or 0.004 error/100,000 doses Nursing hours < 6.1 HPPD Pharmacist hours < 0.22 HPPD Cost of patient-day < $275 < 10% verbal orders TAT < 2 hours for first dose, nonstat medications

and nonsupporters. Supporters see the value of assessing multiple perspectives. Nonsupporters prefer one metric—usually a financial metric—that provides the essential information in a simple and straightforward manner. It is always important to identify the critical variables, build the case for the selected combination of variables and their associated metrics, and document the results.

BOX 8-5 CASE STUDY

Scenario One represents optimal conditions for medication administration. However, when analyzing trends over time, during the last two years, the months of February, July, and August spiked from the average of 4 PADEs per month to an average of 10; none of the other metrics changed during that time. Discuss processes and tools you could use to evaluate this variance and plan for the coming year.

Scenario Two represents conditions that are not optimal for medication administration. This scenario is a procedural nursing care area that has recently had a number of nurses transfer from the inpatient nursing area. The inpatient nursing area has optimal conditions for medication administration, and the nurses are frustrated that the same resources and expectations are not available in the new work area, particularly patient/medication barcoding. Discuss how the team can work to obtain the resources. Include a comprehensive list of factors in the plan to present to administration.

Variance Management

It is rare for desired outcomes to perfectly match actual outcomes. Once the pertinent outcomes data are gathered, available, and displayed on a dashboard, they can be interpreted and applied for potential course correction action. Variance between needs and resources reflects the difficulties inherent in forecasting human behaviors. Important information can be gained from analyzing, monitoring, and adjusting system elements in a timely manner.

Variances occur routinely in all of the major resource categories: personnel, finances, technology, equipment, and time. Information specific to the variances or differences between desired outcomes and actual outcomes is essential to ensure effective system evaluations. Variances may occur at the individual, unit, and system levels, depending on the type of analysis. Once a significant variance is identified, one must determine if this variance is natural or artificial. According to Long (2002), natural variances occur in levels of competence, responses to treatments, timing of interventions, and communication styles. In contrast, artificial variances are those that one wants to eliminate, such as errors, lack of knowledge, or ineffective scheduling. The goal is to minimize the natural variances and eliminate the artificial variances to improve forecasting accuracy.

Examination of the required staff needed for care and the actual staff available is a routine activity of nurse leaders. What is not routine is the systematic

CRITICAL THOUGHT

One must ask if variance is indeed a forecasting problem or merely a normal aspect of a living system.

documentation of the difference between required and actual hours and the interventions undertaken to address and mediate the variance or gap. Note that both positive and negative variances need to be addressed and documented in such a scenario.

Staffing variances are of great concern to caregivers. In spite of the efforts to plan and project adequate numbers of staff, such variances persist. The identification and management of the variance between needed staff and actual staff hours can be helpful in improving and decreasing future variances. At some point in time, a team discussion of this kind of variance should take place to ensure inclusion of issues from the direct caregivers' perspective as well as the manager's perspective. Managing the difference between actual hours of staff and required hours of care requires analysis of individual caregiver variances and total variance hours. **Figure 8-4** presents a variance analysis template that displays the actual and required hours of an evening shift and the variances. When a significant

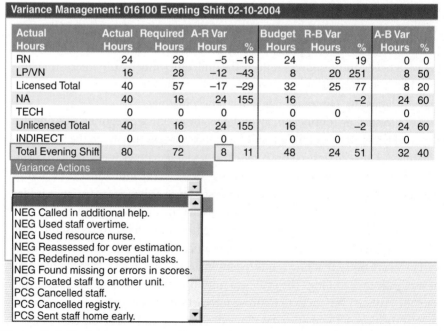

Variance Management: 016100 Evening Shift 02-10-2004

Actual Hours	Actual Hours	Required Hours	A-R Var Hours	%	Budget Hours	R-B Var Hours	%	A-B Var Hours	%
RN	24	29	−5	−16	24	5	19	0	0
LP/VN	16	28	−12	−43	8	20	251	8	50
Licensed Total	40	57	−17	−29	32	25	77	8	20
NA	40	16	24	155	16		−2	24	60
TECH	0	0	0		0	0		0	
Unlicensed Total	40	16	24	155	16		−2	24	60
INDIRECT	0	0	0		0	0		0	
Total Evening Shift	80	72	8	11	48	24	51	32	40

Variance Actions

NEG Called in additional help.
NEG Used staff overtime.
NEG Used resource nurse.
NEG Reassessed for over estimation.
NEG Redefined non-essential tasks.
NEG Found missing or errors in scores.
PCS Floated staff to another unit.
PCS Cancelled staff.
PCS Cancelled registry.
PCS Sent staff home early.

Figure 8-4 Variance management

variance is determined, variance actions are implemented and documented. Most organizations select a reaction point at which action will be taken, such as plus or minus 5% or 10% variance. Staffing variance data provide valuable trend information for nurses as they continually work to create effective workload management systems.

Eliminating non-value-added work is an intervention that is often overlooked. Typically, new interventions and processes are added to work lists without removing outdated processes. Also, system inefficiencies are often not recognized and continue to require time that does not add value to the outcomes. Efforts to identify and minimize time spent in searching for supplies and equipment, inefficient hand-offs at shift change, waiting because of lack of response, and waiting for transportation are areas where innovation can improve nursing care. Workarounds are also important in increasing efficiency and effectiveness and reducing the gap between required and actual staff (Korner, Hartman, Agee, & McNally, 2011; Storfjell, Ohlson, Omoike, Fitzpatrick, & Wetasin, 2009).

Several strategies to address staffing variances have been developed. Examples of interventions to address the variance or gap between needs and actual staffing include the following:

- Work as a team, not as individuals, when there is a gap. Be proactive together. Working as an individual can be isolating, impulsive, and highly stressful.
- Prioritize together as a team. Identify patient care issues that require immediate attention and those that can be safely postponed until later in the shift or until the next shift. Postpone nonemergent patient care.
- Delegate and supervise to the best of your ability.
- Communicate regularly during the shift. Arrange for short, frequent updates with the team to assess how well things are going and reassign and reprioritize as needed.
- Postpone admissions. Adding more work to an out-of-balance unit is unsafe.
- Float existing staff to the unit in need.
- Call in additional staff.
- Reevaluate patient acuity ratings.
- Document variance management, including actions taken, patient care concerns, safety issues, and other events.

In summary, managing the difference between what was projected or anticipated and what actually occurred is an essential step in managing resources. Variance analysis for all resource categories is important and strengthens the forecasting and planning process. Variations typically occur in finances, personnel, and/or supplies; practice and geographic variations are also significant. Variations in finance can result from greater or lesser revenues and greater or lesser expenses. Analysis of variances is best focused at the micro level—the point at which a meaningful interpretation can be made and a focused intervention implemented. The goal of variance analysis is to strengthen the accuracy of predictions and minimize crisis management and intervention when a gap exists between what was available and what was needed.

Everything that has a target will have a variance. Zero variances, as previously noted, are most unlikely. In most cases, variation that exceeds resources is problematic. The delicate and dynamic challenge to balance variation and standardization is forever present. Expert clinicians must determine which basic principles should be standardized and when to vary in the application of those principles.

Variations in practice patterns also have an impact on price, supply, and demand. Wennberg, the principal investigator and series editor of the *Dartmouth Atlas*, has documented significant geographic variations in medical practice since the early 1970s. According to Wennberg and colleagues (Wennberg, 2014; Wennberg et al., 2004), Medicare-insured patients with similar chronic conditions receive strikingly different care, even within hospitals identified as "best" for geriatric care. Their studies show that the frequency of physician visits, the number of diagnostic tests, and the rate of hospital and intensive care unit (ICU) stays vary markedly (**Table 8-4**). Moreover, a higher intensity of care and higher level of spending are not associated with better quality or longer survival times, even in the most renowned teaching hospitals.

Table 8-4 Comparison of Provider Services for Cancer, Heart Failure, and Chronic Obstructive Pulmonary Disease (Risk Adjusted)

	Lowest	Highest	Percent variation
Days in the hospital	8.5	32.3	25%
Days in ICU	0.6	13.4	45%
Physician visits	13.0	99.0	37%

Data from Wennberg, J. E., Fisher, E. S., Stukel, T. A., Skinner, J. S., Sharp, S. M., & Bronner, K. K. (2004). Use of hospitals, physician visits, and hospice care during last six months of life among cohorts loyal to highly respected hospitals in the United States. *British Medical Journal, 328,* 607–612.

The variation documented by Wennberg and colleagues (2004) is difficult to explain or justify. The same analysis of caregiver variation is also needed to identify which standards of care represent best practices and best outcomes. In light of the variations in provider practices, the work of caregivers must necessarily vary in response to differences in length of time in the facility, in the ICU, and in assisting the physician during rounds.

Concluding Thoughts: The Role of the Clinical Nurse Leader in Resource Management

Managing healthcare resources is a complex and sometimes unwieldy process. The goal of having the right resources for the right patient can present overwhelming challenges for healthcare providers. The clinical nurse leader is ideally positioned to regularly identify and share needs with those managing resource processes; such a nurse is able to provide the content of these resource needs. In many organizations, staff create a documented process to communicate the effectiveness of the various resource categories—financial, staffing, equipment, technology, and time—for managers and leaders. This is a vital process because clinical leaders are the only ones who can identify the specific impact of resources on patient care processes; managers and leaders can only infer and speculate based on the observations of clinical leaders. Nurse leaders should provide both positive and negative feedback on resources—the team needs to know both when things are going well and when they are out of range.

SCENARIO

The emergence of care centers in drugstores reflects a shift in supply, demand, and price for the care of patients. Patients who once sought care at an emergency center or physician office are now using clinical services at these venues.

Discussion Questions

1. Identify all of the issues or factors related to each of the three major categories of supply, demand, and price for the drugstores' clinical services.

(continues)

(continued)

2. Based on your analysis, do you believe that supply of healthcare services and the demand for services has been equalized? Why or why not?

3. Are there additional changes in price, supply, or demand that would further equalize the economic dynamics of supply–price–demand?

SCENARIO

Adding technology resources to an organization requires careful consideration. There must be a clear understanding of the potential value of the technology specific to time savings for employees, quality improvements for patients, improvements in patient safety, cost savings, and overall satisfaction.

Several nurses just returned from attending a large national conference at which they saw robots for delivering pharmacy supplies, delivering and picking up medical records, and delivering and picking up food trays. The nurses believe that all three types of robots would benefit the unit in a variety of ways. The nurse executive is very interested and requested the nurses to identify the potential value for the organization.

Discussion Questions

On the basis of this information, develop a value-based proposal for each of the three types of robots and prioritize which robot should be purchased and why. Identify your rationale as belonging to one or more of the following categories:

1. Improvements in patient care outcomes

2. Time savings for specific caregivers

3. Costs/cost savings including technology, maintenance of technology, and patient reimbursements

4. Changes in space needs: increases or decreases in storage space

5. Education required for this technology (include all skill categories requiring new information)

6. Satisfaction of patients, caregivers, and providers

CHAPTER TEST QUESTIONS

Licensure exam categories: Management of care: concepts of management, establishing priorities

Nurse leader exam categories: Business skills: human resource management, financial management, strategic management; Knowledge of the healthcare environment: delivery models and work design

1. The interactions among price, supply, and demand in health care are

   a. Usually linear and driven by prices.

   b. Highly interactive and unpredictable.

   c. Currently driven by the demand for technology.

   d. Unrelated to healthcare quality.

2. Healthcare economics provides

   a. Guidance for healthcare reform

   b. Information about the current status of national spending.

   c. An overview of the study of supply, price, and demand interactions.

   d. Information about the motivations for spending in the United States.

3. Calculation of the demand for nurses is

   a. A state function.

   b. A national function.

   c. Still to be done accurately.

   d. Essential for funding of national legislation.

4. Uninsured populations are the result of

    a. Excessive costs for coverage.

    b. Excess demand for insurance coverage.

    c. Lack of employment.

    d. Immigration status.

5. Time resources

    a. Can be controlled with time management training.

    b. Are not as important to understand and manage as human and financial resources.

    c. Will never be adequate given the complex world of health care.

    d. Are needed to adequately plan, analyze, and provide services.

6. The current U.S. healthcare system

    a. Provides health care that is costly and inconsistent in quality levels.

    b. While costly, provides the most accessible care in the world.

    c. Would benefit from a national healthcare system.

    d. Has an imbalance of price, supply, and demand.

7. Productivity monitoring is intended to provide

    a. A snapshot of the quality of care being delivered.

    b. One metric specific to efficiency of output to total work.

    c. The cost of current supply and demand for healthcare services.

    d. A metric used by the financial services department.

8. Dashboards are

   a. Management tools created to display multiple metrics specific to an area of interest.

   b. Limited to executives because of patient privacy regulations.

   c. Another management fad that will soon be replaced by another fad.

   d. Difficult to create because of the extensive amount of data available.

9. Variance analysis

   a. Is additional work that takes place after the shift has ended and is often forgotten.

   b. Results in useful information about performance specific to a target.

   c. Requires high-level financial experts to complete adequately.

   d. Should be completed at least monthly.

10. Value measurements are intended to identify

   a. The cost–benefit ratio of dollars expended.

   b. A record of process measurements and outcome measurements.

   c. The positive change in a patient's health status or functionality based on expenditures of resources.

   d. The savings resulting from excess demand over supply.

References

Agency for Healthcare Research and Quality. (2012, September). Value portfolio. Rockville, MD: AHRQ. Retrieved from www.ahrq.gov/cpi/portfolios/value/index .html

Arrow, K. (1963). Uncertainty and the welfare economics of medical care. *American Economic Review, 53*(5), 941–973.

Buerhaus, P. I. (1998). Milton Weinstein's insights on the development, use and methodologic problems in cost-effectiveness analysis. *Journal of Nursing Scholarship, 30*(3), 223–228.

Change Healthcare. (n.d.). The actionable cost transparency solution. Retrieved from www.changehealthcare.com

Consumer-Purchaser Disclosure Project. (2011). About the Disclosure Project. www .consumerpurchaser.org

D'Amour, D., Dubois, C., Dery, J., Clarke, S., Tchouaket, E., Blais, R., & Rivard, M. (2012). Measuring actual scope of nursing practice. *Journal of Nursing Administration, 42*(5), 248–255.

Dietrich, M. O., & Anderson, G. D. (2012). *The financial professional's guide to healthcare reform.* Hoboken, NJ: Wiley.

Dunham-Taylor, J., & Pinczuk, J. (2014). *Financial management for nurse managers: Merging the heart with the dollar* (3rd ed.). Burlington, MA: Jones & Bartlett Learning.

Feldstein, P. J. (2012). *Health care economics.* Clifton Park, NY: Cengage Learning.

Finkler, S. A., Jones, C., & Kovner, C. A. (2012*). Financial management for nurse managers and executives.* St. Louis, MO: Saunders Elsevier.

Foland, S., Goodman, A. C., & Stano, M. (2012). *Economics of health and healthcare* (7th ed.). Upper Saddle River, NJ: Prentice Hall.

Getzen, T. E. (2010). *Health economics and financing* (4th ed.). Hoboken, NJ: Wiley.

Harper, M. G., & Maloney, P. (2016). *Nursing professional development: Scope and standards of practice* (3rd ed.). Chicago, IL: Association for Nursing Professional Development.

HealthReform.gov. (n.d.). About HealthReform.gov. Retrieved from healthreform.gov /about/index.html

Hinson, T. D., & Spatz, D. L. (2011). Improving nurse retention in a large tertiary acute-care hospital. *Journal of Nursing Administration, 41*(3), 103–108.

Kennedy, K. (2011, June 30). Health care costs vary widely, study shows. *USA Today.* Retrieved from web.archive.org/web/20160927191831/http://usatoday30 .usatoday.com/money/industries/health/2011-06-30-health-costs-wide -differences-locally_n.htm

Ko, C. (2012, July/August). The critical importance of good data to improving quality. *Patient Safety Quality and Healthcare*. Retrieved from https://www.psqh.com /analysis/the-critical-importance-of-good-data-to-improving-quality/#

Kohlbrenner, J., Whitelaw, G., & Cannaday, D. (2011). Nurses critical to quality, safety, and now financial performance. *Journal of Nursing Administration, 41*(3), 122–128.

Korner, K. T., Hartman, N. M., Agee, A., & McNally, M. (2011). Lean tools and concepts reduce waste, improve efficiency. *American Nurse Today, 6*(3), 41–42.

Li, Y., & Jones, C. B. (2013). A literature review of nursing turnover costs. *Journal of Nursing Management, 21*, 405–418.

Long, M. C. (2002). *Translating the principles of variability management into reality: One physician's perspective*. Boston, MA: Boston University School of Management, Executive Learning.

Malloch, K., Davenport, S., Hatler, C., & Milton, D. (2003). Nursing workforce management: Using benchmarking for planning and outcomes monitoring. *Journal of Nursing Administration, 33*(10), 538–543.

Mick, J. (2011). Data-driven decision making: A nursing research and evidence-based practice dashboard. *Journal of Nursing Administration, 41*(10), 391–393.

Pappas, S. (2013, April/June). Value, a nursing outcome. *Nursing Administration Quarterly, 37*(2), 122–128.

Porter, M. E. (2010). What is value in health care? *New England Journal of Medicine, 363*(26), 2477–2481.

Serb, C. (2011, June). Effective dashboards: What to measure and how to show it. *Hospitals & Health Networks*. Retrieved from www.hhnmag.com/display/HHN -news-article.dhtml?dcrPath=/templatedata/HF_Common/NewsArticle/data /HHN/Magazine/2011/Jun/0611HHN_Feature_Gatefold-EffectiveDashboards

Shaha, S. H. (2010). Nursing makes a significant difference: A multihospital correlational study. *Nurse Leader, 8*(3), 36–39.

Shi, L., & Singh, D. A. (2014). *Delivering health care in America: A systems approach* (6th ed.). Burlington, MA: Jones & Bartlett Learning.

StateHealthFacts.org. (n.d.). Total number of professionally active nurses, 2017. Retrieved from www.kff.org/other/state-indicator/total-registered-nurses/?currentTime frame=0&sortModel=%7B%22colId%22:%22Location%22,%22sort%22:%22asc% 22%7D

Storfjell, J. L., Ohlson, S., Omoike, O., Fitzpatrick, T., & Wetasin, K. (2009). Non-value-added time: The million dollar nursing opportunity. *Journal of Nursing Administration, 39*(1), 38–45.

Wennberg, J. E. (2014). Forty years of unwarranted variation—and still counting. *Health Policy, 114*(1), 1–2.

Wennberg, J. E., Fisher, E. S., Stukel, T. A., Skinner, J. S., Sharp, S. M., & Bronner, K. K. (2004). Use of hospitals, physician visits, and hospice care during last six months of life among cohorts loyal to highly respected hospitals in the United States. *British Medical Journal, 328*, 607–612.

Young, D. W., Barrett, D., Kenagy, J. W., Pinakiewicz, D. C., & McCarthy, S. M. (2001). Value-based partnering in healthcare: A framework for analysis. *Health Affairs, 46*(2), 112–132.

Zelman, W., McCue, M. J., & Glick, N. D. (2009). *Financial management of health care organizations: An introduction to fundamental tools, concepts and applications.* San Francisco, CA: Jossey-Bass.

Appendix A

Common Financial Reports

Balance Sheet (Statement of Financial Position)

A **balance sheet** is a financial statement that includes assets, liabilities, and equity. It provides a snapshot of the organization's financial position at a specific point in time. Current assets include cash, accounts receivable, inventories, income taxes receivable, investments, intangible assets, and other. Property and equipment assets include property, land, buildings, equipment, construction in progress, and accumulated depreciation. Liabilities include accounts payable, accrued salaries, long-term debt, professional liability risks, and other. Equity is the difference between assets and liabilities.

Income Statement

An **income statement** is a financial statement that includes information about revenue sources and expenses at a specific point in time.

Cash Flow Operating Activities

Cash flow operating activities is a financial report that shows the cash inflow and outflow activities or financial stability of the organization.

Reproduced from Dunham-Taylor, J., & Pinczuk, J. (2010). *Financial management for nurse managers: Merging the heart with the dollar* (2nd ed.). Sudbury, MA: Jones and Bartlett Publishers.

Appendix B

Staffing Effectiveness: Scorecard

Evaluation of resources and their impact on outcomes is an essential attribute of cultures supportive of professional accountability. In this analysis, the human resources indicators reflect the inputs that produced the clinical outcomes on the right side of the table.

Human resources indicators	Clinical indicators		
Hours of care: % registered nurses	850 hours/62% RN	Number of patient codes	8
Hours of care: respiratory therapy	125 hours/2% RT	Patient falls with injury	2
Hours of care: social worker	50 hours/0.5% of patient hours	Medication omissions	30
Hours of support: advanced practice nurses	150 hours/10% APN	Medications late (more than 60 minutes)	55
% core staff	80%	Surgical-site infections	0
% registry staff	20%	Patient satisfaction with skill of nurses	88th percentile
Admission support	55% admissions completed prior to unit	Employee satisfaction	75th percentile

Appendix C

Evolving Metrics

In this table, the evolution of documentation from the paper and pen to the mass storage device or memory stick, associated expectations of the innovation, and the metrics to evaluate the innovation are identified. Each evolving change or innovation requires reconsideration of the expected metrics to accurately identify the real value of the innovation. Continuing to maintain the same expectations and use the same metrics for paper-and-pen handwriting as for voice recognition would be an incomplete recognition of the benefits of voice recognition; that is, the metrics must reflect the expectations.

Innovations to improve the process, quality, and storage of information have evolved over time. Each new documentation innovation is associated with new expectations and new metrics. The continuing challenge is to review and revise the expectations and then modify the metric to reflect the outcomes.

Innovation	Expectation	Metric
Paper and pen to record information/ handwriting	Documentation of the information that can be retrieved	Amount of paper/ink used Amount of time to document
Electronic writing/ typing	Documentation of the information Retrievable from paper file Legible Correct spelling	Amount of paper Cost of device/keyboard technology Decreased time for documentation
Computer programs for data/word processing to include storage devices 3-inch floppy disk Zip drive/CD/DVD Mass storage device/ memory stick	Large file data storage Portable High-speed access Retrievable from multiple access points File backup device Device compatibility	Data storage capacity Cost of hardware, devices, and software Size of devices Productivity; number of pages produced
Voice recognition documentation	Elimination of typing Device compatibility Increased speed for documentation	Productivity Number of pages produced Cost of recording/interface devices

Critical Thought, Leader Tip, and Scenario icons made by Freepik from www.flaticon.com; Callout icon made by Yannick from www.flaticon.com; Team Tip icon made by Chanut is Industries from www.flaticon.com

Leadership is a noble calling. In addition to meeting well-defined strategic objectives, leaders must also help their organizations make meaningful contributions to social issues, economic growth, and political stability. That's why effective organizational leadership plays a vital role in shaping our world. — Robert L. Johnson

CHAPTER OBJECTIVES

Upon completion of this chapter, the reader will be able to do the following:

» Understand the fundamental networks and organizations that support professional practice.

» Define ways that structure, profession, practice, and the individual relate and reflect contemporary and emerging structures for health care.

» Enumerate the elements of complex adaptive systems and the frames they create for professional practice.

» Outline the characteristics driving a stronger fit between the demands of the external environment and the internal organization facilitating health transformation.

» List at least five major elements of shared governance that advance professional practice.

» Identify problematic issues related to structures that support professional practice and the interface among those structures, individual behavior of the professional, and the requirements of the profession.

Navigating the Care Network: Creating the Context for Professional Practice

Leadership is about more than just changing things; it is about changing the world. Our world today is in the midst of a major social transformation, one that extends to every component of our sociocultural experience, including health care (Kaufman, 2011). All of this change is unfolding at a time when the principles and processes associated with complexity in systems and relationships are deepening our understanding of what it takes to make meaningful and sustainable change. These emerging concepts are often difficult and challenging to grasp, but are essential to the expression of effective leadership and the realization of meaningful change. The nurse leader at every level of the organization must be increasingly aware of these forces and incorporate them into both lifelong learning and leadership practice.

The U.S. healthcare system has come to the major work of transformation much later than other segments of the social and global community. It is now deeply in the throes of a dramatic shift away from a vertically oriented, tertiary care, pay-for-procedure, illness-focused system and toward a system that represents the social value of health, engages every citizen, and provides access to the most basic of health services (McClellan, McKethan, Lewis, Roski, & Fisher, 2010). It is this system within which the nurse leader operates and must now demonstrate competence in navigating its landscape.

CRITICAL THOUGHT

Leadership is about more than just changing things; it is about changing the world.

Although the political process within which transformation unfolds is noisy, messy, competitive, and challenging to work through, people of every political stripe recognize that the old system is no longer viable or relevant for the future. The design, structuring, funding, and operation of the transformed system will go through many iterations as we struggle to determine what works and what is sustainably effective. Along the way, the changes in the healthcare system will be clarified and validated through the process of experimentation, application, and evaluation.

Much of the effort to move toward a transformed generative healthcare model involves creating a system whose foundation is grounded in general access, service synthesis, critical health impact, resource and service value, impact on sustainable social health, and research-based evidence. Each of these small components of the broader dynamic shift in health care will transform the way in which the healthcare system is organized and structured and, ultimately, the way healthcare services are delivered. Although broad disagreement exists as to which strategies would best achieve this outcome, the effort to move toward that goal is clearly under way.

As the healthcare system works to recalibrate itself in a way that supports a more viable and relevant future, every clinical professional will play a role and has a stake in both the process and the outcome of this change. Changing service means adjusting the structure needed to support that service. Building access and equity into the service framework requires that every professional role incorporate equity, ownership, and engagement as an interdisciplinary design emerges. Indeed, interprofessional teamwork will serve as one of the nonnegotiable elements that underpins all efforts at building truly effective, value-based health care (Pauly, 2010) (**Figure 9-1**).

The structures that will best support this effort and the role characteristics of healthcare leadership that will guide its implementation focus on role clarity, autonomy with integration, professional team-based performance, shared decision making, and the means to ensure that the clinical work is resource effective, timely, value based, and works to advance the mission and vision of the healthcare system. Good clinical structure requires that leaders establish an expectation that evaluation will be ongoing, work will be continuously modified based on the evidence, and the structure necessary to support work will be flexible and

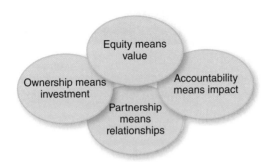

Figure 9-1 Four professional requisites

adaptable enough to meet the demand for change that evidence requires (Rapp et al., 2010).

As the vision and value of a health-based future unfold, become more clearly articulated, and achieve a level of agreement, new structure will evolve to support it. Historically, leadership was based on the idea that form or structure follows function; however, the reality is that both structure and function are dynamically intertwined and constantly work to affect each other. In **complex adaptive systems**, this relationship between the environment and the system is like a continuous dance; each brings something to the partnership, and both are dependent on the actions of the other. Ultimately, synthesis is the product of the actions of both environment and structure. Rather than overtly mandating deliberation, decisions, or work processes, structure should provide a framework for dialogue, deliberation, gathering, deciding, and acting on the part of the stakeholders. Leaders can then represent, through both their collective wisdom and their individual contributions, a synthesis between structure and decisions that demonstrates a sound reflective process, effective dialogue, evidence-driven decision making, integrated action, and coordinated effort in evaluating impact in changing practice. This network of intersections, interactions, and interrelationships is the place where the vast majority of the work related to deliberation, design, and doing occurs (Miller & Page, 2007; Robbins & Judge, 2010).

Structure is the format within which the dynamics of human interaction unfold. Structure either supports that confluence of activities or impedes it. Like the work itself, effective structure evolves and is constantly re-created to adjust to changes in the relationship between the environment and the organization. This relationship is not fixed but rather reflects all of the vagaries and dynamics of the continuous development and advancement of the human community. In turn, the mechanisms involved in this evolution focus on changing who people are and what they do. Organization calls for constant alignment among power, authority,

REFLECTIVE QUESTION

Is collective deliberation and decision making always better than individual decision making? The answer is "no"—but why? In which circumstances is collective deliberation wise, and in which circumstances is collective decision making not appropriate?

decision making, innovation, control, roles, work processes, and the mechanisms for evaluating effectiveness (Tolbert & Hall, 2009). These more fluid structures (networks) for contemporary healthcare organizations now necessarily consider the work of healing and health as a transdisciplinary, integrated, partnership activity. Such networks accommodate the efforts of each member directed toward reinforcing the commitment that all providers have to positively influence health. The people who populate these networks ensure that those who are served in the healthcare system realize the best values of health possible in their own life and experiences. The network structure supports this level of integration, collaboration, and the therapeutic interactions that advance the achievement of individual and population health.

Complex Adaptive Systems

Complex adaptive systems theory is grounded in research conducted in the fields of biology, mathematics, physics, and complexity science (Miller & Page, 2007; Schwandt & Szabla, 2013). Complexity science, as applied to human behavior, entails the study of various approaches to understanding the relationship among behavior, organizations, and the larger systems that form the context for work. Many of the underlying principles within complexity science that apply to human behavior and health care have been derived from research into behavioral economics, networks, evolution and adaptation, pattern formation, systems theory, nonlinear dynamics, and game theory. Although they share many foundational principles, each of these arenas of study focuses on a different element of complex patterns, networks, interactions, intersections, and processes that represent how systems behave.

Of special interest to the study of organizations is an understanding of sociotechnical systems and their impact on human dynamics. Because health care is one of the strongest representations of the interaction of social and technical forces, it is clear that a direct link exists between those forces and organizational design and performance (Resinicow & Page, 2008; Vakili, Tabatabaee, & Khorsandi, 2013). Although linear cause-and-effect relationships are certainly possible, the predominant relationships are nonlinear, complex, unpredictable, and highly interactive. In the past, failure to build organizational structures that recognize these complex sets of interrelationships and to design work models that reflect them has dramatically impacted work processes, patient care, quality, and health outcomes (Paley, 2007; Sturberg, Martin, & Katerndahl, 2014). According to complexity science, focus on either social (organizational) or technical (functional/applied) processes actually increases the unpredictable, uncertain, uninformed, unstable forces affecting systems, organizations, and work groups. In contrast, optimization in a system is a reflection of the strong "goodness of fit" between the human organizational dynamics and the technological functional processes that constitute the overall structure of the work environment.

The traditional compartmentalization in organizational structures has, paradoxically, contributed to their own decline in productivity and effectiveness (Rouse, 2008). That is, despite improvements in technology, organizations' systems, productivity, benefits, value, and outcome have diminished measurably over the long term. Unless goodness of fit exists between the structure of the organization, the dynamics of human behavior, and the processes and tools used to undertake work, any one of these elements taken alone can negatively diminish the value and outcome of the organization's work. This is especially true in systems where the predominant activity is knowledge work (Bennet & Bennet, 2010), and health care is clearly one of those arenas.

Structuring and organizing for knowledge work is one of the fundamental functional capacities of complex adaptive systems. This has not always been true, however, and leaders have not always been able to look at structure as a driver and source of support for behavior and work. Healthcare organizations are fundamentally driven by the application of complexity science, as evidenced by the breadth and depth as well as the variability of complex clinical activity and the intersecting impact of systems and structures that either support or impede this activity. The heavy interdependence associated with knowledge work also indicates the need for an organizational structure that supports and advances interactivity and integration of activities around a common user (the patient) in an environment where the outcome reflects the convergence of the effort of many stakeholders, rather than the efforts of any one stakeholder (Leon, 2011). Remember, clinical work is essentially team work, and the effort of any individual is successful only insofar as it "fits" with the activities of those with whom the individual interacts.

CRITICAL THOUGHT

The strong interdependence of all knowledge workers implies a powerful need for organizational designs and structures that support collaborative relationships.

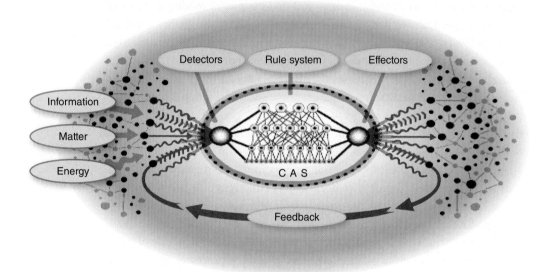

Figure 9-2 Complex adaptive systems network

Complex adaptive systems are living organisms with structures that very much share the same characteristics as biological systems (Ang & Yin, 2008). Although they are not directly linked and are certainly not exact replicas, these complex living systems serve as a model of an organization in which dynamic and interacting forces influence systematic and individual human behavior (**Figure 9-2**). In the past, the organizational structures of hospitals and healthcare systems presented organizations as great machines in a way that reflected the central themes of Newtonian physics (Kelly, 2005). Complex adaptive systems, in contrast, reflect a deeper understanding of complexity science and quantum mechanics as applied to human behaviors and human organizations (Palombo, 2013). This more living, fluid, relational approach to dynamic systems serves as a better metaphor within which organizational structures unfold and provides a more salient characterization of how complex systems actually operate (Bjorn & Persson, 2009). We can readily identify complex adaptive systems in our broader society. From stock markets, to societal networks, to information systems, to every level of biology of living things, the "adaptive" in "complex adaptive system" implies the ability to continuously and dynamically change when the relationship between the system and its environment shifts or is altered by either action in the relationship or circumstances beyond it (Marshall, 2011). Any such system contains a number of interdependent things, which are identified as agents. A complex adaptive system, then, is a densely linked, intersecting, and interacting connection of agents, each making its own contribution and acting both independently in making that

contribution and interdependently in linking that contribution to the indepen-
dent-but-related contributions of other agents (Shanine, Buchko, & Wheeler,
2011).

Placing Power Where the Action Is

In complex adaptive systems, power is relocated out of the formal structure and
is more closely aligned with the point-of-service decision making (Styer, 2007;
Van Beurden, Kia, Zask, & Dietrich, 2013). Although this sort of decentralization
of power occurs in many organizations, it is especially important in healthcare
systems. As these organizations begin to move away from a strong, clearly defined
hierarchical infrastructure and management-only-driven frame for decision making, and toward more clearly knowledge-driven and point-of-service models, they
will have to reformat their strategic, operations, and services processes to become
more effective (Malloch, 2010). Increasingly, short-term and responsive actions
must occur at the point of service in a way that can quickly adjust to changes in
strategy, tactics, programs, policies, and practice so as to respond more effectively
to the needs of the user.

Recalibrating decisions to be more effective means changing the design and
operation of the organizational infrastructure by moving structure and supporting decisions to the point of service (e.g., to support what nurses do with patients;
Box 9-1). In complex adaptive approaches, integration of services and provider

---

BOX 9-1 ORGANIZATIONAL STRUCTURE

The framework for clinical excellence begins with a structure that supports work processes that are fluid, flexible, and supportive of practice
excellence in the organization. Building excellence into the fabric of an
organization requires a supportive structure for caregivers as well as the
commitment and engagement of individuals to the work of healing. Today's nurses are seeking work environments in which excellent patient care
is supported, effective communication occurs, and caregivers are acknowledged for their positive behaviors and negative behaviors are addressed
quickly.

A structure that allows for change and supports efficient work processes
and satisfaction is essential to achieve the desired excellence. A flat, flexible decentralized structure is the hallmark of organizations that have
achieved Magnet accreditation and high levels of excellence (American
Nurses Credentialing Center, 2014).

relationships along the user's continuum of care requires that organizations recalibrate their infrastructure; revise service delivery, interdisciplinary relationships, and work processes that demonstrate the effective convergence of their efforts; explicitly recognize the relationship of effort to outcome; and evaluate practices and their impact to create sustainability.

These changes in the organizational structure and relationships call for full engagement of all stakeholders in the elements of design, partnership, accountability, and ownership of effort and outcome (Porter-O'Grady, 2009). The new frames of references and terms of engagement must reflect the measured effects on delivery, impact, and outcome, creating a clear relationship between the structure process and the outcome of work in a manner that represents their synthesis. As organizations move into digitally driven documentation and clinical systems, for example, their new ways of practicing, interacting, communicating, working, and evaluating impact will require modified vertical constructs, altered lines of authority, more localized locus of control, stronger unit-based collaborative models of deciding and acting, and better intersections and hand-offs among providers and with users (Anderson et al., 2013; Gunter, 2005).

Understanding How Clinical Work Changes

Emerging clinical leaders must be increasingly clear about changing aspects of the environment that suggest the need for a different calibration of work, workplace, and relationships (Davidson, Weberg, Porter-O'Grady, & Malloch, 2017). They must be willing to explore self-directed, seamless, and integrated mechanisms for practice, interdisciplinary relationships, delivery of care, and evaluation of relationships with users (patients). In today's just-in-time dynamic, current real-time practice serves as a baseline for changing next-time practice. Thus, for the practitioner, "the work I did today" informs "how I will do that work differently tomorrow." Much more horizontal and collaborative interaction around this work and how it is performed will be a fundamental expectation of all professional healthcare workers. Furthermore, individuals at the point of service will need to be more self-directed and will require more integrated and supported unit structures. Staff will need a stronger, more seamless, and horizontal set of relationships, interactions, and structures to support the collaborative point-of-service models of decision making, care delivery, and impact evaluation. These much more self-directed, relational structures will require a different management capacity and framework for advancing effective and integrated patient care.

SCENARIO

Mary Cumming, RN, is trying to implement the use of texting for communicating changes in patients' conditions between registered nurses and physicians. The medical and nursing staffs are both thrilled with the idea because it makes communicating so much easier and response times to changing conditions quicker and more efficient.

However, Mary is receiving a lot of pushback from the administration, legal, and quality departments because of the potential for Health Insurance Portability and Accountability Act violations related to confidentiality, consistency, and appropriateness. An additional problem is that younger staff are already texting in the workplace regarding patient care, whereas the more mature staff have not engaged with this practice and are not thrilled with the idea.

The shared governance leadership has asked you and your colleagues to form a texting task force to consider this issue and to discuss all the variables and complexities that influence making a wise decision about what to do. They have asked you to establish a texting standard for the organization and present it to the practice council.

Discussion Questions

1. Discuss the issue with your colleagues, sort through the complexities, and construct a protocol/standard that could be presented to the practice council.

2. With your team, present and defend the protocol/standard to your classmates by citing your supporting rationale and evidence.

Transforming the Nature of Clinical Work

In the contemporary transformation of health care, traditional approaches to clinical delivery of service are no longer supported. Instead, clinical work is being reenvisioned in ways that provide new support for a different understanding of clinical work and healthcare service, information management, definitions of quality, delineations of outcomes, kinds of clinical relationships, and the necessary intersections required to advance effective, evidence-based delivery of care (Chalkidou et al., 2009). These changes will no doubt lead to modifications of the traditional organizational structure, altering the numbers and roles of managers in significant ways. Furthermore, clinical leadership will become increasingly important as more point-of-service decisions, actions, and relationships form the centerpiece of the activities directed toward patient care (Eliopoulos, 2013; Solow & Szmerekovsky, 2006).

Indeed, a number of significant shifts are already underway in the healthcare realm that the clinical leader must incorporate into his or her understanding of leadership in practice:

- Tertiary care is slowly being deconstructed as the focus of health care turns toward providing a full range of services to every citizen in a much stronger primary-care-driven model.
- Accountability and value are requiring a much stronger goodness of fit among services around patient populations in a way that demonstrates a net improvement in the health of these populations.
- Digital technology is making it possible to create an increasingly portable diagnostic, therapeutic, and interventional environment, thereby making the provision of healthcare services increasingly mobile, fluid, and flexible.
- Organizational and management models are expected to reflect a higher degree of engagement and ownership of professional teams at the point of service because much of the ownership and the locus of control for effective decision making, practice, and measurement are being driven from that point of service.
- Increasingly, systems are competing on the basis of value and quality; these systems will be measured according to their health impact, the health status of the populations they serve, and their effective use of resources.
- The fundamental value of practice is no longer embedded in volume measures of how much an individual has done in the interests of patients. Instead, measures now focus on what difference and impact an action had and the efficiency and effectiveness of the relationship between the clinical action and the patient impact.

Many critical influences are driving these specific shifts in function activity and health care. In particular, changes in the environment are driving changes in the healthcare system. Creating a stronger fit between the emerging environmental conditions and the required organizational changes in health care will be important in healthcare services if organizations are to thrive and demonstrate their real value in the lives of those whom they serve:

- Change forces are now global; changes in the greater environment create the need for changes in the local setting. Clinical leaders must be aware of these environmental demands.

- The infrastructure and organization for health care must reflect a lean relationship between management, support, and providers in a network that represents their intense interaction and the need for sustaining their relationship.

- The healthcare financial model now reflects a strong emphasis on value rather than volume. Doing more does not mean doing better. The most effective mechanism for doing better depends on the judicious use of time and resources, as using more resources does not necessarily lead to better outcomes.

- The focus of healthcare system structures, processes, and evidence is reflected in dynamics that clearly demonstrate their impact, effectiveness, and significance in terms of levels of health. Enabling and sustaining health is a social, structural, and functional aim of all healthcare services.

- Evidentiary dynamics and improvement science guide practice within the context of a strongly interfaced digital information infrastructure. Human action and digital infrastructure are now so critically aligned that one cannot proceed without connection to the other.

- Clinical leadership is mostly derived from the point of service and is directed toward advancing decisions, relevant work action, changes in practice, and evidence of positive impact on health (Davidson et al., 2017).

REFLECTIVE QUESTION

Can behavior be changed in any sustainable way simply by inviting people to change? Reflect on your answer carefully. How does structure influence behavioral change, and how does the impact of structure on behavior alter your approach to undertaking change?

From a Medical Model to a Health Model

The medical model requires an organization; the health model requires a network (Liebler & McConnell, 2012). The very foundations of the structure that supports the creation of true and sustainable health are so different from the existing infrastructure that radical organizational surgery will be required to create an effective health model. This future healthcare delivery system, which is emerging now, will be characterized by a growing dependence on a primary infrastructure and, ultimately, a preventive health service structure. Primary service models require that health providers access the user earlier in the cycle of health—long before the traditional high-intensity, high-intervention, high-cost, illness-based system normally addresses the needs of patients. Just imagine the complexity and detail of leadership work that must be undertaken to create this type of truly effective health-based delivery system for the whole nation (**Figure 9-3**).

All of this transformation of health care is occurring within the context of a broader social shift—one that is predominantly user driven (McStay, 2010). In user-driven systems, individual users hold the primary obligation for access, use, accountability, and full participation in the actions that affect their lives and, in this case, their health at every level of society. User-driven models reflecting many of the principles of behavioral economics are emerging in support of this user-driven societal construct. Digitalization, information, and social networks have all created the underpinning for translation of these approaches into a broader sociopolitical model that reflects a growing preference for individual choice and social action. The natural and normative response to this sociocultural shift is greater intensity of interaction, integration, sharing, and social interdependence. The user-driven system is dependent on the individual being inquisitive about the nature of work and new ideas, vulnerable and open to the limit of one's own knowledge, inclusive of multiple points of view, and proactive in thinking about the future and what might become (Davidson et al., 2017).

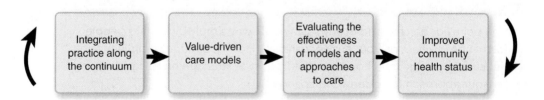

Figure 9-3 Contextual/environmental shifts

Ending Medical Separatism

Historically in the United States, medical practice was the predominant paradigm for the health system. Physicians were unilaterally directive and controlling, serving as the sole managers of medical and health decision making (Joint Commission, 1991; Mazur, 2003; Rivington, 1879; Taylor, 1974; Waddington, 1984). When unilateral control remained in the hands of physicians, broad-based, specific, and personal performance and outcome accountability were necessarily relatively subjective. In this model, the public viewed medicine as cloaked in the mystery of the incomprehensible, scientifically inarticulate, professionally protective, and compartmentally shrouded practices that could be communicated effectively only from one physician to another (Mazur, 2003). Further enabling this protective pattern were broadly permissive state medical practice acts that served to codify these mysteries and practices, protecting them from encroachment, question, or compromise. Over the years, a wide range of laws and regulations of every stripe emerged from the states that insulated physicians further from external influence or compromise and frequently shielded them from questions about and challenges to patterns of practice and professional behavior (Nelson, 2006a).

Although much of this environment has now changed as a product of the emergence of the digital age, the effort to break through the medical separatism shield remains challenging and fraught with difficulty. Nevertheless, the U.S. legal system is slowly chipping away at the brick and mortar of professional entitlement, protectionism, and social nonaccountability (Nelson, 2006b). Adding to the effort to ensure broader accountability is the increasing transparency created by the availability of digital information and the increasing access and knowledge available to people who seek it and use it to make healthcare decisions.

Value-Driven Health Care

Within the context of the digital age, the transparency and availability of information serve as daily reminders of the increasing user-focused locus of control (Granados & Gupta, 2013; Kamae, 2010). In a healthcare world where a digital infrastructure makes it possible for evidence-based, value-driven decisions to be made, conditions are now ripe for reorienting the delivery system to a much stronger point-of-service construct, thereby making it more functional, cost effective, and increasingly service sufficient (Aziz, 2006). The demand for quality now invariably includes a requirement for value, thereby focusing on the relationship between performance and achievement. The achievement of value from the perspective of the user requires a stronger integration and linkage between providers—one that clearly defines expectations from the perspective of the user. Individual provider-driven expectations for outcomes mean nothing to the user if

CRITICAL THOUGHT

In the near future, the U.S. health system will be reconfigured to focus on achieving health values for the community. The nurse leader must put value at the center of practice and ask the question "Why?" before responding to the question "What?"

they are not coordinated well and synthesized in a way that has an overall positive impact on the patient's experience.

This user-driven service model requires a stronger linkage and integration among the various healthcare disciplines, reflecting a deeper value and understanding of other professionals' contributions to the complex interaction positively affecting the patient experience. Achieving this organizational structure requires that interdisciplinary team-based relationships be constructed and that the work of the disciplines be integrated in a way that is mutually supportive. Equity and value of the unique contributions of each discipline at the point of service must be clearly articulated, and every element must converge around particular patient or population groupings in a way that demonstrates its ability to promote better health (Wright et al., 2008).

Traditional organizational structural models cannot support this much more fluid, flexible, user-driven, provider-related model of health service delivery. Consequently, these structures must be carefully deconstructed and newer frameworks created to help organize human action into a positive, systematic, linked, and integrated pattern of practices and behaviors that come together to make a significant difference in the health of those served.

To achieve this goal, the traditional, highly vertical, structured, department-oriented, silo-based models for clinical work must disappear as new constructs are created. The challenge here will be the confrontation of old rituals and routines, patterns and practices, that reflect the long history of people's accommodation to such structures and organizational frameworks. The demand for healthcare providers to be flexible, accountable, and evidence driven will create much noise in the system as the various professions navigate the process of building truly equity-based, balanced relationships. This transformation will be fraught with its own contentions and challenges as new kinds of relationships are configured (Malloch & Porter-O'Grady, 2009a). The resulting structural and political noise will result in some organizational unrest as clinical work groups attempt to move forward and confront those things that tended to move them backward in the past. However, new roles will unfold, new intersections and interactions will

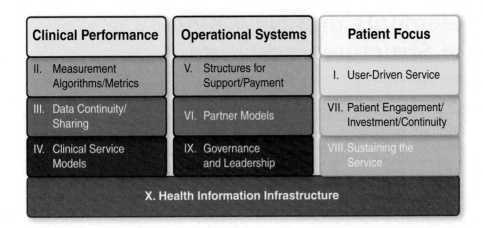

Figure 9-4 Accountable care systems

emerge, and interdisciplinary team-based dynamics will ultimately become the normative pattern of behavior at the point of service (**Figure 9-4**).

The nurse leader will be at the center of this journey to new relationships. Indeed, this leader will likely coordinate, integrate, and facilitate the journey just by virtue of his or her position and role in the new organizational construct. The nurse leader will be central to the shift because of the unique nature of the nursing role and the central position it holds at the point of service (Shifflet & Moyer, 2010). This leader will require a different focus with regard to his or her self-perception, role characteristics, and willingness to engage in the development of new models of relationships, interaction, communication, and clinical practice. More emphasis will be on the clinical leader, requiring the nurse with the bachelor of science degree to be better prepared in understanding these organizational shifts; interacting with other disciplines; more clearly delineating functions, roles, and expectations among the members of the clinical team; and more fully utilizing the digital tools necessary to facilitate and to advance the relationships and practices of these many professionals. The new structure will create a demand for the clinical leader to act as a catalyst and an agent of a much more collateral, collaborative, and horizontal set of relationships that creates an environment for shared decision making, mutual accountability, interdisciplinary practices, and integrated evaluation of the collective impact on the patient experience and the quality of health. This professional shared governance, shared decision making, and shared interaction will then become the framework for structuring the delivery of healthcare services in a much different way.

Elements of a New Kind of Structure

In a professional organization where integration partnerships are critical, vertical structures and command and control management methodologies are no longer relevant frames for organizational design (Zerwekh & Garneau, 2012). In such an organization, the unique contribution of each member of every discipline is critical to the value of the work and to creating the context for service. This criterion is especially important in a patient care environment. The wide-ranging number of disciplines having something to do with patient care must, at some point, intersect, interact, and create a convergence of effort that positively impacts the patient's continuum of care.

As part of this integrated professional organization structure, there must be a framework that supports activities at the point of service and sustains the clinical work processes of the professions in a meaningful way. Integrated value-based services across the continuum of care requires strong partnerships and collaborative foundations. Autonomous nursing practice is dependent on the following attributes for quality patient outcomes: accountability, professional obligation, collateral relationships, and decision making. These driving principles are essential to creating sustainable interactions among the professionals in a way that respects the contribution of each person, the value of each team member to the others, the interdependence represented in the collective work, and the commitment of each discipline to working with all disciplines in an integrated way that successfully addresses the issues of patient care. These founding principles of the organizational structure are commonly referred to as professional governance, and they create a framework that supports the various professions, their interaction, and their collective obligation to advance the interest of health care (Clavelle , Porter O'Grady , Weston , & Verran, 2016).

Several specific reasons explain why a professional governance organizational structure operates effectively in complex adaptive systems such as a healthcare environment. First, the sustainability of healthcare services fully depends on how the point-of-service professionals function individually and collectively. Complex adaptive systems are user driven and require the inclusion and ownership of users as the system addresses their needs along their healthcare continuum. The traditional healthcare model, with its compartmentalized, nonintegrated, unilateral role characteristics, no longer works to support the necessary relationships between disciplines in a way that advances the health needs of the user. Professional governance, by comparison, serves to build a stronger, more effective framework for operating in this more integrated environment (Bednarski, 2009).

Clinical knowledge is forever changing, growing, adapting, and improving. The structures of complex adaptive systems and the components necessary to operate effectively within them call for interdisciplinary equity and collective engagement with all stakeholders in the decisions and actions that represent the life of the system. In a complex organization, participants' willingness to take ownership of their roles amply demonstrates the organization's ability to adapt and thrive and respond to the call for change and transformation (Liang, 2013). In contrast, the compartmentalized, vertically oriented, and unilateral operating systems often found in traditional organizational models cannot support the kinds of relationships and infrastructures needed to provide and improve health care. Membership in professions implies a personal and collective level of ownership in the work of the profession. It requires a structure that recognizes and engages this ownership, invests in decisions and actions of the system, and provides the demand for and integration and coalescing of efforts at the point of service around the needs of those people whom the system serves (Batson, 2004; Jawadi, Daassi, Favier, & Kalika, 2013). This linkage from all members who contribute to this work operates at a level beyond simple and arbitrary hierarchical and position-oriented structures and decision models; that is, it favors a collateral, integrated, invested model of ownership and engagement in which providers and users converge in dynamic interactions geared toward meeting the purposes of the system.

Second, the emergence of knowledge organizations demonstrates that knowledge is not fixed or finite and does not operate simply as a capacity. Knowledge is a utility, so putting distance between the needs of knowledge workers and the supporting knowledge system and the design and structure of the organization can create significant impediments to the creation, generation, utility, and evaluation of that knowledge (Bennet & Bennet, 2010). In a value-driven health system, narrowly vertically controlled structures must evolve into multimodal, multidirectional integrated systems that can accommodate the growing need for interdependence, integration, and building the capacity for judgment on the part of knowledge workers. This growing importance of the character of the professions' collective work and the increasing complexity of healthcare delivery will require congruence and confluence among the organizational structures of healthcare systems, the contributions from and coordination of the professions, and collective effort in creating the conditions for sustainable health.

SCENARIO

Frank Taylor, RN, is the discharge planning coordinator on the geriatric diabetic services team. He is also chair of the service's Practice Council. Because of the changes stimulated by healthcare reform, the unit leadership has begun working on developing a continuum of care geriatric diabetic services model to ensure adequate services are available to these patients across their continuum of need. Focusing on this population's continuing healthcare needs requires Frank and his colleagues to reflect on which model of service might integrate the disciplines and link a variety of geriatric services in a model that would support geriatric diabetic patient care needs along the health continuum. The task appears complex and challenging, but Frank and his colleagues sense that it is the right priority to address.

Discussion Questions

1. Because this task will require interdisciplinary team deliberation and decision making, who should be at the table? How do those individuals reflect the continuum of care for this patient population?

2. Because Frank and his team are building a continuum of care service structure for a specific patient population, which services will be provided for that population? How do they reflect the continuum of care for this population?

3. What is the specific role of the nurse both in development of this continuum of care model and in its coordination, facilitation, and integration once the team has designed and formulated their desired approach for this population?

After responding to these questions, create a map of the continuum of care services for this population, then identify who the key players are at the various stages of the continuum and which services they might provide for this population.

For these complex adaptive systems to thrive and for the professions within them to cooperate within an effective shared decision-making framework, the following principles must be in place:

- The whole is always greater than the parts but also serves to define the parts.

- Every element and component of the system is a part of the whole system and must collectively support that system.
- A problem in any one part of the system ultimately affects the whole system.
- An effective user-driven system always operates from its point of service, where the system lives and where the forces converge to have an impact and fulfill the purposes of the system.
- All disciplines serve the user and/or serve someone who serves the user.
- In complex adaptive systems, form and function interact with each other; otherwise, they are not a dependent relationship.
- In a complex adaptive system, all members have ownership of their work and contribute to the system. The structure of the system provides opportunity for full engagement of the owners and representation of the stake they hold in the work of the system.
- In a complex adaptive system, the managers are facilitators, integrators, and coordinators of the system, providing resource support and enabling the stakeholders to be successful in fulfilling the purposes of the system.
- Impact and outcome are always the locus of value. Decisions and actions are directed toward fulfilling and supporting a systems value.

In evidentiary dynamics and improvement science, evidence-based health practices require a more intensive and relational set of interactions that form a fundamental part of the processes and work of determining, applying, and validating the value of health care and of services provided (Malloch & Porter-O'Grady, 2009b). This evidence of value and impact is provided through the aggregation and integration of data that support the contribution of each professional and the collective integration of those contributions in a manner that clearly demonstrates the difference they make for the patient's outcomes. This evidence-driven effort will not be successful unless it takes place in a context that supports these collective, integrating, collaborative trends and professional processes. In a digital infrastructure, information structures and data generation require that the collation, integration, and generation of relevant information reflect the evidence-based orientation of the organization and the processes and functions that lead to action and advance the evidence's impact in the system. The accuracy of the relational work of the disciplines, its effective integration, and its outcome in terms of the health of the population become the source point that demonstrates data utility, value, and impact on health (Parmelee, Bowen, Ross, Brown, & Huff, 2009).

CRITICAL THOUGHT

In the postdigital age, everything will move toward more control by the user. Such user-driven service structures will include health services. The nurse—indeed, all providers—now must focus on constructing patient-driven, user-friendly clinical models and service processes in a way that empowers users to manage their own health.

Third, in a continuum of care approach, no single healthcare organization can own, control, or unilaterally mandate all of the service linkages and connections necessary to fully serve a specific population at any level of adequacy. Partnership, relationship, interaction, and collective correlation of effort along the horizontal continuum, therefore, will be key to delivery of comprehensive and integrated population service. Increasingly, maintaining and improving the health of the population will demand relevant partnerships across the continuum of care, coordination and integration of the service continuum across partnerships, and shifts or changes in the comprehensive provision of services as the health demands of the population change. In turn, healthcare systems and the professionals within them must be fluid, flexible, focused, portable, and mobile. These organizational and behavioral characteristics will provide the contextual framework for the effective delivery of population health care and complex adaptive systems within which that service can be provided.

These three frames of reference enable shared decision making to emerge within a shared governance structure that supports it. Regardless of which terms are used to describe shared governance in an interdisciplinary environment, the structures must reflect the principles of partnership, equity, accountability, and ownership if the behaviors, practices, and clinical activities necessary to fully achieve an integrated, evidence-driven, valued-based health system are to be realized.

In complex adaptive systems, the interdisciplinary intersection calls for clinical reformatting of the organizational design in a way that supports decisions made and actions taken at the point of service. The place where the patient and the provider meet is the critical juncture in the healthcare organization; it is the centerpiece in the construct around which all structures in the system are built (Patlak, Balogh, & Nass, 2011). However, for this transformation to operate effectively, organizational structures must be reconfigured in a way that allows the system to actively operate from the point of service. While redesigning the system in this way, the following considerations must be addressed:

- The primary driving point of decision making in a complex clinical delivery system is the place where the provider and the user meet.

- Complex adaptive system providers are integrated in a collaborative and linked relationship that coalesces around the needs of the user.
- In complex service-based approaches, the provider and the user need freedom to make the necessary clinical decisions that will positively advance the user's potential for health.
- A full and appropriate range of data must be collected and made available at the point of service to support the collaborating decision makers, inform their clinical activities, and evaluate the impact and value of those activities.
- The purpose of organizational structure in a complex adaptive health system is to ensure that there are no impediments to the seamless interface of people, data, and systems supporting the value of health delivery at the point of service.
- Point-of-care linkage and interface in a complex adaptive system are structured in a way that ensures the engagement of all members, stakeholders, and users and encourages them to undertake relevant processes that result in meaningful and sustainable value.
- The complex adaptive clinical system is constructed from the core point of service outward into the system, such that all structures, formats, processes, supports, operations, and clinical systems serve the primary purpose of the organization as exemplified by the activities that occur at the point of service.

Clearly, the transformation of existing control-structured organizational systems alone will not suffice to configure or support an integrated, continuum-based, value-driven healthcare system (**Figure 9-5**). Although some might question the importance of structure in a complex system, it is central to creating a framework for patterns of sustainable interactions, intersections, and collaborative behavior as represented by the action of that system's members. The primary purpose of structure in a complex adaptive system is to provide a broader framework for the relationships and interactions among human systems behavior, digital systems behavior, patterns of supporting resource distribution, and the various elements of the system that inform the work done at the point of service. Indeed, the capacity to create sustainable patterns of interactions and behaviors depends on the veracity and consistency observed between the system structure and the interfacing human, with their synergy being essential to advance the patient along the continuum of health care (Molter, 2007). A well-defined and fluid system infrastructure provides the framework—that is, the vehicle within which best practices and behaviors are exemplified. This dynamic relationship between structure and action supports the essential range of

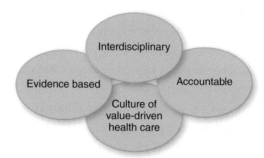

Figure 9-5 Value-based system drivers

necessary connections and behaviors that converge to contribute to the purposes of the system and the work that reflects them.

The Premises of Professional Governance in Health Care

Professional governance represents a structure of relationships in a complex adaptive healthcare system that enables knowledge work and advances the interaction, collaboration, and action of the disciplines in advancing health care. It serves to delineate role accountability, clinical performance expectations, and health impact of individuals, professions, and teams (Clavelle et al., 2016) It relies on the following premises:

- All structures must serve the purposes of the organization and directly support the work that fulfills those purposes. Any part of the organizational structure that does not specifically support the organization's purposes and work automatically impedes it.
- What actually goes on at the point of service defines the reality of the organization's life and reflects its real purpose.
- The power of every profession is embedded in its practice, and its practitioners represent the expression of that power. Organizations must be configured in a way that empowers the profession to fully express the obligations of its practice—that is, that allows them to demonstrate the critical attributes of autonomy:
  - Professional knowledge and skill
  - Defined area of practice
  - Desire for autonomy
  - Responsibility and authority to make decisions based on professional knowledge and skill and the ability to execute these in practice

- An environment that supports professional practice and respects the professional's individual and collective right to challenge circumstances and decisions
- Clinical value and impact are the product of the convergence of effort requiring the confluence of transdisciplinary work and the synthesis of the collective contribution of each discipline to impact health outcomes.
- In any knowledge-based system (such as a professional organization), all knowledge workers contributing to the value of the system have both the right and the obligation to fully participate in the life of the system—to own their own decisions and to control the factors that advance their work. Nothing in an effective complex system should ever arbitrarily or capriciously moderate, remove, or impede the rights and obligations of the knowledge worker to fully express the contributions that they make in partnership with other stakeholders in fulfilling the purposes of the system.
- In a multimodal system (multidirectional flow), emphasis is placed on interface, intersection, integration, and relationship. Consequently, a multimodal complex adaptive system must adapt to a structure that facilitates real autonomy through interaction, communication, partnership, collaboration, and the confluence of effort around a mutually derived value. Real autonomy has the following characteristics:
  - Structural and work autonomy: The worker's freedom to make decisions based on role requirements.
  - Attitudinal autonomy: The belief in one's freedom to exercise judgment in decision making.
  - Aggregate autonomy: Attitudinal and structural dimensions of autonomy, including the socially and legally granted freedom of self-governance and control of the profession without influence from external sources. Autonomy is viewed as self-determination in practice according to professional nursing standards.
  - Professional nurse autonomy: The belief in the centrality of the patient, when making responsible decisions both independently and interdependently, that reflect advocacy for the patient.
- Three major components of convergence in a structure are necessary to ensure structural integrity in the system: governance, operations, and service. In a complex adaptive healthcare system, each of these components is seamlessly linked to the others in a way that supports

the purposes of the organization, the needs of the service, and the values to which it is directed to advance (Klein, 2008). A complex adaptive health system's predominant purpose is to address the health of the populations it serves; it demonstrates this purpose at the point of service where the living community of the system needs to fulfill the values of the system. The provider–user relationship has the same constituents at the point of service as does the community–system relationship at the level of the systems environment. Therefore, the mandates, principles, processes, and values that govern the relationship of the point of service are precisely the same as those that govern the relationship at the environment–system level.

- An effective, complex, adaptive health system is an open system. It is characterized by seamless connections among decisions, decision makers, purpose, and value, representing essential membership in the system, ownership of its values, and full and active participation in its decisions related to strategy, tactics, goals, and practices directed to fulfilling the purposes of the system and obtaining its defined values.

- Management roles in the system reflect both stewardship and servant leadership. The primary role of management in a complex adaptive system is to ensure the existence of a seamless interface between the system's purpose and its resources, which are directed toward advancing that purpose and obtaining its full value.

- Accountability drives the work of professionals in complex adaptive systems and serves as the foundation for all knowledge work performance. Every member of a complex adaptive system has both rights and obligations that stem from the member's full participation in the life and activities of the system. Every member of the system must fully contribute to the extent of his or her capacity in a way that ensures that the system thrives and fulfills its essential value.

- Effective complex adaptive health systems provide a sustainable format for the essential work of the system. Every system creates its own structural scaffolding, which serves as the framework for the intersecting structures, processes, relationships, and behaviors in a seamless and intersecting dynamic flow whose effectiveness is continuously demonstrated by its fulfillment of purpose and advancement of value.

These premises underlie the foundational understanding of knowledge work in a complex adaptive health system. They also reflect the transformative notion of the relationship between components of the system and elements of its impact within the context of a shared purpose. A shared purpose is evident when the following criteria are met:

- The purpose evolves from the accountabilities sustaining it.
- The purpose is enhanced by its full accessibility to all members of the organization.
- The purpose grows along with commitment and ownership.
- The purpose becomes more central with staff involvement.

Furthermore, "systemness" redefines the relationship of the stakeholders to the system and to each other. The direction in which each of these premises points the system leads to the construction of a complex adaptive organization that operates synergistically to fulfill its purpose and to advance its value in the larger social environment.

The Individual and the Organization

In knowledge-work-driven organizations, the complex relationship among individuals, knowledge work, and team integration becomes obvious. Within this framework, the contemporary professional worker must demonstrate the fluidity, mobility, flexibility, and portability that characterize the emergent role of the clinical provider (**Figure 9-6**). Individual human behavior is a complex and dynamic process that emphasizes the different role each individual plays in the community of relationships. Nevertheless, knowledge workers can perform effectively only if leaders recognize the essential autonomy they need to make decisions and to fully act on those decisions. Without this sense of economy and ownership of the work, leaders will receive the benefit of only a small portion of the capacity knowledge workers have to offer in making a difference in their organization. The challenge for an effective knowledge-driven organization lies in successfully matching the knowledge worker with the work, with colleagues, and with the organization (Alvesson, 2004; Ung & Hye, 2013). In a complex adaptive system, the ideal situation includes careful onboarding and analysis of the relationship

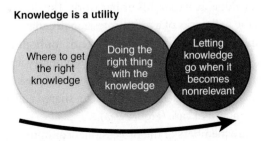

Knowledge is a utility

Where to get the right knowledge

Doing the right thing with the knowledge

Letting knowledge go when it becomes nonrelevant

Figure 9-6 Components of effective knowledge work

between the individual and the defined knowledge work expectations. Foundational expectations call for the individual to demonstrate full accountability for the products of work and specific competence necessary for the process of work.

Inherent in individual contributions is the strength of the enriching and supporting environment that facilitates individual contribution, inclusion, and demonstration of impact. This synergy of forces is essential for the activation of the various elements that might potentially advance the individual's role in relationship to the team and the organization. In complex adaptive systems, a fluid and dynamic interface among the network, the individual as agent, and the obligations of the impact on the outcome are critical to effectiveness. Clearly, the abilities of the individual and the capacity of the organization to use them are important factors that facilitate the goodness of fit and enhance the value of the individual in the work system. Knowledge workers have a unique role to play and specific contributions to make to the organization within the context of the knowledge they bring to the organization and the expectations that the individual and the organization have with regard to its applications and impact (Bennet & Bennet, 2004; Moerschell, Banner, & Lao, 2013). Clinical leaders must always recognize the critical nature of the notion of "fit" when assessing the work and role of an individual within the complex array of factors influencing and moderating that person's success.

All individuals in the healthcare organization must know that they are accountable for advancing the work of the organization. Through their membership in the work community, they must agree to participate in individual and collective deliberations and actions in applying the work of their specific profession, thereby advancing the patient care aims of both the profession and the organization. This partnership between individual and profession, and between profession and system, represents the critical context for ensuring fit, effectiveness, and sustainability. If individuals are not committed to the work of the discipline and the goals of the organization with regard to advancing the health of the community both serve, that lack of commitment will be readily apparent as nonenergy, lack of convergence with the standards and expectations for performance, objections to full participation in the work of the profession, and limited expression of the gifts and talents the individual brings to his or her work. The dramatic opposites of these behaviors are the hallmarks of a true professional: collaboration within and between the disciplines, effective use of data systems for both decisions and actions, grounding of practice in evidence, use of contemporary and relevant standards of care, professional nursing efforts that result in a positive impact on the patient's health experience, and demonstration of a shared collaborative relationship across the continuum of care (**Figure 9-7**).

Knowledge workers are members of the professional community; they do not merely "do a job." Despite shift work, hourly pay, and varying uses of

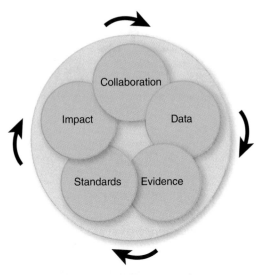

Figure 9-7 Integration of effort to advance values

protocol-based care, nursing work is knowledge work. As professionals, nurses must recognize that the expectations for their individual behavior are defined by the professional community in which they have the right to fully participate. When an individual has that right but not fully exercise it, the fault does not lie with either the profession or the organization. Instead, the individual professional has an obligation to make a contribution through his or her membership, as evidenced by his or her unique contribution to the work of the profession and the goals of advancing the health of the community. The profession always maintains the role of defining the parameters of practice; the individual does not. When the individual exercises his or her personal practice standards in a way that unilaterally operates outside the context of those standards defined by the professional community, that person holds the community hostage and fails to demonstrate personal commitment to advancing the work of the profession. If an individual gains insights and competencies that can advance the work of the profession, that person is obligated to join his or her effort with that of the larger professional community by incorporating those insights into the deliberations that define the parameters of practice for all community members. Failure to do so creates fragmented, discordant, and fractured clinical practices that fail to demonstrate an evidence-grounded effort to advance and improve clinical care.

Professional governance provides the opportunity for individuals to be fully empowered in the deliberations, decisions, and actions undertaken both by the professional and in collaboration with the team. The structure of professional governance clarifies and distinguishes between the accountability that belongs to the

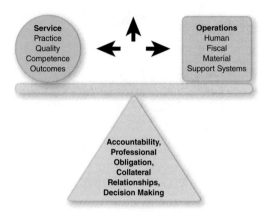

Figure 9-8 Clarity and convergence of system's accountability

system and the accountability that belongs to the practitioner. The structure of professional governance, reflecting the principles of accountability, professional obligation, collateral relationships, and decision making, clearly identifies the locus of control for practice accountabilities and for organizational (management) accountabilities (**Figure 9-8**) (Clavelle et al., 2016). The expectation of shared governance is that every individual will demonstrate personal accountability by fully engaging and participating in decisions affecting the practice of the profession in advanced clinical care for the patients (**Table 9-1**). If individuals do not render as much care for the profession as they do for their patients, both will suffer, and the standards necessary to truly advance the delivery of care become deficient. Collectively, the mechanisms available to each professional staff member act in the aggregate to

Table 9-1 Differentiating Between Responsibility and Accountability

Responsibility (20th century)	Accountability (21st century)
Process	Product
Action	Result
Work	Outcome
Do	Accomplish
Task	Difference
Function	Fit
Job	Role
Incremental	Sustainable
Externally generated	Internally generated

empower the profession as a whole in ways that demonstrate equity, value, and contribution. Behaving in a way that demonstrates professional characteristics, interactions, and demonstrations of impact creates the conditions for equity and establishes a framework for value-driven interdisciplinary models of effective patient care. The resulting congruence and partnership between professional caregivers and the shared decision-making structure through which they operate create a means for sustainable collaboration; cross-disciplinary, evidence-based practice; and ultimately a positive impact on advancing the quality of health of the community.

SCENARIO

The new manager on the surgical unit recently met with the unit's staff. In that meeting, she outlined some of her goals and objectives for the unit and spent a good deal of time talking about her leadership approach and her strong belief in full engagement and empowerment of the professional staff. The manager stated her belief that nurses need to be fully involved and engaged in decisions that affect their practice and that she would act as the facilitator of those decisions. The new manager made it clear that she saw her role not as directing or controlling decision making and practice, but rather as creating an environment that would enhance the ability of individuals to mutually engage each other in decisions that affected both their practice environment and their work.

The unit had a number of staff who had been on the unit for a significant number of years. The recently departed manager had been in her role for more than 25 years and had been generally directive and controlling of decisions. She set the agenda, determined the direction, gave specific indications of what she wanted to happen, and challenged the staff to meet organizational goals and objectives. The senior staff were a little uncertain as to how they should respond to these new management directions set by the recently appointed manager.

You have been appointed as the new unit team leader on the day shift and are responsible for helping all staff members become more engaged in unit decisions, participate more fully in planning and programs for managing patient care, and undertake meaningful change for the unit. Some of the staff members whom you are expected to lead have been on board for a number of years. Your challenge is to engage them in owning and participating in the decisions and changes for the patient care unit.

(continues)

(continued)

Discussion Questions

1. Which conversations do you need to have with your new manager at the outset before considering approaches that you might take to engage long-term staff for the unit?

2. What are some of the specific barriers to obtaining engagement and investment of your staff colleagues as they try to differentiate the more traditional management approach of the previous manager from the new manager's style of empowerment and engagement?

3. You have noticed a general lack of enthusiasm on the part of the longer term staff members to become involved and personally invested in changes that affect their practice and patient care for the unit. What are some of the steps you might undertake to address their capacity to engage new leadership approaches?

4. What are some of the behaviors you need to be aware of in your own leadership practice that might affect your relationship—either negatively or positively—with your staff colleagues as you attempt to engage them in decision making and change?

5. In your learning team, discuss and then role-play a conversation you might have with the long-term staff about their becoming more fully invested and engaged in a particular change process. How might you recognize their contributions, yet simultaneously challenge them to contribute to future changes? How might you demonstrate your recognition of their significance and value as well as their contributions and still challenge them to engage in future change?

 ## SCENARIO

Jan Connor, RN, BSN, recently completed a learning program on complex adaptive systems and their impact on patient care. While Jan got a tremendous amount out of the program, her greatest insight related to the necessity to integrate the efforts of all people in all parts of the organization around the process of patient care. She learned the critical nature of managing the intersections of patient care and assuring that the efforts of all the stakeholders worked in concert to positively impact the patient experience.

Jan slowly began to realize that much of the care offered on her unit was predominantly incremental and compartmentalized: The physicians did their diagnosis and treatment; the nurses coordinated the care team and rendered patient care clinical activities as required; the pharmacy, physical therapy, social work, and other professional services intervened in the patient care periodically as required or requested to meet specific needs. While all of these professional services were offering their best care, their efforts were largely uncoordinated and not specifically integrated around the unique and individual needs of each patient. Much of the work of the disciplines had become ritualized and routine without much team planning, interaction, or face-to-face time between providers.

Jan wants to change this model of care to more strongly emphasize the integration of clinical services, and more specifically intersecting care, in a well-communicated interdisciplinary plan of care that involves increased interaction, relationship, and engagement between the disciplines around individual patient needs. Furthermore, she wants to more fully engage patients in these dialogues so the care offered by the team can be more specifically aligned with the unique individual needs of each patient. Jan is not sure where to begin but she knows it is important to begin this work soon.

Discussion Questions

1. With whom does Jan need to discuss this situation first, and what should be the content of this dialogue?

2. Who is the stakeholder community here, and how should they be gathered around this issue?

3. What would be some of the first elements of discussion and dialogue with the stakeholder group? Are the questions and issues that the group should initially concern itself with more about the group's interactions or the group's relationship to the care of the patient?

4. For this interdisciplinary relationship to work and integration to interdisciplinary care to thrive, which three or four principles must all the disciplines agree upon as a way of guiding their work together?

5. With the colleagues on your learning team, develop a plan for this interdisciplinary group as its members begin the work of building their relationships with one another and implementing an interdisciplinary approach to managing and integrating patient care.

CHAPTER TEST QUESTIONS

Licensure exam categories: Management of care: ethical practice, professionalism, concepts of management

Nurse leader exam categories: Knowledge of the healthcare environment: governance; Professionalism: personal and professional accountability, ethics, advocacy, career planning

1. Building access and equity into the service framework requires equity, ownership, and engagement. What is the role of the professional nurse in this framework?

2. Unless there is a goodness of fit between the structure of the organization, the dynamics of human behavior, and the processes and tools used to undertake work, any one of these elements taken alone may negatively diminish value and outcome. True or false?

3. Discuss how the technology revolution has influenced interprofessional relationships and the role of the professional nurse in building collateral relationships across the digital divide.

4. Discuss how the healthcare world's digital infrastructure now makes it possible for providers to make evidence-based, value-driven decisions at the point of service.

5. Describe how the knowledge worker is essential to complex adaptive systems.

6. Clinical value and impact are the product of the divergence of effort requiring the deconstruction of transdisciplinary work and effort emphasizing the unilateral contribution of each discipline. True or false?

7. Describe how professional governance can create a framework for sustainable interactions, intersections, and collaborative behavior in an organization.

References

Alvesson, M. (2004). *Knowledge work and knowledge-intensive firms.* Oxford, UK/ New York, NY: Oxford University Press.

American Nurses Credentialing Center. (2014). *Magnet recognition program manual.* Silver Spring, MD: ANCC.

Anderson, R., Plowman, D., Corazzini, K. N., Pi-Ching, H., Lnderman, L., & McDaniel, R. R. (2013). Participation in decision-making is a property of complex adaptive systems: Developing and testing a measure. *Nursing Research & Practice, 16*(1), 1–16.

Ang, Y., & Yin, S. (2008). *Intelligent complex adaptive systems.* Chicago, IL: IGI.

Aziz, S. M. (2006). *Citizen e-readiness for digital society.* New Delhi, India: Corniche Books.

Batson, V. (2004). Shared governance in an integrated health care network. *Association of Operating Room Nurses, 80*(3), 493–512.

Bednarski, D. (2009). Shared governance: Enhancing nursing practice. *Nephrology Nursing Journal, 36*(6), 585.

Bennet, A., & Bennet, D. (2004). *Organizational survival in the new world: The intelligent complex adaptive system.* Boston, MA: Butterworth-Heinemann.

Bennet, A., & Bennet, D. (2010). Multidimensionality: Building the mind/brain infrastructure for the next generation knowledge worker. *On the Horizon, 18*(3), 240–254.

Bjorn, J., & Persson, P. (2009). Reduced uncertainty through human communication in complex environments. *Cognition, Technology and Work, 11*(3), 205–215.

Chalkidou, K., Tunis, S., Lopert, R., Rochaix, L., Sawicki, P., Nasser, M., & Xerri, B. (2009). Comparative effectiveness research and evidence-based health policy: Experience from four countries. *Milbank Quarterly, 87*(2), 339–367.

Clavelle, J. T., Porter O'Grady, T., Weston, M. J., and Verran, J. A. (2016). Evolution of structural empowerment: Moving from shared to professional governance. *The Journal of Nursing Administration, 46*(6), 308–312. doi: 10.1097/NNA.0000000000000350

Davidson, S., Weberg, D., Porter-O'Grady, T., & Malloch, K. (2017). *Leadership for evidence-based innovation in nursing and health professions.* Burlington, MA: Jones & Bartlett Learning.

Eliopoulos, C. (2013). Affecting culture change and performance improvement in Medicaid nursing homes: The Promote Understanding, Leadership, and Learning (PULL) program. *Geriatric Nursing.* doi: 10.1016/j.gerinurse.2013.02.015

Granados, N., & Gupta, A. (2013). Transparency strategy: Competing with information in a digital world. *MIS Quarterly, 37*(2), 637–641.

Gunter, B. (2005). *Digital health: Meeting patient and professional needs online.* Mahwah, NJ: Lawrence Erlbaum.

Jawadi, N., Daassi, M., Favier, M., & Kalika, M. (2013). Relationship building and virtual teams: A leadership behavioral complexity perspective. *Human Systems Management, 32*(3), 199–211.

Joint Commission. (1991). *Medical staff.* 99–119. Retrieved from www.jointcommission.org/assets/1/18/MS_01_01_01.pdf

Kamae, I. (2010). Value-based approaches to healthcare systems and pharmacoeconomics. *Pharmacoeconomics, 28*(10), 831–838.

Kaufman, N. (2011). Changing economics in an era of healthcare reform. *Journal of Healthcare Management, 56*(1), 9–13.

Kelly, K. (2005). *Out of control: The new biology of machines, social systems, and the economic world.* New York, NY: Perseus.

Klein, J. T. (2008). Evaluation of interdisciplinary and transdisciplinary research: A literature review. *American Journal of Preventive Medicine, 35*(Supp. 2), S116–S123.

Leon, R. (2011). Creating the future knowledge worker. *Management and Marketing, 6*(2), 205–222.

Liang, T. (2013). Edge of emergence, relativistic complexity and the new leadership. *Human Systems Management, 32*(1), 3–15.

Liebler, J. G., & McConnell, C. R. (2012). *Management principles for health professionals*. Burlington, MA: Jones & Bartlett Learning.

Malloch, K. (2010). Creating the organizational context for innovation. In T. Porter-O'Grady & K. Malloch (Eds.), *Innovation leadership: Creating the landscape of health care* (pp. 33–66). Sudbury, MA: Jones and Bartlett Publishers.

Malloch, K., & Porter-O'Grady, T. (2009a). *Introduction to evidence-based practice in nursing and health care*. Sudbury, MA: Jones and Bartlett Publishers.

Malloch, K., & Porter-O'Grady, T. (2009b). *The quantum leader: Applications for the new world of work*. Sudbury, MA: Jones and Bartlett Publishers.

Marshall, E. S. (2011). *Transformational leadership in nursing: From expert clinician to influential leader*. New York, NY: Springer.

Mazur, D. J. (2003). *The new medical conversation: Media, patients, doctors, and the ethics of scientific communication*. Lanham, MD: Rowman and Littlefield Education.

McClellan, M., McKethan, A., Lewis, J., Roski, J., & Fisher, E. (2010). A national strategy to put accountable care into practice. *Health Affairs, 29*(5), 982–990.

McStay, A. (2010). *Digital advertising*. Houndmills, UK/New York, NY: Palgrave Macmillan.

Miller, J. H., & Page, S. E. (2007). *Complex adaptive systems: An introduction to computational models of social life*. Princeton, NJ: Princeton University Press.

Moerschell, L., Banner, D., & Lao, T. (2013). Complexity change theory: Improvisational leadership for complex and chaotic environments. *Leadership & Organizational Management Journal, 13*(1), 24–47.

Molter, N. (2007). *AAC and protocols for practice: Healing environments*. Sudbury, MA: Jones and Bartlett Publishers.

Nelson, R. (2006a). Protecting patients or turf? The AMA aims to limit nonphysician healthcare professionals. *American Journal of Nursing, 106*(8), 25–26.

Nelson, R. (2006b). The politics of prescribing: In Georgia APRNs seek more authority. *American Journal of Nursing, 106*(3), 25–26.

Paley, J. (2007). Complex adaptive systems and nursing. *Nursing Inquiry, 14*(3), 233–242.

Palombo, J. (2013). The self as a complex adaptive system. *Psychoanalytic Social Work, 20*(1), 1–25.

Parmelee, P. A., Bowen, S. E., Ross, A., Brown, H., & Huff, J. (2009). Sometimes people don't fit in boxes: Attitudes toward the minimum data set among clinical leadership in VA nursing homes. *Journal of the American Medical Directors Association, 10*(2), 98–106.

Patlak, M., Balogh, E., & Nass, S. (Eds.). (2011). *Patient-centered cancer treatment planning: Improving the quality of oncology care: Workshop summary.* Washington, DC: National Academies Press.

Pauly, M. V. (2010). *Health reform without side effects: Making markets work for individual health insurance.* Stanford, CA: Hoover Institution Press.

Porter-O'Grady, T. (2009). *Interdisciplinary shared governance: Integrating practice, transforming health care.* Sudbury, MA: Jones and Bartlett Publishers.

Rapp, C., Etzel-Wise, D., Marty, D., Coffman, M., Carlson, L., Asher, D., . . . Whitley, R. (2010). Barriers to evidence-based practice implementation: Results of a qualitative study. *Community Mental Health Journal, 46*(2), 112–118.

Resinicow, K., & Page, S. (2008). Embracing chaos and complexity: A quantum change for public health. *American Journal of Public Health, 98*(8), 1382–1390.

Rivington, W. (1879). *The medical profession.* Dublin, Ireland: Fannin.

Robbins, S. P., & Judge, T. (2010). *Essentials of organizational behavior* (10th ed.). Upper Saddle River, NJ: Prentice Hall.

Rouse, W. (2008). Healthcare is a complex adaptive system: Implications for design and management. *The Bridge, 38,* 1–2.

Schwandt, D., & Szabla, D. (2013). Structuration theories and complex adaptive social systems: Inroads to describing human interaction dynamics. *Emergence: Complexity & Organization Complexity & Organizations, 15*(4), 1–20.

Shanine, K., Buchko, A., & Wheeler, A. R. (2011). International human resource management practices from a complex adaptive systems perspective. *International Journal of Business and Social Science, 2*(6), 6–11.

Shifflet, V., & Moyer, A. (2010). Staff nurse to nurse leader: Steps for success. *MedSurg Nursing, 19*(4), 248–252.

Solow, D., & Szmerekovsky, J. (2006). The role of leadership: What management science can give back to the study of complex systems. *Emergence: Complexity and Organization, 8*(4), 52–60.

Sturberg, J., Martin, C. M., & Katerndahl, D. (2014). Systems and complexity thinking in the general practice literature: An integrative historical narrative review. *Annals of Family Medicine, 12*(1), 66–74.

Styer, K. (2007). Development of a unit-based practice committee: A form of shared governance. *Association of Operating Room Nurses, 86*(1), 85.

Taylor, L. C. (1974). *The medical profession and social reform,* 1885–1945. New York, NY: St. Martin's Press.

Tolbert, P. S., & Hall, R. H. (2009). *Organizations: Structures, processes, and outcomes.* Upper Saddle River, NJ: Pearson Prentice Hall.

Ung, H., & Hye, K. (2013). Determinants of organizational citizenship behavior and its outcomes. *Global Business & Management Research, 5*(1), 54–65.

Vakili, G., Tabatabaee, F., & Khorsandi, S. (2013). Emergence of cooperation and peer-to-peer systems: A complex adaptive system approach. *Systems Engineering, 16*(2), 213–223.

Van Beurden, E., Kia, A., Zask, A., & Dietrich, U. (2013). Making sense in a complex landscape: How cynefin framework for complex adaptive systems theory can inform health promotion practice. *Health Promotion International, 28*(1), 73–83.

Waddington, I. (1984). *The medical profession in the Industrial Revolution.* Dublin, Ireland: Gill and Macmillan.

Wright, M. C., Phillips-Bute, B. G., Petrusa, E. R., Griffin, K. L., Hobbs, G. W., & Taekman, J. M. (2008). Assessing teamwork in medical education and practice: Relating behavioural teamwork ratings and clinical performance. *Medical Teacher, 30*(6), 1–9.

Zerwekh, J. G., & Garneau, A. Z. (2012). *Nursing today: Transition and trends.* St. Louis, MO: Elsevier Saunders.

Appendix A

Shared Decision-Making Requisites

- Shared decision making is point-of-service driven.
- Stakeholders are involved in their own decisions.
- Decisions are made where the work gets done.
- Staff focuses on population/patient care.
- Managers focus on empowering staff and creating a supportive work environment for staff decisions and practice accountability.
- The goal is to make the right decision as close to the point of service as possible.
- The structure of the organization is built to support point-of-service decision making and empower staff to decide and to act in a way that advances the exercise of their practice accountabilities.

Values

Values are expressed through behavior and can often be elicited from observation. It is important to see values congruent with shared decision making, in the

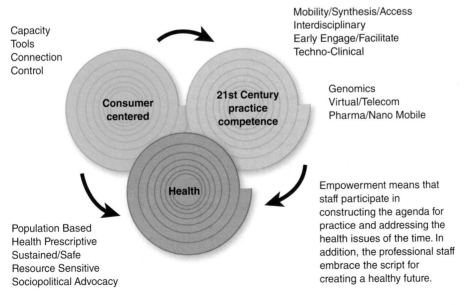

21st Century Practice-Based Accountability of the Clinical Staff

Capacity
Tools
Connection
Control

Mobility/Synthesis/Access
Interdisciplinary
Early Engage/Facilitate
Techno-Clinical

Consumer centered

21st Century practice competence

Genomics
Virtual/Telecom
Pharma/Nano Mobile

Health

Population Based
Health Prescriptive
Sustained/Safe
Resource Sensitive
Sociopolitical Advocacy

Empowerment means that staff participate in constructing the agenda for practice and addressing the health issues of the time. In addition, the professional staff embrace the script for creating a healthy future.

conduct of everyone, if shared governance is to work. Strong leadership plays a key role in nurturing desired behaviors. Committed leaders remain objective on the road to change, model empowered behaviors, and encourage and praise mature behaviors that correspond to a professional practice environment. The norms, rules, and rituals of the past are scrutinized to filter out those behaviors that do not match the envisioned environment. Initiating forums for discussion or an educational process may be necessary to bring a level of awareness to negative behaviors that have been ingrained in past practice and historical relationships.

The implementation of shared decision making changes organizational culture, which is defined by the organization's values. The organizational systems and structures assist in supporting the desired values and behaviors. Concurrently, values and behaviors shape the development of empowerment. As the organization moves toward changing values, the structure and support systems are redesigned to match those values.

Transformation of the culture involves diligence, careful planning, and time. Requisites for change include a firm, consistent set of values, long-term commitment, constant evaluation and reevaluation of each element in the system, and education of all parties to keep the vision alive. Role expectations affect behavior, as do skill and knowledge. Increasing knowledge and skills to support changing values and behavior is helpful. Effective leadership guides behavioral changes, which in turn change culture.

The change leader recognizes that empowerment is a journey for both manager and staff. Building change on a well-defined set of values with established parameters for behavior creates a firm foundation upon which to unfold new empowerment processes and actions.

Empowerment Values

- Confirm and commit to new values.
- Create a vision and enlist others.
- Role model management changes first.
- Promote and set expectations.
- Build skills along the way.
- Change structure and systems to support the new values.
- Define specifically the value of roles and link them to outcomes.

Values in Shared Decision Making

- Free-flowing information
- Mutual respect

- Diversity-infused collaboration
- Accountability for outcomes
- Empowered actions reflecting ownership
- Professional nursing model
- Shared decision making

Influence of Culture

It is important to acknowledge the influence of environmental culture on employees and work because of the powerful force it exerts. Staff are not typically familiar with management skills and practices. Historically, managers have assumed accountability for all the areas of the practice system, including many of the decisions regarding patient care. Structure and education are necessary to achieve the smooth transfer of accountability from managers to staff. In addition to unfamiliarity with managing groups and systems, staff members are likely to have some level of fear related to change; this fear represents another added element with which they must cope during a time of change. Many employees are afraid to ask questions and take positions. There often is an underlying culture that reinforces staff fear to initiate or act. This fear in a professional system severely hampers the organization's efforts to innovate and change.

Culture can either magnify or ameliorate the trepidation of caregivers upon encountering new expectations for accountability. For example, an individual, hearing encouragement to participate, might summon the courage to speak up in a meeting, only to be rebuffed. In such a case, a discrepancy exists between the system's message of openness and the old culture of suppression. The culture sends a contradictory message by communicating, "This is not the way things work around here." Culture begins to change when peer pressure is brought to bear to extinguish unwanted behaviors. Trust, or lack of it, has enormous consequences for organizations. Consolidated and integrated actions are needed to counteract the effect of old culture until it is changed to reflect more professional behaviors. Leaders who develop strategies to address changing culture are more likely to obtain their colleagues' support because of their willingness to take risks and confront past habits and practices.

Changing Culture

- Is possible with a plan and creative and committed leadership.
- Requires planned time for change to take hold; staff need to mourn losses, embrace the new.
- Leaders create conditions for desired environment.

- Feedback, immediate and continual, combats immature behaviors.
- Needs recognition of key moments, celebration, and evaluation of incremental changes.

Changing Historical Culture

- Is unclear or uncertain about quality.
- Inhibits creative behaviors; it values rituals and routines.
- Diminishes the loftiest goals.
- Challenges what is formally communicated in an organization.
- Can create a powerful influence.
- Requires laborious effort to alter.

Context for Staff Work in Shared Governance

- Authority and responsibility for professional practice is invested at the clinical point of service.
- Individual accountabilities and expectations are clearly delineated in role descriptions.
- Shared decision making is embedded in relationships and structures that intersect with role descriptions.
- Knowledge workers' decisions and participation at the point of service have prime importance to an organization's success.

One of the roles of the manager is to conceive ways to help staff recognize how their work integrates with the whole and perpetuates the mission of the organization. Placing competence, authority, and **responsibility** for practice at the point of service is the purpose of shared decision making. The manager explains how the proposed decision fits with the work of others in the organization. Authority and responsibility for professional practice are invested with the staff in shared decision making. The knowledge and skills that staff bring to their roles are applied to the goals of the organization. Knowledge possessed by these workers is a major medium of value and exchange in the workplace. Goals rarely get acted upon or fulfilled at the highest reaches of the organization. Instead, it is where the work is done, action is applied, and outcomes are achieved with the purposes and values of the organization that value is most clearly exemplified. Managers recognize this context and work to build the infrastructure that supports it and create congruent leadership behaviors that advance and sustain it.

Shared decision making facilitates the creation of an effective organization based on a new professional practice paradigm. When empowerment takes

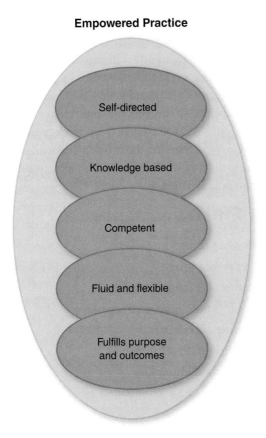

Empowered Practice

Self-directed

Knowledge based

Competent

Fluid and flexible

Fulfills purpose
and outcomes

hold, the relationship between work and the result of work is better defined. This reduces the waste of human energy and other resources because the more streamlined system focuses on integration, ownership, and outcomes. Structural characteristics that sustain the empowered processes of shared decision making and leadership also provide a framework supporting work and worker flexibility. This flexibility is key to the viability of an organization confronting change. Responsiveness to change comes from the successful integration and goodness of fit between the environment and the willingness of staff to alter and adjust their work. Relationship-based integration and interactions will strengthen the clinical system and promote continual improvement. Successful adaptation in the organization is accomplished through application of the competency-based framework supporting the shared decision-making process.

The structure and culture of an empowered environment enables individuals to combine autonomy and teamwork to fulfill expectations and roles and achieve the desired clinical outcomes. Shared decision making reflects the values espoused by the profession and the professional, while creating a real partnership between the professional and the organization. Effective shared decision making creates and maintains a structural format for facilitating staff participation in decision making and dialogue related to decisions, requirements, and actions related to clinical practice. Additionally, interactions are relationship based, which enhances information flow and communication—a fundamental indicator of success. Shared decision making asserts the staff's right to control their practice and make decisions that influence practice, thereby advancing the mission and work of the organization. The result is a more satisfying work environment, more fulfilled professionals, and a more successful organization.

The Power of Empowerment

- System is strengthened through integration.
- Role of every player is recognized.
- System design ensures effective functioning.
- Structure instills and sustains empowerment.
- Flexibility is key to cost-effectiveness.
- Order is a result of freedom to self-organize.
- Delivery system supports all disciplines.
- Optimal levels of performance and outcomes are achieved.
- Ownership cultivates desire for excellence.
- It depends on staff competence and judgment.

Empowered Staff Behaviors

- Openness to new realities
- Sound practice standards
- Engagement with the issues
- Emerging curiosity
- Ability to express concerns
- Commitment to competency
- Growing involvement
- Demonstration of creativity
- Willingness to change
- Clear sense of ethics
- Fundamental honesty
- Consensus seeking

- Structured risk taking
- Willingness to abide by consensus
- Increasing self-esteem
- Initiating partnerships

Appendix B

Shared Governance Staff Assessment Instrument

Instructions: This instrument provides you with an opportunity to assess your work roles and behaviors within the context of a shared governance organizational framework. You can then determine the impact of shared governance on your work and role.

To use this instrument, read the statements carefully. Choose your answer by selecting the response that best matches your personal feelings and the extent to which you agree with the statements. Mark the corresponding space on your response sheet. Please complete all the items and remember that you cannot be identified, so be frank in selecting the response that matches as closely as possible to your own view.

Part A: Survey

ACT>(1 = disagree; 5 = strongly agree)

1. Shared governance is a system of management that allows staff participation.   1 2 3 4 5

2. Shared governance changes the way we related to each other.   1 2 3 4 5

3. In shared governance, staff members make more decisions.   1 2 3 4 5

4. Our organization sincerely wants shared governance to work.   1 2 3 4 5

5. Staff will never let shared governance work here.   1 2 3 4 5

6. I believe in shared governance.   1 2 3 4 5

7. Shared governance is the key element in what keeps me working here.   1 2 3 4 5

8. Shared governance is just a fad that won't last long.   1 2 3 4 5

9. The processes associated with shared governance are consistent with my manager's style of management.   1 2 3 4 5

Part B: Attitudes

On a scale of 1 to 10, where 1 = lowest and 10 = highest, please rank the following:

1. I believe the overall commitment to shared governance in this organization ranks _____ .

   a. I believe the quality of interpersonal relationships in this organization ranks _____ .

2. I believe the overall leadership ability in this organization ranks _____ .

3. I believe the emphasis on effective problem solving in this organization ranks _____ .

4. I believe the concern for the process of shared governance ranks _____ .

5. My level of satisfaction with this organization ranks _____ .

Any question you do not understand or for which do not have sufficient information to answer, please leave blank.

Part C: Demographics

1. My current role here is:
   - ☐ Staff
   - ☐ Specialist (not a manager)
   - ☐ First-line manager (responsible for one unit)
   - ☐ Other manager (responsible for more than one unit)
   - ☐ Senior manager (responsible for entire division)
   - ☐ Other _____ .

2. My regular unit is _____ .

3. My regular shift is _____ .

4. I have worked this shift for _____ years.

5. I have worked for this organization for _____ years.

6. I work here primarily because: (Select only one.)
   - ☐ It is convenient.
   - ☐ The pay and benefits are good.
   - ☐ I find the work environment and relationships satisfying.
   - ☐ I need to work and this is as good a place as any.
   - ☐ I do not like working here.
   - ☐ Other _____ .

7. If I left here, it would be primarily because: (Select only one.)

☐ Offered a better job.   ☐ Unhappy working here.

☐ Better pay and benefits.   ☐ Spousal transfer or domestic situation.

☐ More work satisfaction.   ☐ Need a change.

☐ Other _____ .

8. I typically work ___ hours per week.

9. My age is _____ years.

10. My highest level of formal education is: (Select only one.)

☐ High school.   ☐ Diploma program.

☐ Vocational or technical school. ☐ University degree.

☐ Community college program.   ☐ Graduate degree.

11. I am currently taking classes: (Select only one.)

☐ yes   ☐ no

If yes, then please answer the following question. I am studying:

_____.

12. I have participated or been involved in shared governance in the following ways:

_____

_____

13. If my involvement in shared governance has been minimal or not at all, it is because:

_____

_____

14. Please comment about this questionnaire. Feel free to include anything you think will improve it or will address your issues more fully:

_____

_____

15. If you feel an important question was not asked, please write it for us so that we might assess it for future preparation.

_____

_____

Appendix C

Survey of Shared Leadership Practices

Instructions: This survey focuses on your manager's practices and whether he or she engages in behaviors that allow you to do your best work in a shared leadership organization. You may also use this tool to evaluate your council or shared decision-making group leaders, as well as to facilitate the group to do its best work.

Managers and leaders in empowered organizations purposefully engage in behaviors that enable staff members to effectively meet their professional accountabilities. The items in this survey have been carefully selected as representative of these shared leadership practices. Please examine each scenario and reflect on how characteristic it is of your manager or group leader by thinking about how frequently he or she engages in this behavior.

To the right of each scenario, you are asked to make two sets of ratings:

Actual: Your assessment of how frequently your manager is actually engaged in shared leadership behaviors

Desired: Your assessment of how often, to help you to meet your professional accountabilities, you would like your manager to use a certain shared leadership practice

Read each scenario and record both an actual and a desired assessment in the boxes located in the right margin of this survey.

Use the following scales in making your own assessments:

1. Always
2. Nearly always
3. Frequently
4. Half the time
5. Sometimes
6. Hardly ever
7. Rarely

		1 2 3 4 5 6 7
1. Actively seeks opportunities to help staff groups who are trying to achieve a goal. Eases groups through a process to accomplish goals. Remains neutral and helps the groups stay focused.	Actual Desired	☐ ☐ ☐ ☐ ☐ ☐ ☐ ☐ ☐ ☐ ☐ ☐ ☐ ☐
2. Recognizes that the work of groups is based on each staff member's attitudes, commitment, values, and skills. Enthusiastically works to bring these into the problem-solving process.	Actual Desired	☐ ☐ ☐ ☐ ☐ ☐ ☐ ☐ ☐ ☐ ☐ ☐ ☐ ☐
3. Clearly spells out his or her own facilitator roles and responsibilities to shared leadership groups.	Actual Desired	☐ ☐ ☐ ☐ ☐ ☐ ☐ ☐ ☐ ☐ ☐ ☐ ☐ ☐
4. Observes the various roles that group members play in groups, the methods that they use in decision making, and their communication patterns. Freely shares this information with the group to help them work together better.	Actual Desired	☐ ☐ ☐ ☐ ☐ ☐ ☐ ☐ ☐ ☐ ☐ ☐ ☐ ☐
5. Always protects individuals and their ideas from attack by other staff members. Through his or her own words and actions, communicates the dignity and the individual worth of each person and confidence in his or her ability to make a contribution.	Actual Desired	☐ ☐ ☐ ☐ ☐ ☐ ☐ ☐ ☐ ☐ ☐ ☐ ☐ ☐
6. Assists staff to develop their skills but does not direct or take responsibility for people's skill development. Encourages staff to try new ways of working without fear of failure.	Actual Desired	☐ ☐ ☐ ☐ ☐ ☐ ☐ ☐ ☐ ☐ ☐ ☐ ☐ ☐
7. Suggests to staff members the opportunities to expand their skills. Conveys to each person that his or her work is central to the success of the organization.	Actual Desired	☐ ☐ ☐ ☐ ☐ ☐ ☐ ☐ ☐ ☐ ☐ ☐ ☐ ☐
8. When coaching people, the manager's conversation makes sense, follows logic, and communicates that the manager is giving the staff his or her undivided attention.	Actual Desired	☐ ☐ ☐ ☐ ☐ ☐ ☐ ☐ ☐ ☐ ☐ ☐ ☐ ☐

9. Sets time aside to assist staff members and work groups to develop their skills. Is approachable and available when needed. Does not remain aloof.	Actual ☐☐☐☐☐☐☐ Desired ☐☐☐☐☐☐☐
10. Clearly communicates to staff members any performance problems. Focuses on solutions rather than problems. Does not become emotional or critical when confronting staff. Protects people's self-esteem when discussing performance problems.	Actual ☐☐☐☐☐☐☐ Desired ☐☐☐☐☐☐☐
11. Really listens to staff. Asks questions to clarify understanding of other people's points of view. Does not interrupt or let mind wander during conversations.	Actual ☐☐☐☐☐☐☐ Desired ☐☐☐☐☐☐☐
12. Stimulates reluctant staff members to participate by drawing them out and engaging them in active dialogue.	Actual ☐☐☐☐☐☐☐ Desired ☐☐☐☐☐☐☐
	Dimension I ☐ Total Score Actual ☐ Total Score Desired

	1 2 3 4 5 6 7
13. Works hard to gain support for his or her own ideas. Does not manipulate or withhold information to advance his or her own ideas.	Actual ☐☐☐☐☐☐☐ Desired ☐☐☐☐☐☐☐
14. Spends little time worrying about what the "higher-ups" are thinking. Bravely represents people and groups, even if the issue is unpopular with senior management.	Actual ☐☐☐☐☐☐☐ Desired ☐☐☐☐☐☐☐
15. Always puts people first. Is fair and consistent in treatment of others. Shows no favoritism. Helps people avoid conforming to social pressure at work.	Actual ☐☐☐☐☐☐☐ Desired ☐☐☐☐☐☐☐
16. Can be counted on to follow up. Keeps commitments and is respected for honesty. People know what he or she believes.	Actual ☐☐☐☐☐☐☐ Desired ☐☐☐☐☐☐☐

17. Solicits feedback about impact on others. Responds nondefensively to criticism about his or her own actions.	Actual ☐ ☐ ☐ ☐ ☐ ☐ ☐ Desired ☐ ☐ ☐ ☐ ☐ ☐ ☐
18. Communicates a leadership vision in a way that inspires others to act. Has a strong sense of purpose. Can describe how his or her own work and the work of others contributes to the achievement of the organization's mission.	Actual ☐ ☐ ☐ ☐ ☐ ☐ ☐ Desired ☐ ☐ ☐ ☐ ☐ ☐ ☐
19. Communicates self-respect and personal commitment to doing the best job possible. Openly works to resolve staff difficulties with his or her leadership style.	Actual ☐ ☐ ☐ ☐ ☐ ☐ ☐ Desired ☐ ☐ ☐ ☐ ☐ ☐ ☐
20. Sees power as available to everyone rather than as a limited resource. Assumes that staff members are accountable, with the necessary freedom and authority to do their work. Affirms the personal power of each individual.	Actual ☐ ☐ ☐ ☐ ☐ ☐ ☐ Desired ☐ ☐ ☐ ☐ ☐ ☐ ☐
21. Frees staff members to collaborate and share in decision making. Gets staff personally involved in the work to be done. Accepts staff's control of the content and pace of their own work.	Actual ☐ ☐ ☐ ☐ ☐ ☐ ☐ Desired ☐ ☐ ☐ ☐ ☐ ☐ ☐
22. Works hard to eliminate policies, procedures, or systems that interfere with getting the job done.	Actual ☐ ☐ ☐ ☐ ☐ ☐ ☐ Desired ☐ ☐ ☐ ☐ ☐ ☐ ☐
23. Translates the principles of empowerment to staff through role modeling and fulfilling expectations of staff decision-making groups.	Actual ☐ ☐ ☐ ☐ ☐ ☐ ☐ Desired ☐ ☐ ☐ ☐ ☐ ☐ ☐
24. Questions staff members regularly regarding their understanding and participation in empowerment activities.	Actual ☐ ☐ ☐ ☐ ☐ ☐ ☐ Desired ☐ ☐ ☐ ☐ ☐ ☐ ☐
	Dimension II ☐ Total Score Actual ☐ Total Score Desired

		1 2 3 4 5 6 7
25. Communicates to everyone well-defined and clear goals for change. Freely provides information for the duration of change.	Actual Desired	□□□□□□□ □□□□□□□
26. Establishes and then coaches staff work groups to manage the changes that affect their work.	Actual Desired	□□□□□□□ □□□□□□□
27. Ensures that change is not disconnected from organizational realities by obtaining the necessary commitment, people, materials, and financial support before embarking on change.	Actual Desired	□□□□□□□ □□□□□□□
28. Assists staff in using project management processes to set timelines, allocate resources, prioritize actions, and assign responsibilities.	Actual Desired	□□□□□□□ □□□□□□□
29. Helps staff identify specific and measurable outcomes to track successes and failures. Sees failures as opportunities for learning. Facilitates staff's progress in evaluating themselves and unit outcomes.	Actual Desired	□□□□□□□ □□□□□□□
30. Acts consistently on the belief that every person helps design his or her own work. Instead of the manager informing people of a better way to do their jobs, staff members are coached by the manager to invent their jobs themselves.	Actual Desired	□□□□□□□ □□□□□□□
31. Rethinks work from the customer's focus. Helps staff design systems of work that are flexible, reflect what customers desire, and provide meaningful work for each person that is cost effective.	Actual Desired	□□□□□□□ □□□□□□□
32. Encourages staff on different units, departments, or different shifts to organize their work differently, depending on skill mix, people availability, and so on. Recognizes that there is more than one way to "skin a cat."	Actual Desired	□□□□□□□ □□□□□□□

33. Avoids rigid or fixed ways of doing work. As conditions change, helps the staff reinvent the way work is performed as they learn and as the world changes.	Actual ☐ ☐ ☐ ☐ ☐ ☐ ☐ Desired ☐ ☐ ☐ ☐ ☐ ☐ ☐
34. Confronts negative staff members with the truth about changes in work expectations and empowerment activities.	Actual ☐ ☐ ☐ ☐ ☐ ☐ ☐ Desired ☐ ☐ ☐ ☐ ☐ ☐ ☐
	Dimension III ☐ Total Score Actual ☐ Total Score Desired

	1 2 3 4 5 6 7
35. Directly addresses objections to participation in decision making, countering staff members' objections to participation in this process.	Actual ☐ ☐ ☐ ☐ ☐ ☐ ☐ Desired ☐ ☐ ☐ ☐ ☐ ☐ ☐
36. Staff decision-making meetings are held at least monthly to deal with staff accountability issues.	Actual ☐ ☐ ☐ ☐ ☐ ☐ ☐ Desired ☐ ☐ ☐ ☐ ☐ ☐ ☐
37. Provides staff members with access to information, resources, and time, at least weekly, regarding organizational changes. Asks for response and feedback from staff.	Actual ☐ ☐ ☐ ☐ ☐ ☐ ☐ Desired ☐ ☐ ☐ ☐ ☐ ☐ ☐
38. Incorporates people from every staff role into discussions about patient care and staff work.	Actual ☐ ☐ ☐ ☐ ☐ ☐ ☐ Desired ☐ ☐ ☐ ☐ ☐ ☐ ☐
39. Communicates budget and financial information regularly to the staff. Keeps them informed about changes in finance affecting their work and lives.	Actual ☐ ☐ ☐ ☐ ☐ ☐ ☐ Desired ☐ ☐ ☐ ☐ ☐ ☐ ☐
40. Always helps the staff include financial or resource components in every decision.	Actual ☐ ☐ ☐ ☐ ☐ ☐ ☐ Desired ☐ ☐ ☐ ☐ ☐ ☐ ☐

41. Provides staff members with the time to attend staff decision-making group meetings. Actively and enthusiastically embraces their participation in staff decisions.	Actual ☐ ☐ ☐ ☐ ☐ ☐ ☐ Desired ☐ ☐ ☐ ☐ ☐ ☐ ☐
42. Shares with staff his or her own accountabilities and performance expectations as a manager. Seeks feedback regarding leadership performance.	Actual ☐ ☐ ☐ ☐ ☐ ☐ ☐ Desired ☐ ☐ ☐ ☐ ☐ ☐ ☐
43. Communicates activities, concerns, manager's role, and issues with the medical staff. Has an ongoing and regular pattern of communication with physicians.	Actual ☐ ☐ ☐ ☐ ☐ ☐ ☐ Desired ☐ ☐ ☐ ☐ ☐ ☐ ☐
44. Creates an environment where staff feel connected to their manager and feel great working and relating to him or her.	Actual ☐ ☐ ☐ ☐ ☐ ☐ ☐ Desired ☐ ☐ ☐ ☐ ☐ ☐ ☐
45. Unit runs well. Staff and management generally relate well. Together, they confront change positively, with good results.	Actual ☐ ☐ ☐ ☐ ☐ ☐ ☐ Desired ☐ ☐ ☐ ☐ ☐ ☐ ☐
	Dimension IV ☐ Total Score Actual ☐ Total Score Desired

Instructions for Scoring Your Self-Assessment of Shared Leadership Practices
Part I

The self-assessment of shared leadership practices assesses your managerial or leadership practices along four core dimensions, including whether they are productive. A total score for the survey can be computed as well as a separate score for each dimension.

1. Please total the scores on your self-assessment for each component, and place them in the boxes.
2. Add your dimension scores together to get a total score.

☐ Dimension I:	☐ Dimension III:
Facilitating and Coaching	Change Management
☐ Dimension II:	☐ Dimension IV:
Empowerment	Shared Leadership Principles
☐ **Total**	
Dimensions I–IV	

Part II

1. Total the performance scores from your staff survey.
2. Record your self-assessment scores in the appropriate boxes.
3. For each dimension, add together the staff actual scores for all of your staff surveys. Divide this number by the number of surveys returned. Enter the mean score in the appropriate box. Repeat this exercise for the staff desired scores.
4. Record total scores by adding the dimension scores you had recorded in the previous steps.

	My self-assessment	Staff actual	Staff desired
Dimension I Facilitating and Coaching	☐	☐	☐
Dimension II Empowerment	☐	☐	☐
Dimension III Change Management	☐	☐	☐
Dimension IV Shared Leadership	☐	☐	☐
My total scores **Dimensions I–IV**	☐	☐	☐

How does my staff feedback compare with my self-assessment of shared leadership principles?

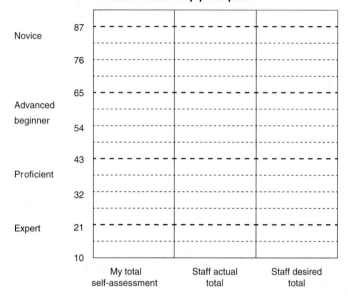

Instructions: Plot your self-assessment, staff actual, and staff desired scores for Dimension IV on the graph.

How does my staff feedback compare with my self-assessment of my empowerment skills?

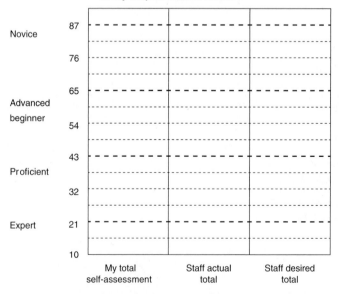

Instructions: Plot your self-assessment, staff actual, and staff desired scores for Dimension II on the graph.

How does my staff feedback compare with my self-assessment of change management?

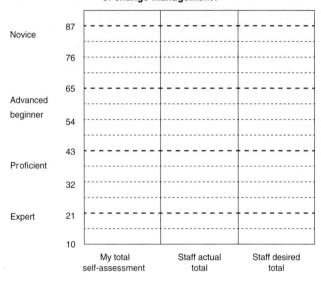

Instructions: Plot your self-assessment, staff actual, and staff desired scores for Dimension III on the graph.

How does my staff feedback compare with my self-assessment of my facilitation and my coaching skills?

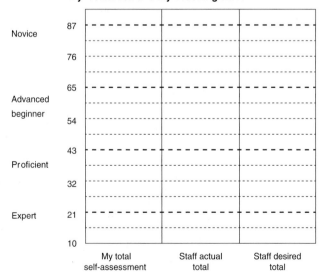

Instructions: Plot your self-assessment, staff actual, and staff desired scores for Dimension I on the graph.

> For us who nurse, our nursing is a thing, which unless in it we are making progress every year, every month, every week, take my word for it, we are going back. —Florence Nightingale

CHAPTER OBJECTIVES

Upon completion of this chapter, the reader will be able to do the following:

» Describe the essential components and responsibilities of the nursing professional role.

» List at least five options for career advancement.

» Outline the challenges and opportunities in creating effective continuing competence models for nursing.

» Understand the implications of violations of the nurse practice act and their relationship to continuing competence demonstration.

» Describe the challenges of integrating technology advancements into the role of the professional nurse.

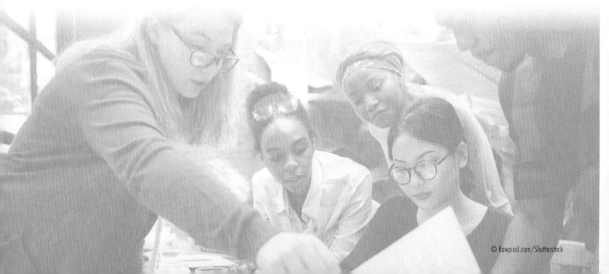

Chapter

10

Managing Your Career: A Lifetime of Opportunities and Obligations

"Nursing is a scientific process founded on a professional body of knowledge; it is a learned profession based on an understanding of the human condition across the life span and the relationship of a client with others and within the environment; and it is an art dedicated to caring for others. The practice of nursing means assisting clients to attain or maintain optimal health, implementing a strategy of care to accomplish defined goals within the context of a client-centered healthcare plan, and evaluating responses to nursing care and treatment. Nursing is a dynamic discipline that is continually evolving to include more sophisticated knowledge, technologies, and client care activities" (National Council of State Boards of Nursing, 2011).[1]

Once a nurse, always a nurse! Nursing is a calling. The nature of the caregiver calling focuses on the innate desire to offer comfort, to contribute to healing, and to alleviate suffering of another human. Once an individual has embraced the professional caregiving role of nurse by completing nursing education and obtaining a license, his or her DNA is altered forever: The call to promote health and care for the sick is ever present in varying degrees. No matter how many hours the nurse works, or even if the nurse does not work, the public expects full engagement in this role. In the United States, the public continues to see nursing as the most trusted profession in the country (Gallup, 2017).

The professional role and accountability of an individual who chooses nursing as a profession and a career can never be removed or used only in selected situations. The professional nurse is more than just a technician with good communication skills: The professional nurse has knowledge of the mission and vision of the organization, an understanding of the culture in which patient care occurs, and an appreciation of the outcomes and cost of care provided.

Understanding the dynamics of patient care services is essential for responsible use of resources. No one is better suited than the professional nurse caregiver to assess the effectiveness of patient care processes and to make recommendations for change when existing processes are no longer effective or when new evidence suggests better ways of providing patient care. Moreover, each and every nurse wants to work in the best workplace on earth (Goffee & Jones, 2013).

This chapter discusses the role of the professional nurse, the challenges of transition from school to practice, the plethora of career opportunities available to nurses, options to demonstrate career progress, the importance of nurse licensure, and ideas on the achievement of work–life balance.

Transition to Practice

The need to support the transition from school to practice for newly graduated nurses has received significant attention, given the high levels of nurse turnover in the first two years of practice. The increasing complexity of the healthcare environment and the reality that a new nurse requires support to ensure a successful transition from school to practice have led to the creation of formalized transition programs. The American Organization of Nurse Executives (AONE, 2010) has developed guiding principles for this process. See **Box 10-1**. These principles clearly outline the importance of a team approach to transition into practice, effective leadership support, willing and competent preceptors, the use and integration of evidence-based processes, stress management, intolerance for lateral violence, and continuing collaboration with educational institutions. In addition, the National Council of State Boards of Nursing (NCSBN, n.d.) has developed a tool kit and research project to further advance the transition process. These resources provide several models or approaches to creating an effective, evidence-based transition plan that integrates the regulatory requirements of state nurse practice acts.

The importance of transition to practice is further evidenced by a formal accreditation program: The American Nurses Credentialing Center Practice Transition Program (American Nurses Credentialing Center, 2014). This program accredits RN residency programs for new graduates, RN fellowships for experienced nurses changing clinical settings, and advanced practice fellowship programs. The criteria for accreditation center around the following domains:

- Program leadership
- Quality outcomes
- Organizational enculturation

BOX 10-1 GUIDING PRINCIPLES FOR THE NEWLY LICENSED NURSE'S TRANSITION INTO PRACTICE

Commitment for newly licensed nurses' transition into practice occurs across all levels of the organization:

- Senior leadership
- Nursing leadership
- Peers
- Medical staff
- Interdisciplinary colleagues

1. The nurse manager must achieve and is accountable for the leadership competencies that support the transition of the newly licensed nurse into his or her professional role.

2. Preceptors demonstrate professional competency and have a strong desire to teach, coach, and mentor.

3. Preceptors are prepared and supported by qualified nurse educators.

4. A structured transition into practice occurs in all settings and for all levels of academic preparation.

   a. A continuous focus on evidence-based techniques and outcomes that foster patient safety and quality is evident throughout the transition process.

   b. Widely diverse ages, ethnicities, backgrounds, and experiences of new graduates are taken into account when developing educational, social, and cultural supports.

   c. The transition process is customized to the specific individual and practice area.

5. Social affiliation supports are in place to mitigate the emotional stressor role.

6. Organizations have in place policies and practices related to zero tolerance of lateral violence.

7. Post-transition support programs are in place to aid in the retention of newly licensed nurses.

8. Collaborative relationships exist with academic institutions that support dialogue to address preparation for practice gaps.

(continued)

Expert: Individual + Content + Other Person + Issue + Organization + Community

The expert forms effective relationships in all areas impacting the work: the community, professional organizations, and internal teams and departments. The expert is able to address adversarial situations effectively, facilitate consensus building, and avoid unnecessary rumination about past events. The expert has fully integrated maxims and rules and uses them as references rather than road maps. The expert sees what needs to be done and then decides how to do it. The expert knows how to perform with calculating and comparing alternatives. The expert is able to form complex and competitive relationships in the most complex and challenging situations with successful outcomes. The expert routinely serves as a coach and mentor for those with less developed relationship skills.

Clinical Advancement

Specific career trajectories include development of expertise in patient care specialties, such as women and children, critical care, surgical services, home care, or community health. Nurses who have an interest in increasing their understanding of disease and health promotion processes for a specialty, increasing the use of evidence, and creating new evidence for practice are particularly well suited for clinical advancement. This pathway requires additional education specific to the area of interest, beginning with continuing education and then moving on to formal educational programs at the master's and doctorate levels. Master's degrees in nursing include these possibilities:

- Clinical nurse leader
- Clinical nurse specialist
- Nurse educator
- Nurse practitioner
- Nurse midwife
- Nurse anesthetist
- Nurse administrator

Doctorate degrees include these four possibilities:

- Doctor of nursing practice: practice emphasis
- Clinical practice
- Leadership practice
- Doctor of philosophy: research emphasis

Leadership Advancement

Management and leadership opportunities are embraced by nurses who seek to become involved in the creation and modification of the infrastructure in which patient care occurs and the implementation of new processes to improve patient care and nurse satisfaction (Habel, 2011). The motivations for advancing to management and leadership positions vary widely; however, the underlying reasons are usually steeped in the desire to advance quality practices, promote excellence, and introduce new ideas for a better work environment. Moving to a management position also requires new knowledge specific to facilitating groups (nurses, therapists, assistive personnel, and support staff) of individuals to achieve shared goals, change and innovation leadership competence, oversight of safety and quality practices and behaviors, creating and managing fiscal resources for both operations and capital equipment, and course correcting when current practices do not meet desired goals (Cipriano, 2011).

Informatics

Informatics and related technology roles represent another career trajectory for nurses. The design and implementation of complex documentation and monitoring systems require computer specialists and nurses as well as nurse informaticists to bridge the disciplines and ensure that the intended goals of effectiveness, efficiency, and safety are met. In addition, electronic monitoring of patients from remote locations is becoming more common and requires nurse clinical oversight. A nurse in these settings becomes a boundary spanner in ensuring team awareness of critical issues and facilitates effective handoffs and transfers and overall relational coordination among team members (Gittell, 2009). Another extension of telemedicine that represents a potential career trajectory for nurses includes school and childcare centers as a means to not only assess child illness but also allow parents to remain at work whenever possible.

Nursing Research

Nursing research is another career path for nurses. In many ways, research is a natural choice for nurses who have been educated to make clinical observations and to evaluate patient progress and outcomes. Learning to become a scientist and nurse scholar requires education at the doctoral level. The National Institute of Nursing Research (NINR, 2010) provides an online course for nurses who are interested in obtaining the practical skills and strategies for preparation as a principal investigator.

Interviewing for New Roles

As one moves through the skill acquisition and development processes, opportunities for new roles present themselves and require applications and interviews. See **Box 10-4**. At some point in most of their careers, nurses will apply for a new position. The risks in doing so include social, political, financial, environmental, and personal risks as an individual chooses to leave a setting in which the policies and practices are known, the salary is fixed and reliable, the physical setting is familiar, and collegial relationships are understood. Moving to a new position will change the individuals with whom the nurse socializes, the nurse's current abilities to manage policies and processes, salary and benefits, the specific location of the work, and the nurse's personal position in an organization. The process of taking risks and applying for a new position necessarily stretches the nurse's boundaries of current thinking and current practices and increases the potential for the nurse to make contributions to the nursing profession as well as to achieve personal growth. Reducing fear in favor of seeing risk as an essential part of creativity and progress further increases the nurse's professional competence.

BOX 10-4 PRACTICAL TIPS FOR CAREER ADVANCEMENT

First steps

- Critically reflect on professional skills, interest, and values.
- Identify areas of interest.
- Seek organizations and positions that fit with reflection and areas of interest.
- Develop a professional social media appearance.
- Record a professional voicemail message.

Resume

- Visually appealing
  - Font
  - Margins
  - Error free
  - Consistency in format and language
  - Comprehensive contact information

- Employers are looking for
  - Leadership
  - Teamwork
  - Communication skills
  - Problem-solving skills
- Brief objective
  - No more than two lines
  - Specific to job and organization; update if applying for multiple positions
- Education
  - Degree
  - Major
  - Graduation date
  - Institution name, city, and state
- Experience
  - Employer name
  - Employment dates
  - City and state
- Awards, honors, and professional affiliations are applicable
- Do not include
  - Marital status
  - Health status
  - Birthdate
  - References
- Cover letter
  - Address to a specific person in the organization.
  - Opening paragraph includes position applying for and what attracted you to the organization and position.
  - Body links individual attributes with job description.
  - Closing mentions interest in interview and directs reader to resume.

(continued)

- Interviewing
  - Prepare and rehearse.
  - Research the organization and be able to describe how you are a good fit.
  - Prepare a list of questions you can ask the interviewer.
  - Determine scenarios where you have past experience that addresses the needs of the employer and the information in the job posting.
  - Refresh yourself about the information in your resume and cover letter.
- The interview
  - Be as rested and refreshed as possible.
  - Dress in conservative professional clothing.
  - Minimize makeup, perfume, and jewelry.
  - Bring a portfolio with your resume, cover letter, questions for the interviewer, and any professional information you wish to highlight.
- Follow-up
  - Thank the interviewer for his/her time and consideration.

Data from American Nurses Association. (2017). ANA career center. Retrieved from http://jobs.ana.org/jobseeker/resources/; National Association of Colleges and Employers. (2017). Career readiness resources. Retrieved from www.naceweb.org /career-readiness/competencies/career-readiness-resources

Several considerations are helpful to make this a positive and rewarding move. Of course, there is always some risk in leaving one position and moving to another. Individuals in the current setting may believe you are abandoning them and your absence will leave an incredible void. Also, there is the possibility that you might not secure the desired position; that is, you might experience rejection. To eliminate or at least minimize the risks in applying for a new position, it is helpful to do an assessment of your motivation for seeking that position. Consider the following questions:

- What are you best at doing? The goal should be to get even better at what you do best.
- What do you most like to do? This could be different from what you are best at doing. Doing what you like is as important as doing what you do best and should be the focus of your career.
- What would you like to learn to do? Consider finding a mentor to assist in this new work.

- Which talents do you have that you have not developed? Being able to develop new talents should be a reason to seek a new job.
- What do others most often say are your greatest strengths? This helps you recognize talents that you might not see as significant.
- Which types of people do you work with best? Worst? Take the time to define those behaviors that facilitate or obstruct your success (e.g., analytical, organized, creative, timely, social).
- Which type of organizational culture brings out the best in you? Controlling and empowering cultures facilitate different work styles. Be sure to consider what works best for you.
- How could your time be better used in your current organization? Identifying certain work that you believe could be valuable should be identified and included in a new position.

Continuing Competence

Maintaining one's competence as a professional nurse includes supporting and enhancing role, licensure, technology, and relationship competencies. While there are many perspectives on professional competency, the professional nursing role deserves special attention (Sandberg, 2001). Each of these competencies is essential for full demonstration of the nurse professional role. The following definitions clarify what is meant by "continued competence" (Hospice and Palliative Credentialing Center, 2011):

- **Competence**: Application of knowledge, interpersonal decision making, and psychomotor skills expected for the practice role; having the knowledge, skills, and ability to practice safely and effectively; the potential ability and/or capability to function in a given situation.
- **Competency**: One's actual performance in a situation. It is "an expected level of performance that integrates knowledge, skills, abilities, and judgment" (American Nurses Association, 2015, p. 86). Competence is required before one can expect to achieve competency.
- **Competent clinical practice**: Situation-specific performance requiring an integration of skills, including cognitive, psychomotor, interpersonal, and attitudinal skills.
- **Continued/continuing competence**: The ongoing synthesis of knowledge, skills, and abilities required to practice safely and effectively in accordance with the scope of nursing practice; the ongoing commitment of a registered nurse to integrate and apply the knowledge, skills, and judgment with the attitudes, values, and beliefs required to practice safely, effectively, and ethically in a designated role and setting.

- **Culture of nursing competence**: The shared beliefs, values, attitudes, and actions that promote lifelong learning and result in an environment of safe and effective patient care.
- **Remediation**: The process whereby identified deficiencies in core competencies are corrected.

Professional Nursing Role

Professional role development is the "identification and development of strategies to facilitate a continuous process of maturation through lifelong learning" (Harper and Maloney, 2016, p. 64). Continuing professional competency following initial licensure as a nurse has been a topic of discussion for many years. Experts have struggled with the content, the areas of focus, and the manner in which continuing competence is determined. As nurses move through different career trajectories, their work becomes increasingly more specialized and difficult to assess using an exam similar to the initial licensure exam (Ulrich & Lavandero, 2014).

In addition, the ownership of continuing competency has been discussed extensively. Leaders have been unable to determine who should be accountable for continuing competency—namely, the state licensing agency, the licensee, or a combination of the agency and the licensee. While boards of nursing have the responsibility to ensure that licensees are safe to practice, experts believe that continuing competence is a shared responsibility between the board and the individual nurse. Once licensed, the nurse is accountable for maintaining current skills and knowledge.

While several methods have been explored for determining and measuring competency, state boards of nursing differ in terms of what they require of licensees. To advance this dialogue, the National Council of State Boards of Nursing (NCSBN) proposed the following principles to guide further development and initiation of pilot projects to identify methods and processes to determine and measure nurse competency (2005):

- Nursing regulation is responsible for upholding licensure requirements, and competence is assessed at initial licensure and during the career life of licensees.
- The individual nurse, in collaboration with the state board of nursing, nursing educators, employers, and the nursing profession, has the responsibility to demonstrate continued competence through acquisition of new knowledge and appropriate application of knowledge and skills.
- A culture of continued competence is based on the premise that the competence of any nurse should be periodically assessed and validated.

- Requirements for continued competence should support nurses' accountability for lifelong learning and foster improved nursing practice and patient safety.
- A continued competence regulatory model for nursing is evidence based and offers a choice of options to address gaps in knowledge, skills, and abilities identified by a diagnostic assessment.
- The regulatory authority for establishing continued competence requirements should remain with the state board of nursing.

These guidelines propose both regulatory and licensee accountability, define assessment frequency, and show integration of evidence.

Licensure Maintenance

In addition to nursing competence, a current license is necessary to practice as a professional nurse. Most states require regular fees, a current address, and notification of any criminal convictions as minimal requirements. A summary of each state's requirements can be found on the NCSBN website (www.ncsbn.org/boards).

In addition to the single state licensure model, 25 states have entered into a multistate licensure agreement in which nurse licenses are recognized across state lines when certain requirements are met. This multistate model allows a nurse to have one license in a primary state of residence and be able to practice in other states with multistate statutes, subject to each state's nurse practice act regulations. The compact allows for physical, telephonic, or electronic nursing practice for nurses with a multistate license. The Nurse Licensure Compact (NLC) defines primary residence in the compact rules and regulations. Sources used to verify a nurse's primary residence for the NLC include, at a minimum, a driver's license, federal income tax return, or voter registration. To be designated a multistate participant, the state must enact legislation to authorize the NLC and adopt administrative rules and regulations to support the compact. The multistate model significantly increases nurse mobility across the United States and decreases the cost of licensure fees when nurses practice in more than one state. The NLC also raises issues specific to different state requirements for criminal background checks and timely communication of discipline.

Technology

Another area of continuing competence for nurses is related to technology. The increasing numbers and types of available software, hardware, and medical devices create challenges specific to personal competence, selection of appropriate systems, boundaries between employer and personal systems, and the use of social media. See **Box 10-5**.

BOX 10-5 SOCIAL MEDIA

The term **social media** refers to the use of web-based and mobile technologies to turn communication into an interactive dialogue. Andreas Kaplan and Michael Haenlein (2010, p. 60) define social media as "a group of Internet-based applications that build on the ideological and technological foundations of Web 2.0, and that allow the creation and exchange of user-generated content." Social media comprise media for social interaction as a superset beyond social communication. Enabled by ubiquitously accessible and scalable communication techniques, social media have substantially changed the way organizations, communities, and individuals communicate.

Ensuring that one is competent with emerging technology is essential as more organizations implement electronic or digital systems for clinical patient monitoring and documentation. Indeed, the effective use of technologies is a core competency for contemporary professionals. What is equally challenging is deciding which technology is appropriate to add and which technology does not offer additional value to one's ability to do work effectively. To be sure, not every new hardware and software product is necessary or affordable for patient care services. Consequently, professionals are now required to develop competence in determining which products will improve quality and safety and, in addition, are affordable. Numerous frameworks for evaluation are available from both proprietary and state and federal agencies.

Another challenge for clinicians is to not become a "digital addict"—that is, to remember these devices and applications are simply tools to facilitate communication and data management. Devices are not intended to eliminate or dominate communication and relationship support. In fact, becoming too digital dependent can be counterproductive to the work of the healer, whose work is steeped in relationships (Thurston, 2013). Professional and patient relationships can suffer when digital devices and technology are overused.

Another technology challenge is the clear identification of the boundaries between employer and personal electronic products. The simplest approach is to completely segregate employer and patient information on one system and personal information and applications on personal computers or devices. Unfortunately, matters are not always that simple and straightforward. To expedite patient care, providers often access patient records from personal computers. While this is not inherently a problem, the confidentiality of patient information must be fully safeguarded by the nurse or user of the system. The blurring of the

BOX 10-6 SOCIAL NETWORKING DOS AND DON'TS

- *Do* use social networking as a tool to broaden your educational and professional horizons.
- *Do* use social networking to stay abreast of employer policies on social networking and Internet use.
- *Do* educate yourself about the privacy settings on websites you use.
- *Do* be aware that current and future employers may see what you post.
- *Do* know that your employer has the right to monitor your online activity on work computers.
- *Don't* use social networking sites at work.
- *Don't* reveal personal details such as your employer, your address, or your date of birth.
- *Don't* use your employer's email address or handle.
- *Don't* upload images or videos of yourself in a clinical environment or uniform.
- *Don't* discuss patients, visitors, vendors, or organizational partners.
- *Don't* talk about coworkers, physicians, your supervisor, or your employer.
- *Don't* discuss clinical events or news stories about your employer.
- *Don't* friend patients, even after they are no longer patients.
- *Don't* give medical advice online.

Data from Prinz, A. (2011). Professional social networking for nurses. *American Nurse Today, 6*(7), 30–31.

boundaries between employer, patient, and personal data has received significant attention in light of recent violations of patient privacy.

In particular, the use of social media (Web 2.0) has presented new challenges. Such interactive technology requires the development of principles for use that can guide professionals in maintaining professional boundaries and protecting patient privacy. Misuse of social media applications in which patient conditions were posted on the Internet and nursing unprofessional conduct was shared has resulted in the creation of guidelines to best use social media. See **Box 10-6**. This so-called dark side of social networking has raised worrisome issues in the healthcare realm. In the digital world, where boundary crossings between employer and personal technologies become possible, the challenge to ensure patient privacy and personal professionalism becomes significant and requires purposeful actions.

The following websites provide additional resources for the application and use of social media:

- NCSBN social media guidelines: www.ncsbn.org/Social_Media.pdf
- American Nurses Association press release dealing with social media and networking for nurses: www.nursingworld.org/ FunctionalMenuCategories/MediaResources/PressReleases/2011-PR /ANA-NCSBN-Guidelines-Social-Media-Networking-for-Nurses.pdf
- American Nurses Association Social Networking Principles Toolkit: www.nursingworld.org/socialnetworkingtoolkit
- Chris Boudreaux's social media policy database: socialmediagovernance.com/policies/

To be sure, there are many positive aspects of social networking, such as the opportunities for career building and knowledge sharing. Social networking worldwide helps nurses to think more globally and connect with colleagues who have similar interests. Most organizations and universities have created social media sites for sharing specific information on coursework, marketing, and outreach tools. Specific policies have been developed for appropriate use of social media.

Performance Management

Demonstrating competence has traditionally been a supervisor-driven process in which the supervisor documents the employee's perceived performance for the year. More recently, nurse professional portfolios and professional demonstration evaluations by the individual nurse have been recognized as more specific and comprehensive for the nurse's evaluation and overall career goals and accomplishments. Shifting from performance evaluation by a supervisor to performance demonstration by the nurse provides information that is more specific and more easily linked to documenting accomplishments and advancing career goals.

Examples of elements of a professional nurse portfolio for the annual performance review include the following:

1. Contributions to the care and safety of patients
   - Numbers, types, and outcomes of patients cared for during the year, including particularly challenging and complex patients
   - Interdisciplinary collaboration effectiveness identifying specific scenarios and the outcomes of the patient care event
   - New practice behaviors based on evidence

2. Continuing education

- Internal and required
- External and voluntary

3. Contributions to colleagues

- Coaching situations and the outcomes

4. Contributions to the organization

- Internal committee contributions and outcomes

5. Contributions to the community

6. Challenges encountered; support received from supervisors and colleagues

7. Assessment of personal life and work balance

- Required support and goals for the next year

Relationship Management

Another area amenable to performance demonstration is relationship management. Relationships in the digital age require a new level of discretion in forming and sustaining connections. Professionals should regularly ask themselves which activities they should be involved in and to what degree they should be involved. The management of vast amounts of information and increasing expectations requires new approaches for work efficiency and time management. When time is limited, purposeful encounters become critical to enhancing and extending relationships and to accomplishing work. Haphazard and unplanned encounters decrease productivity and delay goal achievement.

Interestingly, certain phrases or utterances can undermine one's message and image and should be considered as part of relationship management. Comments such as "I was wondering if perhaps . . . ?" or "May I ask you a question?" are not productive. Instead, you should ask the question directly and avoid the time wasters. The comments "Let's revisit . . ." and "Just to reiterate . . ." also do not add value, but rather provide an upfront acknowledgment that you have nothing new to add. Too much repetition can also be viewed as one-upmanship. The goal with effective communication is to be direct and get to the point.

Be proactive in managing your relationships as a nurse. Professionals proactively develop relationships with colleagues in each discipline impacting the healthcare experience so that when a need occurs, the established relationship serves to facilitate efficient solution finding. To be sure, relationships are built one encounter at a time, over time. When issues arise that need to be addressed by individuals from different perspectives, it is often too late to begin to build the necessary relationships. Such relationships need to be in place before they are needed to be effective in the accelerated technology world.

It is helpful to consider when to enhance, end, and avoid relationships. Individuals should consider enhancing and continuing any relationship that meets the following criteria:

- Supports the overall work of the organization and professional role
- Offers new ideas and information
- Is comfortable in engaging in discussions representing differing values
- Is able to challenge assumptions and beliefs
- Is able to see situations from another's point of view
- Portrays high personal integrity
- Accepts and incorporates feedback in a nonresistant and nondefensive manner
- Accepts responsibility for failure or errors
- Does not need reminders about responsibilities to patients or to other healthcare professionals to complete them
- Is available for professional responsibilities (e.g., required activities, available on clinical service, responsive to pager)
- Takes on appropriate responsibilities willingly (not resistant or defensive)
- Takes on appropriate patient care activities (does not turf patients or responsibilities)

Not surprisingly, the goals and purposes of relationships change over time. Few relationships remain the same year after year. In one's work life, relationships that were once mutually beneficial and facilitative of the work inevitably change when an individual moves to another location or organization. Also, the values and interests of individuals change over time, decreasing the common bonds and goals once shared. This is not to say that the individual is not valued personally but rather that the relationship as a means to effective work processes is no longer present. Consider ending relationships with individuals under the following circumstances:

- Values and goals are no longer congruent.
- The individual is no longer in your area of work interest.

Nurses are encouraged to avoid relationships in which individuals are known to have the following characteristics:

- Bully and harass others
- Engage in routine gossip
- Differ considerably in values/work processes specific to the respect of individuals and integrity
- Are unreliable and need constant reminders to complete work

Nurses should consider forming new relationships to accomplish the following goals:

- Reach out beyond traditional disciplines to disciplines outside of health care but within the community, such as school board members, legislators, and banking professionals to expand knowledge of the community.
- Gain greater insight into one's own discipline through university affiliation or membership in a national organization.

Course Correction: Life After Discipline

In the course of their career, nurses may exceed their scope of practice or commit an error that violates the nurse practice act and be subsequently reported to the board of nursing for investigation. Boards of nursing review complaints and determine if a violation has occurred and what the appropriate actions should be, ranging from dismissal, to letters of concern, to decrees of censure, to probation, to suspension, to revocation of the license.

The reframing of errors within the concept of practice breakdown sheds further light on the complexity of practice errors and the need for a more just approach. When a nurse is under investigation, it is highly stressful and emotional for the nurse. No nurse ever intends to practice beyond the licensure requirements; however, it does occur, and the sooner it is addressed, the sooner the nurse can refocus on acceptable practices. According to Marx (2001), practice errors may be one-time human errors for which discipline is inappropriate or a reflection of high-risk behaviors where the nurse practice needs to be assessed and remediated to ensure public safety.

Excellence Versus Perfection

In our quest for patient quality and safety, the best goals are those focused on excellence, not perfection. Human fallibility is an unavoidable, predictable component of being human. When mistakes occur and lead to negative results, we should give aid to those who are harmed and extend compassion toward the person who made the mistake (Marx, 2009). Further, Marx tells us that in the quandary we face when things go awry, there is a contradictory challenge: We must hold those who caused the event appropriately accountable (perfection) and make fixes to prevent future events (excellence). The goal for any nurse following a report and sanction to the board is for course correction or remediation to occur quickly and effectively. Punishment should be considered when the nurse is willfully negligent and has a pattern of unprofessional conduct.

Personal Balance and Health

Nurses spend their work life taking care of others and all too often forget or ignore the need for personal balance between work and personal life and do not make time for self-care. As the most trusted profession, nurses should set the example for health and self-care. See **Box 10-7**. Self-care should encompass physical, intellectual, emotional, social, spiritual, personal, and professional well-being (American Nurses Association, 2017). According to Shiparski, Richards, and Nelson (2011), it is dangerous to care for others before oneself. Such practices lead to unhealthy, de-energizing work environments. Also, the reality of compassion fatigue—an extreme state of tension and preoccupation with the suffering of those being helped to the degree that it is traumatizing for the helper—is experienced by those helping people in distress. Rest, tranquility, and stress management are essential for those working in the high-stress healthcare environment.

Carving out specific time for reflection and planning for the future can provide enormous support to the nurse's quest to thrive in a chaotic environment. According to Lawrence (2011), taking time for critical reflective practice positively impacts work engagement and decreases moral distress.

Minimizing negative thoughts is another strategy to enhance personal balance. Focusing on what could happen from a positive perspective, rather than a

BOX 10-7 NURSE SELF-CARE

1. Take time to think about yourself.

2. Get off the hamster wheel.

3. Say no without feeling guilty.

4. Avoid negative people and develop skills to extract yourself from contact with them.

5. Eliminate appointments that are not necessary.

6. Create a space for mementos that trigger appreciation, gratitude, and joy.

7. Go on an email diet. Answer email no more than three times a day; text only on the hour.

8. Take time to plan rather than just diving in.

9. Stop watching mindless TV/negative news media, especially before bed.

Data from Richards, K., & Nelson, J. (2011). Overcoming obstacles to create the optimal healing environment. *Nurse Leader, 9*(2), 37.

CRITICAL THOUGHT

With all of the demands and expectations of nurses, maintaining focus is often difficult. Ask yourself the following questions to support focus on your work:

- Do your patients' needs seem to blur across past and present patients? Keeping patients distinct from one another in your mind is a continuous challenge.
- Are you focused on completing checklists before you complete patient care?
- Is it difficult to remember a day when you completed what you wanted to do and handed off your patients to the next shift—and felt good about it?

negative trajectory, is more healthy and productive. According to Stringer (2011), when positive internal dialogue includes self-compassion, stress decreases. Nurses are typically hypercritical of their work, and in spite of the fact that the conditions for care and participation of patients in care are less than optimal, they blame themselves when the outcomes are not perfect.

Developing effective listening skills is becoming ever more challenging in light of the increasing amount of information from both digital and print sources that is thrust upon us. Good listening requires preparation and concentration, and includes sensitivity to both the context in which one is listening and the content of the conversations. Sensing both the location in which one is hearing information and the focus of that information increases the richness of what one is hearing. Listening to dialogue from caregivers in a patient room may lead to perception of a very different message than listening to caregivers discuss patient care in a conference room without the patient. The purpose and goals of the communication can be quite different.

Exercise, Nutrition, and Role Modeling

Two areas that are often challenging for nurses to self-manage are exercise and nutrition. Given that nursing work pertains to health and healthy behaviors among patients, the importance of role modeling takes on a new perspective for nurses. Specifically, nurses should not smoke, should manage their weight, and should participate in exercise on a regular basis. When a nurse is overweight and reeking of cigarette smoke, it is difficult for the patient and family to seriously consider education about smoking cessation and weight control. Health promotion is an ongoing career management activity that is important not only for role modeling, but also for minimizing the nurse's own risk for cardiovascular and respiratory disease (Flannery, Resnick, Galik, & Lipscomb, 2011).

Contributing to the Profession

The role of a professional also includes contributing to the profession through membership in professional organizations, coaching, mentoring, sharing new ideas, scholarly writing, and recognizing the accomplishments of other nurses. Each of these activities serves to advance the profession as a whole and the practices of other nurses.

Professional Organization Membership

The work and oversight of a profession necessarily need to be accomplished by its members. Rates of participation in professional associations have been traditionally low, with only small numbers of the profession engaging with these organizations. According to Reese (1999), the emerging workforce is not composed of joiners, and they do not become involved in professional organizations as members or leaders. Yet, the work of standards setting and expectations for outcomes for each discipline must still be accomplished.

Models of engagement that integrate the values of the profession and the generational values of all members in new ways and include multiple types of communication, multiple media sources, and virtual collaboration and decision making will facilitate increased participation in professional issue discussion. The emergence of sophisticated electronic, audio, and video technology has diminished the value of many face-to-face meetings and large annual gatherings. At the same time, this technology offers promise for rethinking professional

CRITICAL THOUGHT

Avoiding compassion fatigue is essential for all caregivers. Physical and emotional exhaustion can cause a decline in one's ability to feel compassion when taking care of others.

Compassion fatigue is a cumulative result of internalizing the emotions of patients, coworkers, family, and friends. It is about focusing on caring for others and not providing care to yourself (Richards & Nelson, 2011).

organizations and the way in which their work is accomplished. Use of discussion groups, chat rooms, and numerous other online tools can encourage all generations to become involved in the profession's activities. This transformation will be especially important in sustaining the core values of each profession and at the same time linking professions in a virtual world.

Coaching and Mentoring

Coaching or mentoring colleagues in informal or formal ways is equally important in role development. See **Boxes 10-8 and 10-9**. No professional can ever expect to be fully self-sufficient as an isolated individual. Feedback and counsel from trusted, competent colleagues specific to improving the quality of one's work life,

---

BOX 10-8 COACHING AND MENTORING DEFINITIONS

- **Coach**: One who assists others to develop viable solutions, prioritize them, and then act on them. A coach works to assist healthy individuals to achieve their goals; when behaviors are unhealthy, the coach refers the person to counseling. In this relationship, a partnership is being formed between the coach and the one being coached.

- **Mentor**: A wise and trusted advisor and confidant who guides others on a particular journey. A mentor provides support, challenge, and vision.

- **Mentoring**: The process of a more accomplished person assisting others to develop expertise and learn new skills based on the mentor's personal, untapped wisdom, reinforcing their self-confidence, supporting real-life situations, and sharing personal experiences when appropriate.

BOX 10-9 GOALS OF COACHING AND MENTORING

- Assist others to become more accomplished.
- Assist others to be the best they can be with their own knowledge, skills, and talents.
- Instill accountability and confidence in others so they can ultimately teach themselves.
- Assist others in using their own skills and knowledge to make decisions.

CRITICAL THOUGHT

The coach and mentor enable the mentee to find his or her own essence or presence of professionalism as a leader, to become a living vessel representing the character of a strong professional with vision, willingness, capacity, and commitment to the work of the organization.

learning to prioritize effectively, and advancing one's career are essential in the journey to leadership excellence. The role of the coach or mentor is designed to assist leaders in this work. The coaching/mentoring process provides the opportunity to continually seek open, honest, and timely feedback as well as an opportunity to share one's experiences and wisdom. Experts serve regularly in the role of both mentor and mentee; they are always giving of themselves to others and always learning from their interactions with others.

The need for coaching and mentoring is ever present. Initially, new nurses are best served by having a more formalized relationship with a single mentor and making a commitment to a structured process. As the individual evolves over time, less formal and structured support is needed. In turn, new and different levels of mentorship with different emphases are identified. To be sure, the frequency and intensity of mentoring change throughout one's career based on the role and context of the work. Experienced nurses often have mentoring relationships that are not formal; rather, the nurse seeks guidance from many mentors. When experienced nurses assume new roles or responsibilities, the need for more formal mentoring reemerges. At this point, mentoring focuses on enriching and accelerating the integration of the new work into the new role.

Coaches and mentors have learned that all healthcare work is based on relationships and that individuals exist and become successful based on their relationships with others. Successful nurses have also learned that relationships can either enhance one's ability to get the work done or hinder it.

For example, relationships may advance the work of the nurse and the organization, invigorate and renew one's personal spirit and passion, stifle the work of the nurse and the organization, or do nothing to advance or stifle one's overall well-being. Day in and day out, the quality of those relationships serves to either enhance or hinder one's effectiveness and can be considered the lifeblood of sustainable excellence. Coaches and mentors are well positioned to share experiences of both positive and negative relationships and, most importantly, to brainstorm with the mentee to identify future relationships that will support and enhance the work of leadership.

A coach or mentor begins by guiding the individual to develop skills in listening carefully, selecting reading materials, applying ideas, and observing. This effort always focuses on supporting the individual as he or she progresses in the personal development journey to discover and live in the role that is the best fit for the individual, the role in which he or she is most successful.

Individuals approach the coaching experience in different ways. Not everyone is always ready for coaching or to be coached; however, sharing ideas, wisdom, and insights is important for advancement of both individuals and the profession. Some individuals proactively seek out guidance and new ideas; they are adventuresome, visionary, and open to change and innovation. Others require more safety and security prior to a coaching experience. Some individuals remain quite skeptical and reluctant to seek or accept advice. As these differences suggest, prior to formal or informal coaching, it is important to determine an individual's comfort level with new ideas and change. This information can inform the coaching/mentoring process to facilitate more successes than failures.

Coaches or mentors do not encourage individuals to adopt their own behaviors or to emulate their behaviors. Instead, effective coaches or mentors realize that the world is changing too fast to repeat their successful behaviors of the past, and they work with the individual to develop their own style of leadership based on principles and values. Coaches and mentors realize that the future is very different from the present or the past and requires new and creative behaviors for success—behaviors that the mentee is empowered to create.

In addition to professional role behaviors, mentors and coaches typically address the nuances of professionalism specific to appearance, **attitude**, and conflict management. While who and what are professional is always open to discussion, some fundamental expectations specific to attire, communication, and attitude are

CRITICAL THOUGHT

- The mentor must avoid the tendency to create a clone of himself or herself in the mentoring relationship.
- The mentor must avoid moving from the role of mentor to that of therapist; the mentor focuses on guiding healthy behaviors, while the therapist focuses on correcting unhealthy behaviors.
- Communication between the mentor and mentee must be direct and honest, avoiding insincere or inaccurate messages.
- The mentee must be open to listen to new ideas but not to replicating ideas without careful consideration.

associated with the role of the leader. The professionalism of leaders is traditionally exemplified by the degree to which behaviors related to these three areas are demonstrated. Mentors can assist both emerging leaders and experienced leaders in ensuring the highest degree of professionalism through lifelong examination and reflection of these areas.

Attire

Much has been written about dressing for success and professional attire in the workplace. While each individual has developed his or her own understanding of which attire is or is not professional and appropriate for the workplace, the primary consideration must always be the customer, client, patient, or family to be served.

In healthcare organizations, the goal when selecting attire is to ensure cleanliness and control the spread of infections. Another goal is to minimize distractions to the patient and thereby support a patient/family-centered focus rather than draw attention to the dress of the caregiver. Clean, conservative attire best facilitates and supports an emphasis on the patient and family. Wild prints, exposed skin, excessive jewelry, and cologne shift the emphasis and attention to the caregiver rather than the patient.

The workplace should not be considered an appropriate venue in which to make fashion statements or display new fashion styles, expensive jewelry, or strong colognes. The first impression made with patients and their families should be positive, one in which the organization is portrayed as competent, safe, and focused on the work of patient care.

In the mentoring dialogue, mentors and mentees should proactively examine their attire and be assured that personal appearance is not a hindrance to effective communication. Wise leaders ensure their personal presentation to team members continually exemplifies the highest level of professionalism, not only as a mark of respect for one's individual reputation but also as a symbol of a good attitude.

Attitude

In addition to the physical presence of the leader, the attitude of the leader is important. Attitude—that is, the manner, disposition, or inclination as to how one approaches and reacts to situations—further defines one's level of professionalism. One of the simplest descriptions of positive or negative attitudes is often expressed from the perspective of a glass. Is the glass half full, indicating a positive, optimistic, and hopeful attitude? Or is the glass half empty, indicating a negative, pessimistic, and defeated attitude? A mentor can be helpful in assessing and reflecting with the mentee about attitude.

Managing Conflict

Addressing difficult situations filled with conflict is another topic for coaching and mentoring. These tough situations are often encountered in the provision of patient care—situations that are typically relational, recurring, and deeply rooted in personal values issues. Learning to understand and address the trials and tribulations of organizational life requires persistence, commitment, integrity, and a trusted colleague. For some nurses, the ability to respond effectively to difficult situations is straightforward and only minimally stressful. For others, confronting difficult situations seldom comes easy and is usually filled with angst and trepidation.

SCENARIO

Consider the following five categories of tough issues. Do any of these behaviors apply to you? Do you observe them in others? Use coaching and mentoring principles to address each of these areas of concern. Identify specific strategies and timelines to address each issue.

1. Lack of prioritizing

- Fails to meet deadlines
- Repeatedly breaks appointments
- Continually extends beyond the planned time allocation
- Overloads schedules

2. Poor communication

- Inappropriate interpersonal encounters
- Antagonistic and apologetic without results
- Is rude, interrupts, and reacts before all the information is provided

3. Lack of collaboration

- Manipulative, hard bargaining
- Avoids issues
- Tunnel vision

4. Lack of diversity

- Avoids conflict at all costs
- Does not want to consider other viewpoints
- Limits team membership to selected similar colleagues

(continues)

(continued)

5. Lack of integrity

- Fails to address the poor performance of a colleague who has become a friend
- Routinely offers insincere empathy
- Fails to identify the underlying issue before reacting

Coaches and mentors who are competent in addressing these situations can help the individual avoid unnecessary missteps and additional stress. No strategy can ever fully remove the stress associated with such issues; however, strategies to increase understanding of the issue, clarify who really owns the problem, and re-frame the situation can assist in more effective resolution of the issues. Seldom is a difficult situation limited to a single, specific event. Indeed, addressing difficult situations would be much easier to manage if there were no past history with an individual, one did not ruminate about the situation, and all recent experiences with the involved individuals had been positive.

The goal of the coach/mentor–individual relationship in managing tough situations is to transform difficult relationship problems into situations that are managed fairly and in which individuals are treated with decency in a timely manner. Coaches and mentors have experience with what has worked for them in the past, including recognizing the importance of timing, storytelling to address situations directly and humanely, recognizing that individuals are not always positive and receptive, delivering the message despite resistance, and managing responses. These experiences should always be considered informational rather than directional for the individual. The individual needs to integrate the information into his or her personal style and comfort level in a way that is humane, focused, and goal oriented.

Professional Information Sharing

Nurses are regularly involved in many patient care situations in which new and improved processes are identified, the application of new research works well, and, of course, certain practices do not work well. All of this information is needed by other nurses practicing across the profession. Learning to share these experiences early in one's career will greatly enhance patient safety and quality.

One way to share this information is professional writing. Several resources are available to assist nurses in learning to write effectively. Textbooks, workshops, mentors, and online resources all provide guidance in the writing process. According to Sarver (2011), the following tips are helpful in becoming a successful writer:

- Narrow your topic.
- Ask first. Check with a journal or website to determine interest in the topic.
- Follow author guidelines.
- Make a writing appointment with a successful author for guidance.
- Be willing to revise.
- Ask at least two people to review the manuscript before submission.
- Never think you cannot write; you can!

Another way to share information is through a presentation. There are two types of presentations, poster and podium presentations. Nursing conferences depend on you to submit the work you are doing for presentation at conferences. The first step in this process is often writing an abstract that is judged against other abstracts for acceptance at a conference. A good abstract:

- Is clear, concise, and follows all rules.
- Is free of grammatical errors and abbreviations.
- Fits with the theme of the conference.
- Has a dynamic title that denotes the findings of your work.
- Has a consistent structure that is easy to follow, such as background, purpose, methods, results, and conclusions.

Once the abstract is accepted, it is time to move forward to register for the conference, make travel arrangements if necessary, and prepare for the presentation. Regardless of the type of presentation, it is important to convey a professional appearance, following appropriate dress and decorum. For a poster presentation, designing and printing the poster is the first step. Follow the conference rules for poster size and format. Once at the conference, it is likely that a time will be assigned to stand at your poster. During this time, it is important to be able to give a brief overview of the poster to any conference attendees and be prepared to answer questions. The poster is often displayed for the entirety of the conference. The information should be clear and complete so that a viewer can understand the information even if you are not present at the poster. Contact information should be included on the poster so that the audience can follow up if there are questions or desire for further discussion.

If giving a podium presentation, a time will be assigned for the presentation. A template for the presentation and submission in advance of the conference are often required. Guidelines for a visually appealing presentation should be considered, and it is important to practice in order to be prepared with the content and to ensure that the presentation can be completed within the time limit.

Additional resources for podium and poster presentations include:

- Bindon, S. L., & Davenport, J. M. (2013). Developing a professional poster: Four "ps" for advanced practice nurses to consider. *Advanced Critical Care, 24*(2), 169–176.
- Kohtz, C., Hyper, C., & Humbles-Pegues, P. (2017). Poster creation: guidelines and tips for success. *Nursing, 47*(3), 43–46.
- Vanderbilt University Medical Center. (2017). Podium presentations. Retrieved from ww2.mc.vanderbilt.edu/evidencebasedpractice/43350
- Vanderbilt University Medical Center. (2017). Poster presentation resources. Retrieved from ww2.mc.vanderbilt.edu/evidencebasedpractice/50288
- Wood, G. J., & Morrison, R. S. (2011). Writing abstracts and developing posters for national meeting. *Journal of Palliative Medicine, 17*(3), 353–359.

Additional Thoughts

Information is dynamic and ever changing. Managing one's career requires thoughtful evaluation—on a regular basis—of career goals, interests, educational goals, and measurement of success as a professional. This chapter provides an overview of multiple areas for consideration in advancing one's reputation and contributions to the profession of nursing and to the healthcare system.

SCENARIO

Confronting internal negativity is an exercise that begins with identifying negative barriers to moving forward. In a small group, consider the following statements:

- "I've never been able to . . ."
- "It's too late for me to . . ."
- "I'm not very good with numbers."
- "I never have enough time to . . ."

Discussion Questions

1. Are these statements used routinely by any members on the team?

2. Are there other negative statements that are also used by team members?

3. Identify strategies to eliminate or at best minimize these statements both personally and in helping others eliminate internal negativity.

4. To present formally to a supervisor, work with two to three team members—using financial principles, value-driven outcomes, and multilevel measurements—to build a convincing case for decreasing negativity.

SCENARIO

The last 50 nurses hired have reported an unsatisfactory transition to their practice experiences. The majority of the negative responses focused on inadequate coaching and regular feedback. You have volunteered to form a team to explore the situation and provide strategies to decrease the dissatisfaction.

Discussion Questions

1. Which coaching practices should be in place that are specific to positive and negative performance?

2. How frequently should feedback be given? What should be included?

CHAPTER TEST QUESTIONS

Licensure exam categories: Management of care: professionalism

Nurse leader exam categories: Professionalism: career planning; Leadership: succession planning

1. Nursing professionalism is determined by

    a. The length of the nurse's time in the profession.

    b. The length of time the nurse has held a license in good standing.

   c. The role identified by the American Nurses Association and the state nurse practice act.

   d. AONE.

2. The transition from a competent nurse professional to a proficient nurse

   a. Requires time, experience, and knowledge.

   b. Occurs within the first six months of practice.

   c. Occurs in all nurses within five years.

   d. Focuses on the integration of the community into critical thinking.

3. Performance demonstration differs from performance evaluation on the basis of

   a. The time required for sharing performance goals.

   b. The role of the unit-based team with which the nurse works.

   c. The amount of salary increase available.

   d. The creator of the performance document.

4. Nurse licensure

   a. Is not a requirement for continuing education credits.

   b. Is not affected when a nurse is involved in a system error.

   c. Is designed to inform the public that a nurse is safe to practice.

   d. Is suspended when a nurse has multistate privileges.

5. Career trajectories are

   a. Limited by geographic regions.

   b. Defined by local organizations.

    c. Nearly unlimited for nurses.

    d. Highly overestimated for nursing professionals.

6. Continuing competence for professional nurses

    a. Includes integration of skills, including cognitive, psychomotor, interpersonal, and attitude.

    b. Is an accountability assumed by the nursing board.

    c. Is an accountability assumed by the individual licensed nurse.

    d. Is not related to annual performance reviews.

7. Technology competence is

    a. An emerging and essential requirement for competent nurses.

    b. Expected of all nurses providing patient care.

    c. Variable across organizations.

    d. Not regulated by nurse practice acts.

8. Scholarly writing is

    a. Required for graduation from a bachelor of science degree in nursing program.

    b. A challenge based on the style of formatting required by the journal in which the article will be published.

    c. An expectation in nurses' annual performance reviews.

    d. Evidence of commitment to advancement of the profession.

9. Membership in a professional organization

    a. Is optional for a nurse professional in a rural setting.

    b. Is a reflection of commitment to support professional standards review and development.

c. Is seldom effective in supporting professional practice issues.

d. Can be expensive, but it is worth the investment.

10. Discontinuing relationships

    a. Is appropriate in managing professional relationships.

    b. Is unprofessional conduct.

    c. Is best accomplished with a coach or mentor as intermediary.

    d. Increases the amount of conflict a professional nurse must deal with.

References

American Nurses Association. (2015). *Nursing scope and standards of practice* (3rd ed.). Silver Spring, MD: ANA.

American Nurses Association. (2017). Healthy nurse, healthy nation. Retrieved from www.nursingworld.org/healthynurse

American Nurses Credentialing Center. (2014). Practice Transition Accreditation Program. Silver Spring, MD: ANCC.

American Organization of Nurse Executives. (2010). AONE guiding principles for the newly licensed nurse's transition into practice. Retrieved from www.aone.org /resources/newly-licensed-nurses-transition-practice

Benner, P. (2004). Using the Dreyfus model of skill acquisition to describe and interpret skill acquisition and clinical judgment in nursing practice and education. *Bulletin of Science, Technology & Society, 24*(3), 188–199.

Cipriano, P. F. (2011). Move up to the role of nurse manager. *American Nurse Today, 6*(3), 61–62.

Dreyfus, H. L., & Dreyfus, S. E. (2004). The ethical implications of the five-stage skill-acquisition model. *Bulletin of Science, Technology and Society, 24*(3), 251–264.

Flannery, K., Resnick, B., Galik, E., & Lipscomb, J. (2011). Physical activity and diet-focused worksite health promotion for direct care workers. *Journal of Nursing Administration, 41*(6), 245–247.

Gallup. (2017). Honesty/ethics in professions. Retrieved from www.gallup.com /poll/1654/honesty-ethics-professions.aspx

Gittell, J. (2009). *High performance healthcare*. New York, NY: McGraw-Hill.

Goffee, R., & Jones, G. (2013). Creating the best workplace on earth. *Harvard Business Review, 211*(5), 99–106.

Habel, M. (2011). Spread your wings: RNs have what it takes to be effective leaders. *CE Nurse*, 52–57.

Harper, M. G., & Maloney, P. (2016). *Nursing professional development: Scope and standards of practice* (3rd ed.). Chicago, IL: Association for Nursing Professional Development.

Hendren, R. (2011, November 15). Top 5 challenges facing nursing in 2012. *HealthLeaders Media*. Retrieved from www.healthleadersmedia.com/content /NRS-273338/Top-5-Challenges-Facing-Nursing-in-2012

Hospice and Palliative Credentialing Center. (2011, June 8). *Statement on continuing competence for nursing: A call to action*. Retrieved from www.nbchpn.org

Kaplan, A. M., & Haenlein, M. (2010). Users of the world unite! The challenges and opportunities of social media. *Business Horizons, 53*(1), 59–68.

Lawrence, L. A. (2011). Work engagement, moral distress, education level and critical reflective practice in intensive care nurses. *Nursing Forum, 46*(4), 256–268.

Marx, D. (2001). *Patient safety and the "just culture": A primer for health care executives*. New York, NY: Columbia University.

Marx, D. (2009). *Whack a mole: The price we pay for expecting perfection*. Plano, TX: You Side Studios.

National Council of State Boards of Nursing. (n.d.). Transition to practice model toolkit. Retrieved from https://www.ncsbn.org/686.htm/2013_TransitiontoPractice _Modules.pdf

National Council of State Boards of Nursing. (2005). Meeting the ongoing challenge of continued competence. Retrieved from https://www.ncsbn.org/Continued_Comp _Paper_TestingServices.pdff

National Council of State Boards of Nursing. (2011). Nurse practice act, rules & regulations. Retrieved from https://www.ncsbn.org/nurse-practice-act.htm

National Institute of Nursing Research. (2010). Online: Developing nurse scientists. Retrieved from www.ninr.nih.gov/training/online-developing-nurse-scientists

Prinz, A. (2011). Professional social networking for nurses. *American Nurse Today, 6*(7), 30–31.

Reese, S. (1999). The new wave of Gen X workers. *Business and Health, 17*(6), 19–23.

Richards, K., & Nelson, J. (2011). Overcoming obstacles to create the optimal healing environment. *Nurse Leader, 9*(2), 37.

Sandberg, J. (2001). Understanding competence at work. *Harvard Business Review, 201*(3), 24–28.

Sarver, C. (2011). From practice to print: Creating a thriving culture of writing. *Nurse Leader, 9*(3), 23–25.

Shiparski, L., Richards, K., & Nelson, J. (2011). Self-care strategies to enhance caring. *Nurse Leader, 9*(3), 26–30.

Stringer, H. (2011). *Your Own Best Friend: Benefits of Self-Compassion.* Nurse.com/ Advanced Practice. Retrieved from https://www.nurse.com/blog/2010/11/22 /your-own-best-friend-benefits-of-self-compassion/

Thurston, B. (2013). Are you a digital addict? *Fast Company, 177,* 75–77.

Ulrich, B., & Lavandero, R. (2014). Leadership competence: Perceptions of direct care nurses. *Nurse Leader, 12*(3), 47–50.

Appendix A

Writing for Publication

Taking the leap and writing for publication requires content, courage, and resilience. Scholarly writing provides an opportunity to develop critical thinking skills and professionalism. Consider a recent patient care situation that you believe yielded information that other nurses would find useful. The situation could be a positive situation or a negative situation in which you want to warn other nurses to do or not do something.

1. Describe the specific situation in one or two paragraphs.
2. List the key points you are trying to make with your information. Which problem are you trying to address or fix?
3. Review your situation and key points with another nurse in the class. Request constructive feedback to strengthen your article.
4. Complete a literature search in a major search engine (e.g., PubMed, CINAHL, ERIC) and summarize the information for inclusion in your article.
5. Identify at least two online and two paper publications that would be interested in your information.
6. Create a one- to two-page submission for one online and one print publication using the specific author guidelines. (Note: Focus on content of the article, not the article length.)
7. Create a letter of inquiry to the editor for consideration of publication.
8. Be aware of potential copyright violations (Catalano, 2014).
9. Describe your learning from this experience.

Appendix B

Giving a Podium Presentation

Preparation Process

- Abstract
  - Five **C**s of abstract construction (Koegel, 2007)
    - **Clarify** theme and goals.
    - **Compare** with conference theme or goals.
    - **Compose** to be clear, concise, cohesive, and complete.

- ‣ **Comply** with rules.
- ‣ **Confirm** all process-related details.
- Refer to *Ideas to Action: Creating and Presenting a Poster* for more details. Available at https://www.americannursetoday.com /how-to-create-an-effective-poster-presentation
- Presentation types
  - Handouts
    - ‣ Roundtable
    - ‣ Panel
  - PowerPoints
    - ‣ Breakout/concurrent
    - ‣ Keynote address
- Conference guidelines
  - Know and adhere
    - ‣ Presentation type, length, format, handouts, and registration
  - Continuing education credit (Slagell & Headley, 2008)
  - Templates
- Organization (Longo, 2012; Slagell & Headley, 2008)
  - Goals/objectives (Longo, 2012)
    - ‣ Specific purposes
    - ‣ Align with conference goals
  - Ask yourself (Longo, 2012)
    - ‣ Why is this being presented?
    - ‣ What else is on the agenda?
    - ‣ Who is your audience?
      - ◆ Already know
      - ◆ Biases
      - ◆ Need to know
  - Opening
    - ‣ Thank you
    - ‣ Opening hook
    - ‣ Objectives/agenda/flow
  - Q and A
    - ‣ Invite questions
    - ‣ Repeat/rephrase

- ‣ Invite audience if you do not know answer
- ‣ Follow-up
- ‣ Do not argue
- Three to five points
  - ‣ Organized
  - ‣ Clear transitions
- Closing
  - ‣ Transitional cue
  - ‣ End early
  - ‣ Shift B

Example: Print your own medicine (Lee Cronin, TEDGlobal2012)

Media Use

- PowerPoint
  - Prompt not manuscript (Longo, 2012)
  - Seven lines, seven words (Longo, 2012)
  - Colors (Longo, 2012)
  - Contrast
    - ‣ Background
      - ◆ Dark with light font reduces glare
      - ◆ Blue—easy to read
      - ◆ White—hard on eyes
    - ‣ Use white text.
    - ‣ Highlight in yellow.
    - ‣ Avoid red and green.
    - ‣ Be consistent.
  - Font (Longo, 2012)
    - ‣ Size
      - ◆ Heading: 44
      - ◆ Text: 24–42
    - ‣ Type
      - ◆ Sans serif (Arial or Helvetica)
      - ◆ Same font for the entire **presentation**
      - ◆ ALL UPPERCASE TAKES FOREVER TO READ.
        - ‣ Use to emphasize only

- Emphasis
  - Bold
  - Color
- Numbers
  - 657,121.15 *or* 660,000 *or* 660 thousand?
- Symbols
  - Data
    - Bar graph—compare groups
    - Line graph—change over time
    - Pie chart—numerical proportions
    - Scatter chart—relationship
    - Legend
    - Laser pointer
  - Appear function
    - Useful when many points to discuss
    - Avoid most other animation
  - High quality photographs/video
  - Patient permission/confidentiality
  - Copyright
  - Prezi
  - Visuals to enhance, not duplicate
  - Proofread everything

If you have to apologize for a slide, *leave it out or figure it out.*

Delivery

- From the TED stage (Gallo, 2014)
  - Persuasion occurs when there is (Aristotle)
    - Ethos: credibility
    - Logos: logic, data, statistics
    - Pathos: appeal to emotions
  - Emotional—novel—memorable
  - Storytelling
  - Avoid overused buzzwords, cliches, and metaphors
  - Listening is draining

- Brain can consume three chunks of information in short term memory
- 18-minute rule
- Dress (Litin & Ende, 2010)
  - Professional and comfortable
  - Scarves, jewelry, and name badges can interfere with audio
- Credibility (Litin & Ende, 2010)
  - Write your own biosketch, specific to your talk.
  - Provide email address.
  - Present your most professional self.
  - Turn off phones, pagers, tablets.
- Control what you can.
  - Arrive early. (Longo, 2012; Slagell & Headly, 2008)
    - 60/20 rule (Koegel, 2007; Longo, 2012)
      - Arrive 60 minutes before presentation.
        - First 40:
          - Room layout
          - Test/practice with equipment
          - Props
          - Handouts
        - Last 20:
          - Introductions; identify moderator
          - Information gathering
          - Rapport building
  - Use the restroom.
  - Stay hydrated—bring water.
  - Avoid caffeine, carbonation, and gum.
- Voice
  - Rate/volume/pitch/pauses
    - How to speak so that people want to listen: (Julian Treasure, TEDGlobal2013)
  - Microphone
    - Standard
    - Lavalier
  - Sound test

- Body language
  - Posture (Koegel, 2007)
  - Standing
    - Shoulders square to audience
    - Hands at side, elbows away from ribcage
    - Head and eyes up
    - Eye contact—do not forget about the back of the room
    - Seated
      - Hands on table
  - Gestures
    - Strengthen an argument (Gallo, 2014; Koegel, 2007)
    - Power sphere—belly button to eyes
    - Purposeful—versus problematic
- Mind the clock
  - Practice is the only way to know length.
  - Allow time for logistics.
    - At least five minutes
    - Loading of AV equipment
    - Introductions
  - Shift B and wrap it up!
- Nervous
  - Practice
  - Audiences are forgiving
  - Not usually visible
- Practice
  - Deliberate practice (Ericsson, K., Krampe, R., & Tesch-Römer, C., 1993)
  - Makes you more authentic (Gallo, 2014)
  - Mechanics of giving the presentation: do not monopolize.
  - Out loud, not silent
  - Verbal graffiti and condescenders (Gallo, 2014; Longo, 2012)
    - Become aware
    - Recognize patterns
    - Anticipate and pause

- Automatic slide transition feature
- Record yourself
- Ask for help from people who know you and your topic.
- Give presentation
  - Audiences familiar and unfamiliar with topic
  - People who will provide honest feedback

References

Catalano, L. A. (2014). Avoiding copyright violations in educational presentations. *American Nurse Today, 9*(5), l–5.

Ericsson, K., Krampe, R., & Tesch-Römer, C. (1993). The role of deliberate practice in the acquisition of expert performance. *Psychological Review, 100*(3), 363–406.

Gallo, C. (2014). *Talk like TED: The 9 public-speaking secrets of the world's top minds.* New York, NY: St. Martin's Press.

Koegel, T. J. (2007). *The exceptional presenter: A proven formula to open up! And own the room.* Austin, TX: Greenleaf Book Group Press.

Litin, S. C., & Ende, J. (2010). The lecture: Tips to make your next presentation go better than your last. In K. M. Skeff and G. A. Stratos (Eds.), *Methods for teaching medicine.* Philadelphia, PA: American College of Physicians.

Longo, A. (2012). Presentation skills for the nurse educator. *Journal for Nurses in Staff Development, 28*(1), 16–23.

Slagell, J., & Headley, S. (2008). Verbal bourbon: Speaking secrets to intoxicate your audience. *The Serials Librarian, 54*(3–4), 235–238.

TED. (2012). *Lee Cronin: Print your own medicine.* Retrieved from https://www.ted.com/talks/lee_cronin_print_your_own_medicine

TED. (2013). *Julian Treasure: How to speak so that people want to listen.* Retrieved from https://www.ted.com/talks/julian_treasure_how_to_speak_so_that_people_want_to_listen.

Critical Thought, Leader Tip, and Scenario icons made by Freepik from www.flaticon.com; Callout icon made by Yannick from www.flaticon.com; Team Tip icon made by Chanut is Industries from www.flaticon.com

> Compromise makes a good umbrella, but a poor roof; it is temporary expedient, often wise in party politics, almost sure to be unwise in statesmanship. —James Russell Lowell

CHAPTER OBJECTIVES

Upon completion of this chapter, the reader will be able to do the following:

» Define major concepts specific to healthcare policy.

» Appreciate the challenges and nuances of policy development.

» Describe at least three major health initiatives and their impact on nursing.

» Identify future activities of the professional nurse to advance nursing from a policy perspective.

» List the desired competencies of the clinical expert nurse in advancing healthcare policy.

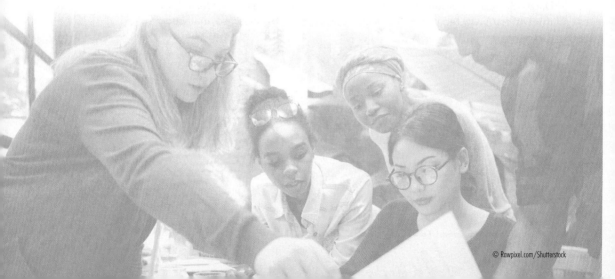

Policy, Legislation, Licensing, and Professional Nurse Roles

The area of healthcare policy often focuses on national or state legislation initiatives and processes. For healthcare workers, however, there is much more to be considered from a policy perspective. Specifically, the study of healthcare policies can be expanded to include those organizational policies necessary for order and progress, external agency, and legislated policies adopted by varying levels of formal processes. Some policies hold the force of law, with designated sanctions for noncompliance. Other policies hold the force of the organization's infrastructure and human resources requirements, with designated disciplinary sanctions for noncompliance. This chapter examines the broader perspective of healthcare policy, including both internal and external policies, along with the role of the professional nurse in policy management, both local and national policy issues, challenges in creating and sustaining effective policy, and thoughts about future healthcare policy.

To begin our discussion, we should consider why healthcare policy is needed. If everyone were equally gifted, equally educated, equally motivated, equally healthy, and equally wealthy, would national healthcare policy be necessary? Even if these equalities did exist, we might wonder if policy issues would arise when funding for health care exceeded

CRITICAL THOUGHT

Four stages of political development have been identified to describe how nursing has evolved to be savvier about policy processes. These stages are applicable to any type of policy development—for example, organizational, public, social, or legislated health policies.

1. Buy-in: There is an emerging interest in policy issues and the relationship to individual nurse performance and ability to practice.

2. Self-interest: Nurses identify specific areas of interest to the profession and the need for formalization for action.

3. Political sophistication: Nurses are recognized by key stakeholders as knowledgeable and necessary for effective policies.

4. Leadership: Specific political agendas and identity are seen as legitimate.

Modified from Mason, D. J., Levitt, J. K., & Chaffee, M. W. (2007). *Policy and politics in nursing and health care* (4th ed.). Philadelphia, PA: Saunders.

certain targets. Or perhaps there would be no debate about how much funding would be needed for healthcare services because any allocation would benefit each individual equally. Nevertheless, we might wonder if access to care would still create policy concerns, given the wide geographic distribution of the population and location of providers for all geographic areas.

The reality, of course, is that the playing field for health care is not level; thus effective policy processes that actively involve key stakeholders are essential. The unequal distribution of citizen knowledge, competence, skills, and physical and mental health in a society that values both pro-individual and pro-market perspectives requires sensitivity to both viewpoints when creating policy. To be sure, the processes can be fragmented, incremental, and incomprehensible, given the competing values (Shi & Singh, 2015). This work is never-ending and continually changing as healthcare needs change and participants change. Embracing the work of healthcare policy creation requires courage, time, persistence, and the ability to form effective and meaningful relationships. As the largest caregiver group in health care, the nursing community is well positioned to provide important input in these processes specific to quality, values, providers, outcomes, safety, patient care delivery systems, technology, and funding.

It is also important to acknowledge the dark side of policy. Not all policy processes are perceived as open, honest, and collaborative. Indeed, some skeptics claim that certain policy processes are quite negative and dishonest. In particular, the label of "politician" has often been associated with behaviors such

CRITICAL THOUGHT

The following caregiver competencies are required to effect healthcare reform:

- Integrating between specialists and teams (e.g., teams addressing care for chronic conditions, medically frail patients, and complex needs of seniors)
- Understanding financial management and getting value for the money
- Overcoming system inertia and moving the patient toward goals
- As clinical leaders, innovating to improve the system
- Developing expertise in communicating and collaborating
- Maintaining information technology skill in documenting, monitoring, and mining data

as controlling information, cajoling others to support issues, coercing others to support issues, being impatient while individuals consider information, being closed-minded to others' ideas, being confrontational and dishonest, and sharing only part of the information or partial truth telling. What is important to remember is that each one of us is part of the policy process, whether or not we want to acknowledge it; there is no reason to engage in these negative behaviors. Further, when these negative behaviors are identified, calling others out on these behaviors is equally important in the work of advancing effective healthcare policy.

Key Concepts

This section presents a selected list of key concepts that lay the foundation for future policy discussions. The list represents a wide range of concepts and is by no means inclusive of all of the healthcare policy concepts of importance to nurses.

- *Federal Register*: The official daily publication that presents rules, proposed rules, and notices of the federal government and serves as an unbiased source of information. The *Federal Register* is an excellent source of current policy activity at the national level (U.S. Government Publishing Office, 2004).
- **Health policy**: Policy directed toward promoting the health of citizens (Mason, Levitt, & Chaffee, 2007); the aggregate of principles, stated or unstated, that characterize the distribution of resources, services, and political influences that impact the health of the population (Miller, 1987).

- **Institutional policies**: Policies that refer to rules that govern the workplace (Mason et al., 2007).
- **Licensure**: The process by which an agency of a state government grants permission to an individual to engage in a given occupation (Aiken, 2004).
- **Nursing certification**: The provision of tangible recognition of professional achievement in a defined functional or clinical area of nursing (Aiken, 2004).
- **Organizational policies**: Policies that pertain to positions taken by organizations to govern the workplace and behavior (Mason et al., 2007).
- **Policy**: The choices that a society, segment of society, or organization makes regarding its resources, involving setting goals and priorities by a society or organization and deciding how and which resources should be used to achieve those goals. Policies reflect the values and beliefs of the leaders of society and/or organizations who make the policies (Mason et al., 2007).
- **Public policy**: An authoritative ruling relating to a decision made by government (Mason et al., 2007).
- **Social policy**: Policy intended to enhance the public welfare (Mason et al., 2007).
- **State Nurse Practice Act**: An act that regulates nursing practice, including requirements to enter into practice, licensure maintenance, scope of practice parameters, and disciplinary action (Aiken, 2004).
- **Statute**: A law passed by the legislature.
- **U.S. Department of Health and Human Services**: The overarching federal administrative agency concerned with monitoring the quality of health care in the United States (Shi & Singh, 2015).

The Policy Continuum: Local to National

While the emphasis of healthcare policy is typically on national issues, healthcare policy is also required at the organizational level. Specifically, organizations providing healthcare services are required to have policies specific to provider roles, patient care procedures, safety practices, equipment management, staffing and scheduling, and many other areas. Nurses are encouraged to become involved in the local policymaking processes in their organizations to better understand the organization and as a precursor to engaging in external policymaking processes at the state and national levels.

Policies are also generated by state legislatures, state agencies authorized by legislation, and state professional associations. These policies and processes are designed to serve the unique needs of the state. Examples include regulatory boards for licensure and state agencies that focus on the needs of children, the elderly, and mentally compromised persons.

At the federal level, policies are generated or enacted by the legislature, designated agencies, and numerous professional associations. Generally, processes to achieve federal legislation or agency policy require more time and energy for consensus building and negotiation to ensure that the intent of the policy is understood and supported. In addition to healthcare reform bills, other examples of federal legislation include the Health Insurance Portability and Accountability Act and the Patient Self-Determination Act.

Numerous national professional associations make recommendations for safe and effective practice; however, these guidelines do not hold the force of law. Examples of such organizations include The Joint Commission, the American Nurses Association, the Institute of Medicine, and the Robert Wood Johnson Foundation. While such associations do not have any legislative authority, they are usually highly regarded and their actions are supported by both organizational and legislative processes.

Contemporary Healthcare Policy Issues and Initiatives

In the United States, numerous healthcare policy issues now face both the states and the country as a whole. Common areas of focus include scope of provider services, provider competence, quality, safety, cost, access to care, timeliness, privacy, ethical issues, effectiveness, evidence, engagement of patients with providers, technology, coordination of care across the life span, waste, fraud, and abuse. In addition to the specific policy issues, numerous initiatives are underway from a variety of sources to address selected policy issues.

The following initiatives are examples of both legislation and professional organization recommendations. These initiatives reflect the wide range of approaches to creating policies to advance health care in the United States.

Patient Protection and Affordable Care Act

The Patient Protection and Affordable Care Act (PPACA or ACA), a federal statute, was enacted in March 2010. It is designed to help replace a broken system with one that ensures all Americans have access to health care that is both affordable and driven by quality standards. The goal of this act is to deliver seamless (digital), high-quality, patient-centered care for Medicare beneficiaries instead of

CRITICAL THOUGHT

The external policymaking process follows these steps:

1. Identify the policy or issue specific to a societal problem for a community, state, or nation.

2. Set the agenda and place it within other policy priorities.

3. Formulate a plan for gaining support and adoption of the policy.

4. Implement or adopt legislation.

5. Evaluate the impact of the legislation.

the fragmented care that preceded it. Two key components of the statute include meaningful use of technology and the implementation of **accountable care organizations** (ACOs) to coordinate and integrate care services.

Meaningful use by users is expected to maximize the use of electronic health records to (1) improve quality, safety, and efficiency and reduce health disparities; (2) engage patients and families; (3) improve care coordination; (4) improve public health; and (5) ensure adequate privacy and security protections for personal health information (Murphy & Alexander, 2010). Medicare incentives are linked to effective, meaningful use, whereas providers who fail to achieve meaningful use will be subject to reductions in Medicare payments.

ACOs consist of networks of providers that are rewarded financially if they can slow the growth in their patients' healthcare spending while maintaining or improving the quality of the care they deliver. The accountable care model emphasizes population care, value-driven outcomes, emphasis on the point of service at which patient care occurs, protocols for effective hand-offs, and inclusion of the family in decision making. An important distinction between health maintenance organizations and ACOs is that in ACOs, the providers themselves (rather than an insurance company) control the diagnosis and treatment decisions. **Figure 11-1** provides an overview of the components of an ACO. It is important to note that the ACO rests on a firm technology foundation.

Among the issues in the PPACA of concern for nurses are changes related to advanced practice nurses. Certified nurse midwives were not included in the federal government's list of ACO professionals. While nurse practitioners were included in the ACO professionals list, the method proposed for assigning beneficiaries to ACOs does not incorporate primary care services provided by

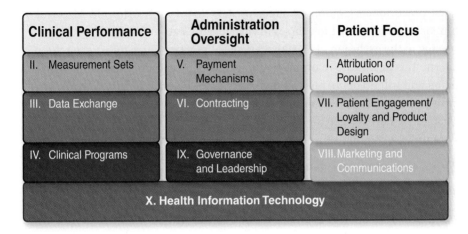

Clinical Performance	Administration Oversight	Patient Focus
II. Measurement Sets	V. Payment Mechanisms	I. Attribution of Population
III. Data Exchange	VI. Contracting	VII. Patient Engagement/ Loyalty and Product Design
IV. Clinical Programs	IX. Governance and Leadership	VIII. Marketing and Communications

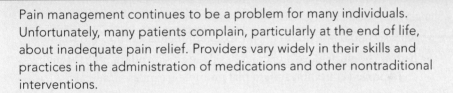

X. Health Information Technology

Figure 11-1 Accountable care organizations

SCENARIO

Pain management continues to be a problem for many individuals. Unfortunately, many patients complain, particularly at the end of life, about inadequate pain relief. Providers vary widely in their skills and practices in the administration of medications and other nontraditional interventions.

Discussion Questions

Given the expectations for an effective ACO, consider the following:

1. Describe the policies that would be needed to correct this problem.

2. Which providers would be involved?

3. What evidence would be used to select interventions?

4. How would the effectiveness be evaluated?

5. How would interventions be documented?

6. Should patients with intractable pain be considered a specific "population group"? Why? Why not?

nurse practitioners (National Council of State Boards of Nursing, 2011). Significant opportunities exist for nurses to engage both state and federal legislators specific to the exclusion of an active advanced practice nurse role in the reform efforts. This healthcare reform legislation continues to evolve in its implementation and will no doubt be modified many times before a stabilized model is created. Regardless of the turmoil created by the passage of the PPACA, such changes are necessary to modify what had been a very ineffective U.S. healthcare system.

The Future of Nursing: Leading Change, Advancing Health (Institute of Medicine Report)

In 2008, the Robert Wood Johnson Foundation and the Institute of Medicine (IOM, now the Health and Medicine Division), two national professional associations, launched a two-year initiative to respond to the need to assess and transform the nursing profession. This work ultimately produced a report specific to the future of nursing, *The Future of Nursing: Leading Change, Advancing Health*, published October 5, 2011. Four key messages were developed by the committee (Shalala & Vladeck, 2011):

- Nurses should practice to the full extent of their education and training.
- Nurses should achieve higher levels of education and training through an improved education system that promotes seamless academic progression.
- Nurses should be full partners, with physicians and other healthcare professionals, in redesigning health care in the United States.
- Effective workforce planning and policymaking require better data collection and information infrastructure.

This report and recommendations from national professional associations do not hold the force of law, but they are widely respected and supported by many in the healthcare community.

Transition of Care Program

Significant concern continues to exist specific to changing caregiver teams (hand-offs) and the nearly 20% readmission rates for several medical diagnoses. To address these challenges, the National Transitions of Care Coalition (www.ntocc.org) was formed in 2006, bringing together leaders, patient advocates, and healthcare providers from various care settings to focus on improving the quality of care coordination and communication. Transfers encompass moving a patient from primary care to specialty physicians; within the hospital, they include moving patients from the emergency department to other departments, such as surgery or intensive care; they also occur when patients are discharged from the hospital and go home, to an assisted living setting, or to a skilled nursing facility.

The initiative addressing transfer issues resulted from a national professional association that established a goal to decrease readmissions. Driven by research evidence, this group was formed to address a significant quality problem. Often initiatives using this approach are more expeditious than those using legislative approaches.

Informed Consent

Informed consent is an essential component of the healthcare process and is generally overseen by state regulations. Specifically, the individual provider performing healthcare services or procedures is required to explain the procedure to be performed, the risks involved, the expected outcomes, potential complications, and alternative treatments that are available (Barrett, 2005).

Patient Self-Determination Act

The Patient Self-Determination Act, which was enacted in 1991, requires organizations receiving federal funding to provide education for staff and patients on issues concerning treatment and end-of-life issues. Specifically, an advance directive signed by a competent individual must be honored if the individual becomes incapacitated in the future (Salmond & David, 2005). This act continues to be of great importance in upholding patient respect and autonomy.

Good Samaritan Laws

Good Samaritan laws state that healthcare providers are protected from potential liability if they volunteer their healthcare skills away from the workplace, provided that the actions taken in that role are not grossly negligent. This protection is limited to emergencies and does not cover nonemergent care or advice given to others outside of the workplace (Brooke, 2004).

Health Insurance Portability and Accountability Act

The Health Insurance Portability and Accountability Act (HIPAA), which was passed in 1996, focuses on the patient's right to confidentiality and the improvement of the portability and continuity of health insurance coverage (Erickson & Millar, 2005). Both issues remain critical to quality healthcare services. In relation to confidentiality, unauthorized release of a patient's information or photographs is not allowed. Written authorization by the patient is required for release of any information about the patient in writing, on the phone, or in person. The insurance portability requirement of this law has proved more troublesome to implement; however, the efforts continue with revisions of rules to achieve the desired goals of simplifying the coding of health information to ease the digital exchange of information among healthcare providers.

Professional Nursing Role and Policy

To use a cliché, if you are not part of the solution, you are part of the problem! Ignoring issues steeped in political drama and conflict will not make them go away—but neither will it bring about resolution. As nurses advance in their professional role competence, involvement in the profession becomes more realistic and interesting. The following six activities should be embraced by all nurses.

First, become competent in the processes of policy development and the differing approaches that are effective at the local, state, and national levels. Competencies begin with basic relationship development and participation on local committees. Recognizing the similarities between internal and external political processes provides support and reassurance that this type of work is, indeed, possible and effective.

The second activity is to develop focused partnerships with stakeholders who know and understand the evidentiary support for policymaking or policy revision. The ability to understand and integrate evidence into policies is desperately needed. In addition, working from an evidence-driven perspective further diminishes the tendency to create policy based on emotions and one-time events. This activity can occur at a unit level when reviewing care delivery policies and informing them with the latest evidence. Additionally, evidence-based policy discussion can take place at the organizational and national level. Clinical leaders can influence the system in many ways.

The third activity is to take a risk and propose a new policy that is of great interest to you. Consider virtual care, patient falls, medication errors, integrating work-arounds, or some area of health care that you believe needs attention. Begin with local policy initiation and progress to the state agency level, such as the board of nursing or department of health services. It is seldom necessary to do this work alone. Engage in discussions in your organization or committees at the board or agency levels to determine interest.

The fourth activity is to examine a current policy—either internal or external—and identify the effectiveness of the policy. This evaluation can often be a challenge; however, it is necessary to determine the pragmatic value of the policy. Some policies may be quite effective, whereas others may not have achieved their intent and may cost time and effort to continue to comply with the policy. Consider pain management or restraint policies for investigation. Many efforts to get to an ideal policy have failed to achieve the desired result of safety and respect.

CRITICAL THOUGHT

The process of building competence as a political expert begins at the local organizational level and then expands to the external local, state, and national arenas. This developmental process requires time, reflection, and coaching from established policy experts if the nurse is to successfully engage in policymaking. Components of the process including the following activities:

- Build working relationships with policy committee members in your organization.
- Participate on committees focused on policy areas of interest, such as critical care or technology areas.
- Participate in professional organizations of interest.
- Develop relationships with local and state legislators.
- Develop relationships with state agency leaders, such as the state department of health services and the state board of nursing.
- Provide input to legislators specific to healthcare issues and other areas of interest.
- Participate on legislative lobby days with state nursing associations.
- Register to vote—and vote in every election.
- Develop relationships with U.S. legislators.
- Get involved with a local political party.
- Share your ideas with leaders and elected officials involved in policy work.
- Run for office!

The fifth activity is specific to integrating evidence into the policy processes whenever possible. The digital age has provided an increasing amount of information that can now be evaluated and integrated into policy when appropriate. The importance of integrating evidence into the policy process cannot be overemphasized. Inclusion of compelling evidence in policymaking at any level is essential; however, this need is not always met given the multiple influences in the policy process. As more information becomes available in digital form, the expectation for higher levels of evidence is appropriate.

Also, given that the values of independence and market forces often come into conflict during the quest to develop the best healthcare policies, nurse leaders

CRITICAL THOUGHT

Specific topics on which to exert political influence include the following:

- Funding for safety initiatives
- Technology implementation and standardization of applications and language
- Mandates for value-based health care and outcome evaluation
- National healthcare funding philosophy for patient care and education of providers
- Provider role clarity
- Healthcare research priorities
- Participation in the National Licensure Compact
- Staffing effectiveness initiatives

must be motivated to get involved in policymaking to ensure that the balance between the marketplace and the individual is as good as it can be. Many relationships focus on influencing local, state, and national public policy as well as organizational policy, but there is not always appropriate evidence in support of these policies. The focus of political relationships, whether internal to the organization or in the public arena, must continue to evolve to ensure that healthcare work is evidence driven, occurs safely, and is affordable.

The sixth and final recommendation deals with increasing nursing presence in healthcare policy discussions. According to Donelan, Buerhaus, DesRoches, and Burke (2011), nurses need to increase their presence at the national policy level by developing well-honed messages and participating in news media, research publications, and advertising forums to advance the issues of nursing supply, workplace safety, and funding for education.

Numerous resources are available to help nurses develop key messages specific to nursing's future. In addition, strategies to contact and communicate with local and national media are encouraged from a proactive perspective. Being prepared for both internal and external inquiries about the challenges, needs, and expectations of the profession is not only proactive but also stress reducing. The Farrah Consulting Group (2003) offers the following guidelines for being "media ready":

- Know the position you want to take and articulate it clearly.
- Proactively reach out to the media whenever possible. Build on relationships so that reporters will contact you with questions or challenges when they are seeking information.

- Avoid reporters who tend to present biased stories with little objectivity.
- Stay on message. Repeat, if necessary!
- Practice your message and presentation with internal staff.
- Minimize off-the-record comments.
- Focus on proactive crisis management with a defined plan as to who the spokesperson will be, as well as preparing for the worst possible questions that someone could ask.
- Respond promptly.

Final Thoughts on Policy

This is only the beginning of your work with healthcare policy as a registered nurse. There are many needs and opportunities for nurses across the spectrum of key stakeholders who participate in making healthcare policy decisions. Often, these key stakeholders *and* legislators have very little, if any, background in health-care issues. These stakeholders need your assistance and are usually very open to collaboration and discussion of emerging issues. For nurses, it is our day and our time to be more widely known and more effective in advancing quality health care.

SCENARIO

According to the Jefferson School of Population Health, the provision of compassionate, quality care for individuals with chronic illness continues to be a challenge. Many patients continue to suffer because pain is not adequately addressed during treatment, and patient preferences are often neglected at the end of life. In particular, hospitalized patients with lung cancer, at the end of their lives, experience barriers to palliative care access and do so on a broad scale, across the United States (Reville, Miller, Toner, & Reisnyder, 2010).

All too often, confusion exists about the difference between palliative care and hospice care and about when to initiate each type of care. Both physicians and nurses have acknowledged their lack of training in end-of-life commu-nication and the point at which to suggest a transition to palliative care. For hospitalized patients with lung cancer, a delay in referral to palliative care until late in the disease trajectory has been documented (Reville et al., 2010), and this service is largely underutilized as a means to address symptoms and psychosocial concerns. Specifically, palliative care professionals were con-sulted for only 8% of all hospital admissions among this patient population.

(continues)

(continued)

Discussion Questions

1. As an experienced nurse, identify and describe the specific opportunities at the institutional, organizational, public, social, and health policy levels to improve palliative, hospice, and end-of-life care.

2. What are the issues at each level that prevent adequate care?

3. Which key stakeholders need to be involved in addressing this issue?

4. How will you evaluate progress at each policy level when changes are made?

5. Describe a plan specific to nursing interventions at each policy level, including the facilitators of and barriers to the policy proposal.

SCENARIO

Given the significant challenges with patient readmissions within 30 days of discharge, there is a need for additional local analysis by nurses providing patient care. Substitute the problems associated with palliative care with patient readmissions and respond to the previous five questions.

CHAPTER TEST QUESTIONS

Licensure exam categories: Management of care: advocacy, concepts of management, ethical practice

Nurse leader exam categories: Communication and relationship building: communicate involvement, influencing behaviors; Knowledge of the healthcare environment: governance, healthcare economics, and policy

1. Healthcare policy is most effectively created

    a. at the state level.

    b. at the state and national levels.

    c. at the national level.

    d. at legislative, association, state, and national levels.

2. Nurse practice acts

   a. focus on discipline of nurses.

   b. are state based.

   c. require endorsement from the federal government to change any statutes.

   d. are consistent from state to state.

3. Nurse input into health policy

   a. is essential because nurses are the largest caregiver group and are familiar with patient care issues.

   b. is seldom recognized or valued.

   c. is best done through a lobbyist.

   d. requires membership on a board of nursing committee.

4. The dark side of politics

   a. is specific to certain types of legislation.

   b. requires competence in negotiation.

   c. is an unfortunate and negative result of negotiating in bad faith.

   d. is the result of extensive experiences in the political processes.

5. Policy is distinguished from politics in that

   a. policy reflects the outcome while politics reflects the human processes to achieve a policy.

   b. policy reflects the desired outcome while politics reflects the guidelines to achieve a policy.

   c. policy reflects the intentions of elected officials while politics reflects the political agenda required to achieve a policy.

   d. policy is the final result of negotiations while politics reflects the seamier side of the negotiations to achieve the policy.

6. Institutional policies

    a. are guidelines that do not have consequences if they are not followed.

    b. are designed to serve the social needs of the community.

    c. are created by state agencies to support healthcare organizations.

    d. are organizational policies designed to ensure effective practices in the workplace.

7. The U.S. Department of Health and Human Services

    a. is a federal agency funded by Congress.

    b. provides funding for both federal and state initiatives.

    c. does not provide funding for Medicare.

    d. requires elected officials to participate on agency committees.

8. Accountability care organizations

    a. are expected to provide improved coordination and documentation of patient care.

    b. are limited to urban areas near universities.

    c. do not require initial funding for their launch.

    d. are recommended in the HIPAA legislation.

9. Nurse licensure

    a. is intended to provide a vehicle for continuing education documentation.

    b. is intended to provide evidence of safe practitioners and to protect the public.

    c. is intended to inform healthcare facilities of those safe to practice.

    d. requires evidence of a negative criminal history.

References

Aiken, T. D. (2004). *Legal, ethical, and political issues in nursing* (2nd ed.). Philadelphia, PA: F. A. Davis.

Barrett, R. (2005). Quality of informed consent: Measuring understanding among participants in clinical trials. *Oncology Nursing Forum, 32*(4), 751–755.

Brooke, P. S. (2004). Stretching the Good Samaritan law. *Nursing, 34*(7), 22.

Donelan, K., Buerhaus, P. I., DesRoches, C., & Burke, S. P. (2011). Health policy thoughtleaders' views of the health workforce in an era of health reform. *Nursing Outlook, 58*(4), 175–180.

Erickson, J. L., & Millar, S. (2005). Caring for patients while respecting their privacy: Renewing our commitment. *Online Journal of Issues in Nursing, 10*(2), 1115.

Farrah Consulting Group. (2003). Polishing the pitch: A primer on effective media strategies. farrahconsulting.com

Mason, D. J., Levitt, J. K., & Chaffee, M. W. (2007). *Policy and politics in nursing and health care* (4th ed.). Philadelphia, PA: Saunders.

Miller, C. A. (1987). Child health. In S. Levine & A. Lillienfeld (Eds.), *Epidemiology and health policy* (pp. 83–89). New York, NY: Tavistock.

Murphy, J., & Alexander, D. (2010). The journey to meaningful use and the impact on nursing. *Voice of Nursing Leadership, 6*(8), 6–9.

National Council of State Boards of Nursing. (2011). APRN consensus model: The consensus model for APRN regulation, licensure, accreditation, certification, and education. www.ncsbn.org/aprn-consensus.htm

Reville, B., Miller, M., Toner, R. W., & Reisnyder, J. (2010). End-of-life care for hospitalized patients with lung cancer: Utilization of palliative care service. *Journal of Palliative Medicine, 13*(10), 1261–1265.

Salmond, S. W., & David, E. (2005). Attitudes toward advance directives and advance directives completion rates. *Orthopedic Nursing, 24*(2), 28–34.

Shalala, D., & Vladeck, B. (2011). Leading change: How nurses can attract political support for the IOM report on the future of nursing. *Nurse Leader, 9*(6), 38–39, 45.

Shi, L., & Singh, D. A. (2015). *Delivering health care in America: A systems approach* (6th ed.). Burlington, MA: Jones & Bartlett Learning.

U.S. Government Publishing Office. (2004). About *Federal Register*. Retrieved from https://www.gpo.gov/help/about_federal_register.htm

Appendix A

Selected Resources for Healthcare Policy

This appendix contains a selected list of references and resources that are helpful in understanding national healthcare policy initiatives and issues. Many other resources can be added to your personalized list of resources as you become more familiar with healthcare policy specific to your particular area of interest.

Agency for Healthcare Research and Quality (AHRQ)

The Agency for Healthcare Research and Quality's mission is to improve the quality, safety, efficiency, and effectiveness of health care in the United States. AHRQ's research focuses on improving decision making as well as the quality of health care. AHRQ was formerly known as the Agency for Health Care Policy and Research.

www.ahrq.gov

American Nurses Association (ANA)

The ANA House of Delegates and the ANA Board of Directors work together to create policy for health care, the workplace, patient care, and many other areas where nurses are engaged. The House of Delegates and the Board of Directors often consider significant issues and address these concerns by way of a position statement or resolution.

www.nursingworld.org/MainMenuCategories/Policy-Advocacy/Positions-and
-Resolutions

American Organization of Nurse Executives (AONE)

The American Organization of Nurse Executives is the national organization of nurses who design, facilitate, and manage care. Since 1967, AONE has served its members by providing leadership, professional development, advocacy, and research to advance nursing practice and patient care, promote nursing leadership excellence, and shape public policy for health care. AONE is a subsidiary of the American Hospital Association.

www.aone.org/resources/future_of_nursing.shtml

Commonwealth Fund

The Commonwealth Fund promotes health care that emphasizes improved access, quality, and greater efficiency, particularly for society's most vulnerable people.

www.commonwealthfund.org/About-Us/Mission-Statement.aspx

Health Affairs

Health Affairs is a monthly journal published by Project Hope. It is a leading journal on health policy and research. This peer-reviewed journal, which was founded in 1981, explores health policy issues of current concern in both domestic and international spheres.

www.healthaffairs.org

Health and Medicine Division

The Health and Medicine Division (formerly the Institute of Medicine) is a division of the National Academies of Sciences, Engineering, and Medicine (the National Academies). This nonprofit organization works outside of government to provide unbiased and authoritative analysis and advice to decision makers and the public.

nationalacademies.org/hmd

Jefferson College of Population Health

The Jefferson College of Population Health serves to foster health policies and forces that define the health and well-being of populations through research, publications, and education in population health, public health, health policy, healthcare quality and safety, and health outcomes.

www.jefferson.edu/population_health

U.S. Department of Health and Human Services

The Department of Health and Human Services is the U.S. government's principal agency for protecting the health and well-being of all Americans through the provision of essential human services, especially for those who are most needy.

www.hhs.gov

Appendix B

Shaping Public Policy: The Nurse Leader's Role

Joey Ridenour and Greg Harris

Nurses learn the skills of politics and policymaking through mentoring, role modeling, and practice. The information in this chapter assists nurses in developing the strategies most likely to garner success in shaping public policy at the legislative level. It explores the core competencies of lobbyists and provides insight into how these roles expand the nurse's knowledge and practice in policymaking.

Core Competencies

Several steps must be taken before a legislative proposal is introduced. Attention should be given to key factors, the legislative climate, and how it could affect the proposal. Stakeholders and other interested parties need to be identified and a judgment made about how they may react to the proposal. In addition, the following 10 fundamental questions should be addressed:

- What problem will the legislation solve?
- Why should this approach be used?
- Who else follows this approach?
- Do solutions exist that are not legislative? If so, have they been tried?
- Has a legislative effort been tried before?
- What costs would be imposed by the proposed solution and who would bear them?
- If the proposal is not undertaken, what costs would be borne and who would bear them?
- Who will sponsor the legislation?
- What coalition building will need to be done?
- Who will support the effort, who will oppose it, and who will sit on the sidelines and remain neutral?

Once these questions have been answered, the nurse leader may begin working with others in the drafting effort, which must take into account the factors certain to be raised during the legislative process.

History Matters

The nurse leader may work or consult with a lobbyist to know the history of the subject that the proposal addresses, including any administrative, legislative, and judicial actions taken. If the legislature has considered a similar proposal before, assume the sponsor of the proposal will be informed of the prior difficulties by those who oppose the bill. If the courts have taken a position on the issue, expect legislative staff or opponents to inform the legislature of the precedent. Also, if another person previously attempted to address the issue administratively and encountered difficulties, anticipate that those difficulties are likely to become the focus of discussion as the legislation progresses.

The experiences of regulatory agencies may be relevant to the nurse's effort. Accordingly, the focus should not be limited to the state's nurse practice act. Instead, attention needs to be given to regulations regarding other health professions and how the legislature, judiciary, and other administrative departments have addressed efforts similar to the proposal.

Importance of Legislative Staff

The legislative staff play an important role. Some staff members focus on drafting the new statutory language and have little need to be concerned about the interests and pressures the legislature may focus on during the session. Others may concentrate on stakeholders and the political strengths and constituencies the various interest groups represent, but may not appreciate the need to define the issues faced by the legislature. The staff assistant who works directly for a legislator plays a key gatekeeper role, communicating messages from the legislator, relaying messages from the lobbyist and nurse leader, and scheduling meetings with parties who have concerns related to the bill.

Each legislative staff member requires a different type of attention. The lobbyist or nurse leader must spend time with legislation drafting staff to make sure they understand the issue, the proposal's objectives, the specific language chosen, and how the proposal fits within existing laws. Be prepared to share an anecdote that illustrates the problem at hand and the need for a policy solution. Also be ready to provide evidence, data, and other relevant facts that show the proposal addresses a problem and not merely an anecdotal incident or isolated event (Foley, 2007).

The nurse leader also must invest time with legislative committee staff so they can appropriately communicate the rationale for the proposal to legislators as it moves toward a committee hearing. A staff briefing will precede the committee hearing. Committee staff will draft a bill summary to explain the bill, the reason for its introduction, and the proposed changes it contains. Throughout this effort, others will comment on the bill to legislative staff and legislators. Typically, these comments and concerns will be raised repeatedly throughout the effort, which will test the nurse or lobbyist expertise, familiarity with the subject matter, and candor.

Framing the Issue

Consider how best to frame the message in support of the proposed bill and how to convey this message to the bill sponsor and legislative staff. Expect to prepare several different messages, each keyed to a particular audience. Anticipate spending more time framing the issue with the bill's sponsor than with a legislator who does not sit on the committee that will hear the bill. Similarly, prepare to spend more time with legislators who have shown an interest in the issue or, conversely, who are known to be skeptical of the proposal. Finally, anticipate spending more time with the legislative staff who will deliver briefings on the bill to legislators than with staff who will not spend time working with the substance of the legislation.

The key to framing the issue successfully is to be brief and to the point. Legislators face hundreds, if not thousands, of proposals in a legislative session. One-page summaries, bullet-pointed memoranda, and tabular references may be the best way to convey key points to them.

Other strategies include:

- Phone calls can be used to leave short messages with legislators or their assistants.
- Email increasingly is the preferred mode for communicating information about legislation. However, it should be used with caution because emails can be easily forwarded to others.
- Letters and attachments often can be persuasive, if for no other reason than their relative novelty in an age of electronic communication.
- Sending a hard copy of a summary or memorandum will save the legislator or staff members the time and expense of printing a document that has been sent electronically.
- Personal visits provide a venue for planned message delivery as well as a chance to address others' comments or concerns.

Preparing for the Legislative Hearing

Once the issue has been framed and the bill has been placed on a committee agenda, the next phase preparing for the **hearing** begins. Like the first phase, this step requires identification of issues that will be raised about the bill before the committee. Assume some unknown issue or question will be raised during the hearing. Work with legislative staff, legislators, allies, and supporters of the bill to help gain a sense of the issues or questions that may be raised.

Adequate preparation also requires knowing the format of the committee hearing process, including how to submit advance written testimony and how bill-related materials are to be distributed to committee members when the bill is heard. The hearing room should be studied, as should the protocol to address the committee chair and committee members during the hearing.

The committee chair, staff, and committee members will provide a sense of their understanding of the bill and what they expect of you at the hearing. With this advance intelligence, listen closely to the committee's questions and reaction to the bill rather than speaking to fill the silence. Use good judgment about whether to participate as committee members engage in dialogue on the bill.

Hearing preparation also should include an assessment of other issues considered by the legislature during the session, bills that have come before the committee during that session, and issues that also will be on the agenda when the bill is heard. This information helps the nurse leader understand the committee's orientation to the subject of the board's bill, the likelihood that the bill will attract attention as it moves forward, and the reason for this attention. Thus, the committee agenda will provide insight into the bill's relative prominence or controversy.

It is not uncommon for a bill to be heard by more than one legislative committee. If the bill already was heard in a committee, its previous reception heightens the need for its supporters to know of any overlap of members between the committees, the nature of the issues raised during the prior hearing, and whether the concerns were resolved.

When several nursing representatives plan to testify on a bill, it is important that the "persons testifying coordinate their testimony, raising different aspects of an issue rather than repeating the same points" (Santa Anna, 2007). It is also helpful to emphasize where there is unified agreement on the issues.

Committee Testimony Process

A senior legislator chairs the committee hearing and usually begins with remarks. Committee members may come and go during this process. Legislative staff will ensure that key testimony is relayed and written documents are provided.

Ten Key Strategies for Success

When undertaking any legislative project, take advantage of opportunities to learn from others' experiences, summarized in the following points.

1. Do not assume anything. Don't assume others will know your intent. Make the policy goal of the bill as clear as possible. You cannot know all of others' concerns about the bill, but clarity will help allay them. Also, do not assume you have the votes you need until the bill is signed into law.

2. Listen not only to what others say but to what they do not say. Sometimes, the things people do not share reveal their true feelings, objectives, or motives. These things may be difficult to observe or find out, so active listening and paying close attention are required. Above all, do not lose sight of the original intent of the proposed bill, and be ready to compromise on noncritical issues.

3. Know the legislative environment. Get to know and understand the other issues currently percolating through the legislative process. These issues almost certainly will affect the bill, either directly or indirectly. Ignoring the legislative environment could undermine your efforts.

4. Remember that everything is connected. Connections exist among many issues, and others' policy goals may coincide or collide with the bill's goals. Being aware of other issues going through the legislative process can help you avoid pitfalls or strike strategic alliances. Political effectiveness in one sphere is influenced by nurses' involvement in other spheres; interaction and interdependence among the spheres occur throughout (Mason, Leavitt, & Chaffee, 2007).

5. Be aware that it is not your bill. Only legislators introduce bills and only legislators vote on them. Speak with the bill's sponsors about amendments that have been discussed, amendments under consideration, and opposition that may be forming. If you allow the bill's sponsors to be surprised or ambushed about the bill, they may stop all work on your effort.

6. Keep the governor's office informed. Communicate with the governor's office about the policy goals and the reason for seeking the legislation. Help the governor's staff prepare for questions that are likely to be raised about the board's efforts.

7. Keep the coalition informed. During the advance work on the bill, spend a great deal of time working on the bill with other interested parties or stakeholders. If changes to the measure become necessary, ensure that the coalition learns of this. The coalition's support will be needed throughout the process; therefore, its members need to know of any new support earned or opposition avoided. Continued negotiation on the bill may cost support from somebody who had previously agreed to promote the legislation. Assume all supporters will want to know about the agreed-upon changes supported or drafted for the measure. Skipping this step risks losing coalition members.

8. Be patient. The legislative process offers many opportunities for both quick action and long periods of inaction. The bill will move at a pace that falls largely outside the nurse leader's control. This means that in addition to being patient, you must be prepared for new questions and for the bill to resume its movement through the legislature at any time.

9. Do the necessary; avoid the unnecessary. Accomplish the steps identified for the legislation to pass. Along the way, other opportunities will develop for unnecessary, gratuitous, or counterproductive steps. Avoid settling grudges or being punitive, disrespectful, or rude. No matter how tempting these behaviors might seem, they will almost certainly come back to haunt the effort. Also, they may become a distraction.

10. Do not lose sight of the goal. The legislative effort should be about getting things right, not simply about "winning." Sometimes, the goal may be reached without a legislative solution. If so, be satisfied. Simply having a bill move through the process is no guarantee of success and may even do more harm than good to your mission of protecting the public.

During testimony, the nurse may be asked an unanticipated question that warrants further research for a factual response. Resist the tendency to guess. Instead, committee members should be told you need to research that question. A wrong guess could impair the efforts and harm the bill's progress. Promising to get back to the committee members or a particular legislator provides both an opportunity to get the answer right and to follow up to be sure all concerns are addressed.

After the Hearing

Once the proposed bill clears its first committee, prepare for additional hearings. Use the experience gained in front of each committee to prepare and improve presentations to subsequent committees.

Legislative staff may require more information to brief legislators who did not participate in the hearing for the bill. Issues may be identified that require amendments to be offered when the entire legislative body debates the bill; this will entail drafting amendments and understanding their meaning. Maintain and continue to cultivate relationships with legislative staff to learn if others have proposed amendments, and be prepared to support or oppose those efforts.

Intelligence Gathering During the Legislative Process

During the legislative session, part of the discovery and intelligence-gathering campaign includes asking direct questions of those with an interest in the bill and, more importantly, obtaining commitment in support of the bill. Legislators and their staff will ask if others support or oppose the bill and the rationale for opposition. Strength of nurse leader efforts will be advanced by candor.

Understanding the legislature's mindset is also important to the bill's success. If the bill will impose costs, determine how those costs can be paid and if a funding source exists. During economic downturns, legislators will view any spending (particularly new spending) with skepticism. Consider whether a proposal that includes new spending should be brought forward at all or whether the measure's cost-generating aspects can be postponed until the budget crisis passes.

Nurses and lobbyists also must understand the policy preferences of the legislature and of individual legislators. Legislators who vote against a given set of bills may be encountered. It is important to understand the reason for their position, as their votes may never be gained and efforts to accommodate them may simply build opposition or unnecessary tension.

Challenges and Opportunities

Working on legislation presents both challenges and opportunities. Preparation in advance of the bill's introduction will enable the nurse leader or lobbyist to anticipate and address these challenges and opportunities.

If the proposed legislation was analyzed at the outset and the bill's policy goal was identified, persons who may have different positions or may oppose the bill will have been identified. Be prepared for the prospect that complete agreement with others involved in the process may never be achieved. For this reason, stay prepared in several areas. First, make sure the bill's sponsor and champion know what arguments will be presented against the bill so they will not be blindsided. Second, work with others who support the bill; this is particularly important in the context of a proposal to demonstrate that support for the measure includes main constituencies and not just the nurse. Inform the sponsor of the positions being taken, as this information will assist the legislator to gauge potential opposition and support for the effort. The legislator will view this additional information as a sign of the extent to which the nurse leader or lobbyist is prepared to address the issues and as an indication that this legislative effort has been fully vetted.

Finally, a differentiated set of rules applies to the legislative process, with its own language and rituals that need to be understood. Although success may come even to those who do not grasp these points, lack of familiarity with them can interfere with the effort and may cause others to view the effort as not being serious. This does not mean the lobbyist or nurse needs to be "seasoned." Instead, it means the individual who leads the legislative initiative needs to understand that success requires homework, teamwork, and preparation.

Future Role of the Nurse in Advancing Public Policy

Nurses must develop specific strategies to make the most of their regulatory expertise and to partner with lobbyists to successfully enact legislative changes that benefit the public. Identifying and developing the core competencies of current and future nurses in shaping public policy is crucial and is best achieved through mentoring, role modeling, and direct practice in the legislative arena.

References

Foley, M. (2007). Collective action in the workplace. In D. Mason, J. K. Leavitt, & M. W. Chaffee (Eds.), *Policy & politics in nursing and health care* (5th ed.). St. Louis, MO: Saunders Elsevier.

Mason, D., Leavitt, J. K, & Chaffee, M. W. (Eds.). (2007). *Policy & politics in nursing and healthcare* (5th ed.). St. Louis, MO: Saunders Elsevier.

Santa Anna, Y. (2007). An overview of legislation and regulation. In D. Mason, J. K. Leavitt, & M. W. Chaffee (Eds.), *Policy & politics in nursing and health care* (5th ed.). St. Louis, MO: Saunders Elsevier.

Joey Ridenour, MN, RN, FAAN, is executive director of the Arizona State Board of Nursing.

Greg Harris, JD, a partner in the law firm of Lewis and Roca in Phoenix, Arizona, served as a public member on the Arizona State Board of Nursing from 2000 to 2005 and on the NCSBN Board of Directors from 2002 to 2005.

Critical Thought, Leader Tip, and Scenario icons made by Freepik from www.flaticon.com; Callout icon made by Yannick from www.flaticon.com; Team Tip icon made by Chanut is Industries from www.flaticon.com

The best executive is the one who has sense enough to pick good men to do what he wants done, and self-restraint enough to keep from meddling with them while they do it. —Theodore Roosevelt

But again, to look to all these things yourself does not mean to do them yourself . . . but can you not insure that it is done when not done by yourself? —Florence Nightingale

CHAPTER OBJECTIVES

Upon completion of this chapter, the reader will be able to do the following:

» Appreciate the complexities of management and clinical delegation.

» Describe the basic concepts of delegation and supervision as they relate to the delegation of nursing work.

» Identify inappropriate delegation processes and the implications for negatively impacting patient care.

» Develop strategies to address the common errors and breakdowns in delegation and supervision.

» Develop skills to manage situations when delegation does not proceed as planned.

Delegation and Supervision: Essential Foundations for Practice

Without effective delegation, an organization might potentially come to a complete standstill. See Box 12-1. In such a scenario, each individual would do his or her work independently of others, with no connections to any other individual. There would be multiple silos working hard and going nowhere.

Delegation is required wherever there is a hierarchal order of individuals working together to accomplish goals. The importance of working with and through others has never been greater in health care, given the increased complexity, new technologies, and innovations in this field. The ability to delegate, assign, manage, and supervise is a critical competency for all healthcare workers, especially nurse leaders. Further compounding the challenges is the nursing shortage and the increasing demands being placed on those nurses who remain in the system. This chapter presents an overview of the basic principles of delegation, key concepts related to delegation and supervision, the challenges of delegating effectively, and strategies to enhance delegation skills. The role of the registered nurse (RN) in using delegation appropriately to ensure a safe and effective care environment is addressed.

The authority for delegation is outlined in the organizational chart of the facility. Included within positional managerial authority are the right and duty to delegate authority. Just as the possession of authority is a required component of any managerial position, the process of delegating authority to lower levels within the hierarchy is required for an organization to have effective managers, supervisors, and employees.

Delegation is both a management concept and a legal concept. As a management concept, it is discussed in terms of authority,

BOX 12-1 NURSING DELEGATION

Nursing delegation involves the transferring to a competent individual of the authority to perform a selected nursing task in a selected situation. The nurse retains accountability for the delegation.

responsibility, and accountability. Delegation begins with and flows from the chief executive officer (CEO) throughout the organization. All work is driven by the oversight of the CEO leader. Formal or organizational authority may be obtained from specific roles. Other formal sources of authority may occur through a position in an organization or through an individual contract. An individual can delegate only the authority that he or she individually possesses. Delegation is about the giving of power, responsibility, and work to another qualified individual.

The legal concept of delegation differs from the management or organizational concept of delegation and is defined in terms of authority and liability. Legal sources of authority come from legislative, judicial, and administrative branches of government. Most frequently, legal delegation is derived from the authority of the nurse licensure or other professional licensure. To empower one person to act for another requires the person doing the delegation to possess legal authority; before delegation can occur, there must be a source of that legal authority, which is licensure. All decisions related to delegation of nursing tasks must be based on the fundamental principle of protection of the health, safety, and welfare of the public.

For effective delegation to occur, the following elements must be present:

- Autonomy: The power to do the job (a job description). An individual must have an organizational job description that identifies the expectation for specific work. For example, the RN job description states the role of the nurse in providing patient care and control over nursing practice.
- Authority: The right to do the job (a license). The RN must also have a current and valid RN license to practice in the state in which patient care is being provided.
- Competence: The skill (knowledge, affective, and/or psychomotor) to do it. The nurse must demonstrate the knowledge and competence to effectively delegate.

If any one of these elements is missing, effective and legally defensible delegation cannot occur.

CRITICAL THOUGHT

Nursing judgment is the essential element in every delegation decision.

Delegation: Definitions and Key Concepts

This section highlights many of the key concepts and definitions specific to delegation (Mueller & Vogelsmeier, 2013).

- Accountability: Being answerable for actions or inactions of self or others; the obligation to account for or explain the events. Both **individual accountability** and **organizational accountability** for delegation exist. Organizational accountability relates to providing sufficient resources, staffing, and an appropriate staff mix; implementing policies and role descriptions; providing opportunities for continuing staff development; and creating an environment conducive to teamwork, collaboration, and client-centered care. Individual accountability is about knowing the requirements and behaviors of effective delegation (**Figure 12-1**).

- Assignment: The distribution of work that each staff member is to accomplish in a given time period. Assignment occurs when the authority to do a task already exists. It means that a nurse designates another nurse to be responsible for specific patients or selected nursing functions for specifically identified patients.

- **Authority**: The legal source of power; the right to act or command the actions of others and to have them followed. Authority is gained

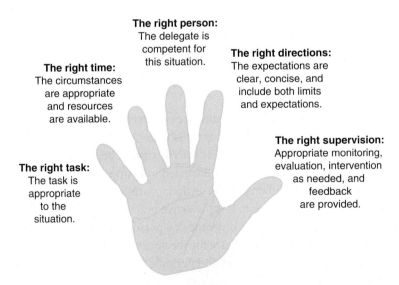

The right person:
The delegate is competent for this situation.

The right time:
The circumstances are appropriate and resources are available.

The right directions:
The expectations are clear, concise, and include both limits and expectations.

The right supervision:
Appropriate monitoring, evaluation, intervention as needed, and feedback are provided.

The right task:
The task is appropriate to the situation.

Figure 12-1 The five rights of delegation

from licensure (law) or by virtue of such characteristics as intelligence, knowledge, moral worth, and leadership ability (personal authority). Authority is a key component in developing a clear understanding and definition of delegation. Through delegation, the delegator transfers a span of authority and responsibility to the delegate, while the delegate is accountable for accomplishment of what has been delegated. The delegator retains final accountability for the delegation decision and for his or her own authorities and responsibilities.

- Critical thinking: Active, purposeful, organized thinking that takes into consideration focus, language, frame of reference, attitudes, assumptions, evidence, reasoning, conclusions, implications, and context when deciding what to believe or do in a given situation.

- Decision making: A complex cognitive process that involves choosing a particular course of action from among alternatives. Decision making is an essential component of the problem-solving process.

- **Delegate**: The individual staff person receiving the delegated task.

- **Delegation**: The transfer of responsibility for the performance of a selected nursing activity or task from a licensed nurse authorized to perform the activity or task to someone who does not have the authority. Delegation is the transfer of authority by one person to another; it is the act of transferring to a competent individual the authority to perform a selected nursing task in a selected situation, meaning the process for doing the work. It is a skill requiring clinical judgment and final accountability for client care. Delegation is the transfer of responsibility for the performance of an activity from one individual to another, with the original owner of the responsibility retaining *accountability of the outcome*.

- **Delegator**: The individual making the delegation.

- **Responsibility**: Reliability, dependability, and obligation to accomplish work.

- **Supervision**: The provision of guidance or direction, evaluation, and follow-up by the delegator for accomplishment of a task delegated to another; watching over a particular activity or task being carried out by other people and ensuring that it is carried out correctly. Supervision includes the initial and ongoing direction, procedural guidance, observation, and evaluation. It is the active practice of directing, guiding, and influencing the outcome of a person's performance of an activity, while providing guidance for the accomplishment of that task or activity, with initial direction and periodic inspection of the actual accomplishment of the task or activity.

As noted in these definitions, while a licensed nurse must be actively involved in and be accountable for all managerial decisions, policymaking, and practices related to the delegation of nursing care, both individual accountability and organizational accountability apply to delegation. Organizational accountability for delegation of licensed or legal functions of nursing requires that the organization provide the infrastructure for the delegation, supervision, and acceptance of delegated tasks by qualified individuals. The organization is accountable for ensuring that the individuals who accept delegated tasks are not only competent in performing the tasks but also are competent in their role in the delegation process.

Organizational accountability for delegation relates to doing the work of the organization based on the involved individuals' hierarchal positions and accountabilities in the organization. For example, it is the responsibility of the organization to ensure that both delegators and delegates have received information specific to the principles of delegation and supervision, including age-specific training, and are qualified to care for the client population specific to the tasks being delegated.

Steps of the Delegation Process: Roles of the Delegator and the Delegate

Learning to delegate effectively requires preparation and practice. See **Box 12-2**. Surely, understanding the concepts involved as well as the basic roles and steps is an important start. Also, understanding the expectations of the delegator and delegate roles in delegation is essential. Basic principles for delegation guide the practice of nursing delegation. See **Box 12-3**.

The delegator is responsible for the following:

- Assessment of the situation
- Ascertaining the competence of the delegate (education, training, skills, and experience)
- Follow-up supervision
- Management of results

The delegate is responsible for the following:

- His or her own actions
- Accepting only tasks or assignments that he or she is qualified to perform
- Providing feedback on tasks according to the guidelines specified by the delegator

BOX 12-2 THE IDEAL DELEGATOR

- Delegates authority whenever possible in areas affecting his or her work
- Consults with employees before making decisions pertaining to their job responsibilities
- Gives employees the reasons for implementing decisions
- Does not play favorites
- Recognizes excellent work
- Counsels employees who fail to observe the proper chain of command relationships and delegation principles
- Never reprimands or disciplines employees in front of coworkers
- Encourages employees to offer their opinions and criticisms of supervisory policies
- Listens to employees' explanations before placing blame in disciplinary situations; accepts reasonable explanations, not excuses
- Role models all the rules that other employees are expected to follow

BOX 12-3 BASIC DELEGATION PRINCIPLES

1. Delegation is considered a part of the nurse's role.
2. When the nurse delegates, the nurse assumes responsibility for supervision.
3. Each nurse is accountable for practicing according to state law. Licensed persons are responsible for providing nursing care in circumstances that are consistent with their training, education, and experience.
4. The nurse delegator is accountable for the acts of delegation and may incur liability if found negligent in the process of delegating and supervising.
5. The person delegated to is accountable for accepting the delegation and for his or her own actions in carrying out the delegated tasks.

It is the nurse manager's legal responsibility, in making assignments, to delegate appropriately and provide adequate supervision.

Once the delegation process occurs, the delegate must ensure that the delegation is within his or her capability based on the following assessments:

1. Determine if the task is within his or her scope of ability, licensure, and job description.
2. Consider the current work assignment.
3. Consider the current situation, such as complexity or potential for harm.
4. Accept graciously, and willingly identify concerns to the delegator.
The basic actions in delegation processes follow six steps.

Step One

Assess the patient or client, the situation, and the appropriateness for delegation. It is important to know your personal delegation strengths and weaknesses as well as those of the members of your team. Decisions to delegate nursing tasks, functions, and activities are based on the needs of the clients, the stability of the clients' conditions, the complexity of the task, the predictability of the outcome, and the available resources to meet those needs and the judgment of the nurse (American Nurses Association & National Council of State Boards of Nursing, n.d.). Be sure to understand the importance and expectations of the state nurse practice act, practice limitations, and job requirements.

Step Two

Assess the patient's needs and appropriateness for delegation. Ensure that the delegate has the legal and organizational permissions or right to perform the delegated task. It is essential for the delegating nurse to have an understanding of what the assistive personnel's credentials are in terms of education and demonstration of skill.

Making the Determination on What to Delegate

Based on nursing judgment, state law, and agency policies, a nurse must determine whether a task is delegable by relying on the criteria established in state nursing practice guidelines, the employing organization, and professional association recommendations. The following list provides guidelines for determining what should be delegated:

- The task is a routine or standardized task with a predictable outcome that is not threatening to the mental health of the patient.
- The task requires no judgment based on nursing knowledge or expertise.
- The results of the task are reasonably predictable.

- The task can be performed safely, according to exact, unchanging directions, with no need to alter the standard procedures for performing the task.
- The performance of the task does not require complex observations or critical decisions with respect to the task.
- No repeated nursing assessments are needed.
- The consequences of performing the nursing task improperly are minimal and not life threatening.

In most states or jurisdictions, a licensed practical/vocational nurse (LP/VN) may delegate tasks to a trained, unlicensed person if authorized by the RN to delegate and if the task is within the LP/VN's scope of practice. An LP/VN may not supervise the practice of an RN because the RN scope of practice is outside the LP/VN scope of practice. An LP/VN may supervise employment activities of an RN that do not constitute the practice of nursing, such as human resources policies.

Examples of common tasks delegated by RNs to nursing assistants include most activities of daily living, bathing patients, feeding patients, ambulating patients, taking vital signs, and performing skin care.

Tasks That Should Not Be Delegated

Supervisory accountability cannot be delegated. Although a supervisor must delegate authority to employees to accomplish specific jobs, the supervisor's own personal accountability cannot be delegated. Assigning duties to employees does not relieve the supervisor of the responsibility for those duties. When delegating assignments to employees, the supervisor remains accountable for the actions of the employees in carrying out these assignments.

Several other specific situations require mention:

- LP/VNs may delegate nursing tasks within the LP/VN's scope of practice, provided an RN first directs an LP/VN to do so.
- Assessment, evaluation, and nursing judgment cannot be delegated.
- Delegation is unnecessary if the particular activity or task is already within the legally recognized scope of practice of the individual who is to perform the activity or task.

CRITICAL THOUGHT

If a delegating nurse makes an acceptable delegation to a competent delegate and an error occurs, then the delegate is accountable for his or her actions in its performance, and the delegator is accountable for supervision, follow-up, intervention, and corrective action.

If the activity or task is not within a nurse's scope of practice, it cannot be delegated by a nurse. You cannot delegate what you do not have! Note that physicians cannot delegate physician work to nurses.

Step Three

Plan for the work to occur. Determine with the delegate when the work is to occur and under which patient circumstances. The following steps provide guidelines for preparing with the delegate:

1. Clearly identify the work that needs to be done.
2. Clearly identify the level of supervision and expected frequency of interactions between delegator and delegate.
3. Clearly identify the importance of requesting assistance when needed.
4. Create a plan for daily feedback between the delegator and the delegate specific to delegation principles performance.
5. Discuss strategies to increase effectiveness of delegation and supervision activities, including frequency of supervision and potential for additional delegation.

Step Four

Provide directions as to what is to be done. Always communicate in a positive, supportive manner. Maintain communication that is clear, complete, and constant. Ensure that the delegate understands what is to be done, when it is to be done, and which feedback is expected. Provide oversight and opportunity for communication during the task assignment time and as agreed upon.

Step Five

Evaluate the patient outcomes; compliance with standards of practice, policies, and procedures; and effectiveness of the delegation. Evaluate what happened and what the results were.

Step Six

Provide feedback to the delegate that includes recognition of work well done and areas of opportunity for improvement.

Protecting Your License: Nursing Liability for Delegation

Prior to learning the principles and processes of delegation, nurses are often concerned as to the potential professional liability specific to their RN or LP/VN license. Nurses initially believe they are responsible for the actual work of the delegate. In reality, the nurse is accountable for selection and delegation of tasks to the delegate. This includes ensuring that the conditions are appropriate for delegation and that the delegate is competent to perform the delegated work. The delegator nurse is not responsible for the actual work performed by the delegate. The delegate is fully responsible for his or her work. Thus the delegator is accountable for the process; the delegate is responsible for the work.

The Challenges of Delegation

The introduction of technology to advance communication has led to new challenges in effective delegation and supervision. The openness of communication channels through the Internet, email, instant messaging, and cell phones provides opportunities for sharing information with little restriction. Often, this openness means that boundaries are crossed beyond the level of authority, autonomy, and competence for the assigned work. Individuals may share information that they are not authorized to share, work may be performed on the basis of online instruction, and competence may not always be established through acceptable channels. Boundary clarity, according to Mackoff (2014), is an important competency through which nurses define and shape limits and responsibilities in their relationships with their colleagues. Accepting one's role and licensure authority as well as regularly reflecting on and reinforcing one's boundaries remains an underlying expectation of effective delegation. Failing to maintain boundaries, becoming overly involved emotionally, and not taking time for reflection almost always have a negative impact on delegation effectiveness.

As we have experienced, not every delegation event is successful. In addition to poor boundary clarity, delegation may fail for several other reasons. Sometimes there is underdelegation, in which not enough work is delegated. Sometimes there is overdelegation, in which, although the work is appropriate to delegate, the workload is beyond what the delegate can reasonably accomplish in the assigned time. Finally, the delegation can be improper, such that one or more of the "five rights" are violated: the wrong task, the wrong time, the wrong patient, the wrong delegate, the wrong supervision.

Oversupervision

Unfair delegation occurs when the delegator is constantly looking over the shoulders of those asked to do the work. This practice is confining and restricts the creativity and problem-solving potential that longs to come of most people. It is also unfair for the delegator to make decisions behind the backs of those to whom work is delegated. Often, the delegator begins to overmanage or add too many unnecessary check-ins, frustrating competent delegates.

Underdelegation

All too often, individuals fail to delegate for a variety of reasons. Some fear losing authority and recognition. It requires courage to turn important work over to others. Dictators never delegate; they just look for the weak-willed to implement their every desire. Another reason for limited delegation is fear of the work being done improperly or poorly—this is the most obvious reason why some people just cannot delegate. While there is always the fear of less than satisfactory results, often the reason for under-delegation is a lack of willingness to allow others to do the work their own way. In many cases, there is no perfect way to do the job.

There are numerous other reasons why delegation does not occur as intended, including the following examples:

- Lack of training and positive experience specific to delegation. A failed experience in delegation requires refocusing on the basics of delegation and working with others to create effective delegation processes. It is a rational risk that is essential to take. There can also be a lack of supervisory skill or lack of ability to direct, or uncertainty may arise regarding how to develop subordinates through the delegation process.

- Not comfortable with risk taking. Delegation inevitably involves risk—in nursing, this translates into fear that if the work is not done by you, a patient could be harmed or a lawsuit could be filed. Some people also have a desire to avoid conflict and confrontation and have a fear of being disliked.

- Unwillingness to take the necessary time to work with others. Task-oriented people want to just get the job done instead of waiting on others to do it through delegation. Some nurses prefer doing rather than managing.

- Fear of work being done better. Some leaders are paranoid about having others do a better job than they themselves could have done. Some also believe there is a lack of support for their decisions.

- Sometimes, delegation is undermined from within. Individuals may find it hard to let go of control and need to feel indispensable. They may have a fear of losing authority or personal satisfaction. Delegation requires trust.

- Fear of depending on others. Being independent reflects strength and competence. Shared leadership is quite different: It requires learning and less aggressiveness, combined with a willingness to depend on others in a team environment where the whole task is not completed until each member does his or her part. Some leaders may have a lack of confidence in their subordinates.

CRITICAL THOUGHT

Thoughts on delegation, supervision, and oversight:

- The RN is accountable for delegation and supervision of assigned patients.
- Oversight is an expectation within the delegation and supervision process. There may be layers of oversight within the process; for example, RN → LP/VN → nursing assistant, or RN → instructor → student.
- Hand-off activities are critical events in the delegation process to ensure continuity of oversight.
- Documentation of delegation and supervision/oversight should never eliminate the accountability or oversight of the work to be done.

- Preoccupation with negative fantasies about what could happen. Such fears block the delegator from working with others to develop effective delegation skills.
- Lack of skill in balancing workloads and disorganization.

Refusal by Delegate

Another challenge in effective delegation is the refusal by the delegate to accept an assignment. Refusal of assignments poses a new challenge to the already overburdened clinical nurse. It is important to determine, as best as one can, the reason for the refusal to accept the assignment. While potential delegates may not freely offer the reasons for their refusal, it is important to consider the following potential reasons:

- Lack of willingness to do the job (lazy, unmotivated)
- Lack of skill (not comfortable with skills)
- Perceptions of unfair assignments (feelings of overwork)
- Physical condition (not able to physically do the work)

Strategies to Support Effective Delegation

In light of the challenges, several strategies may be implemented to address the challenges and improve delegation processes (Day et al., 2014). The first is to gain an understanding of personal delegation competence.

Individuals can consider the following questions to assess their current status with regard to delegation and supervision:

1. Why is it so hard to delegate? Is something blocking an individual from embracing delegation as a means to provide more effective and efficient patient care?
2. How does one know *what* to delegate?
3. How does one know to *whom* tasks can be delegated?
4. How does one know *when* to refuse an assignment?
5. Why don't I delegate? What is blocking this behavior?
6. Why don't I willingly accept delegated tasks? Is it difficult to work on a team and be mutually accountable for team members?
7. What would help me improve my ability to delegate appropriately?
8. What should I do if I identify inappropriate delegation?
9. Should my performance be rated above average if I willingly accept appropriately delegated tasks? If I delegate appropriately?
10. Should I be rated below average if I routinely refuse and/or challenge the nurse when tasks are delegated? If I do not delegate appropriately?

When considering the behaviors in the preceding list, also consider which tasks are or could be involved in delegation of patient care work. Ask yourself the following questions:

1. Can someone else do the task?
2. Should someone else do the task?
3. Do I have to do the job?

Often, these types of challenging questions assist nurses in reevaluating situations and considering new approaches to patient care. They also provide insight into why individuals may be reluctant to accept delegated tasks as well as to delegate.

CRITICAL THOUGHT

Delegation is an elementary act of managing.

Another strategy is to access evidence-based resources for delegation and supervision. As the pressure increases to deliver higher productivity without compromising quality, processes of delegation will become ever more important in health care.

Finally, the strategy of developing and sharing clinical scenarios as a teaching tool is most effective in providing nurses with proactive strategies to address challenging situations. Scenarios may relate to common problems with delegation, to emerging new practices that may be unclear specific to delegation appropriateness, and to high-risk situations that require new perspectives.

Final Thoughts

No individual can complete his or her work without the participation of other individuals. Out of necessity, delegation is required to connect the work of the organization across individuals and departments. Effective delegation is both an art and a science; it encompasses organizational process delegation and legally authorized delegation by specific licensure. It is not about dumping work on another person or abdicating one's own responsibility. Rather, delegation is about accountability—transfer of authority and responsibility to perform work. It is about actively supporting basic work processes in a complex world in order to ensure a safe and effective care environment through appropriate management of care.

SCENARIO

Delegation is often misunderstood and not used as effectively as it could be—even though most nurses recognize that delegation is necessary to function effectively and efficiently as a nurse. Nurses on your unit tend to underdelegate and believe they can do it (whatever the task might be) better themselves.

Discussion Questions

In a small group, respond to the following items:

1. My definition of delegation is _____ .

2. I am reluctant to delegate because _____ .

3. My delegation would be better if _____ .

4. My plan to share this information with my team is _____ .

Share your responses with one another as well as your suggestions to increase your competence in delegation and to assist others to delegate appropriately.

SCENARIO

Charlotte, an experienced nurse, was working with two licensed practical nurses (LPNs) from an external nurse registry. She assigned the LPNs to administer all of the medications, including management of the IVs. The LPNs made several errors.

Discussion Questions

In your group, consider the concepts of autonomy, authority, and competence for both Charlotte and the LPNs.

1. What was appropriate and what was inappropriate?

2. How could this same situation be avoided in the future?

SCENARIO

Yohannes, RN, is the nurse manager at an outpatient clinic. One member of Yohannes's nursing team, Ean, is an LPN. Yohannes learns that another RN in the clinic delegated to Ean taking the initial vital signs on all patients and triaging incoming calls. It comes to light that Ean did not complete the vital signs and triaged a patient inappropriately. Discuss Yohannes's role in this scenario.

SCENARIO

Isabella is an RN on a medical-surgical hospital unit. She has been practicing for two months. However, today her nursing assignment has unexpectedly become busy. She is caring for a patient whose medical status is deteriorating and thus needs multiple medications, infusions, and frequent monitoring. She also has two other patients under her care. Isabella is not able to safely complete all these things in a timely manner. Liam, a certified nursing assistant (CNA), and Jack, an RN, have offered their assistance. Using critical thinking and the steps of delegation, discuss how Isabella can delegate care in this situation.

SCENARIO

Bridget, RN, is working with Jenny, CNA. Bridget delegates the task of using the bladder scan machine to record a post-void residual on a patient to Jenny after the patient is finished toileting. Jenny tells Bridget that she will assist the patient using the bathroom but will not do the post-void residual bladder scan. Upon further discussion, Bridget learns that this is not a task that Jenny is comfortable with and Jenny does not feel like she is competent to do the task even though it is something within her scope of practice. How can Bridget handle this situation?

CHAPTER TEST QUESTIONS

Licensure exam categories: Management of care: delegation/supervision, concepts of management

Nurse leader exam categories: Knowledge of the healthcare environment: delivery models/work design, patient safety, interprofessional practice

1. Legal delegation includes the oversight and delegation of

   a. the work of unlicensed support staff.

   b. the operational and clinical work identified in the organizational chart.

   c. the work of licensed staff in providing patient care services.

   d. specific work of the RN that does not require physician supervision.

2. Supervision as a component of the delegation process

   a. is an essential activity of the delegation.

   b. requires continuing education documentation and verification of competence of the RN.

   c. is designed to ensure hourly follow-up.

   d. is required only when there is an assignment of duties involved.

3. There are several purposes of delegation. Which of the following is *not* a purpose of the delegation process?

   a. increased workload management effectiveness

   b. improvement of patient satisfaction

   c. full use of scope of practice of licensed and unlicensed personnel

   d. increasing the workload of RNs

4. Strategies to increase delegation competence include

   a. personal assessment of delegation abilities.

   b. identification of the need for discipline when delegation does not occur.

   c. regular training sessions that include scenarios for discussion.

   d. increasing the time allocation for delegation work.

5. Challenges for RNs in delegation are significant because

   a. delegation principles are not taught in nursing school.

   b. some nurses believe their nursing license is at risk when delegating to unlicensed personnel.

   c. appropriate delegation is difficult to determine.

   d. there are wide variations in delegation rules set by state boards of nursing.

6. Determining when not to delegate includes consideration of

   a. the patient's condition during the previous shift.

   b. the discharge status of the patient.

   c. the significant potential for harm.

   d. the liability for malpractice.

7. Inappropriate delegation occurs when

  a. effective supervision takes place on site.

  b. medication administration is delegated by a licensed person to an unlicensed person without medication administration authority.

  c. an unlicensed person delegates to a licensed person.

  d. a licensed practical nurse delegates to an unlicensed person.

8. Boundary clarity is an important foundation for effective delegation because

  a. it provides guidelines for making equitable assignments.

  b. the work of the nurse is clearly defined.

  c. the limits and responsibilities of work are defined.

  d. it provides rules to avoid making errors.

9. Accountability differs from responsibility in that

  a. accountability includes expectations to perform authorized work based on licensure or job description.

  b. responsibility is about the provision of resources, policies, and staff development for delegates, while accountability is about using the resources effectively.

  c. accountability is about ensuring adequate resources and staff development for delegation, while responsibility is about ensuring attendance at staff development workshops.

  d. accountability is about being able to answer for and explain actions and results, and responsibility is about doing the task.

10. Assignment differs from delegation in that

  a. neither delegation nor assigning requires authority.

  b. ownership of authority for the tasks belongs only to the RN.

  c. delegation requires authority for tasks, but assignment does not.

  d. delegation does not include authority for tasks, while assignment includes authority for tasks.

11. The RN has delegated the following to other members of the healthcare team. Which delegation is appropriate?

    a. patient ambulation to a physical therapy assistant

    b. administration of oral antihypertensive medications to an LPN

    c. insertion of an indwelling catheter to a CNA

    d. reassessment of pain response after pharmacologic and nonpharmacologic interventions

12. When preparing to delegate an appropriate task, what should the RN do?

    a. avoid delegating to an employee who complains about accepting assignments

    b. communicate the expectation that the delegate ask for assistance when needed

    c. provide clear direction for the work that needs to be done

    d. identify and communicate the frequency of interactions between the delegator and delegate

References

American Nurses Association & National Council of State Boards of Nursing. (n.d.). Joint statement on delegation. Retrieved from www.ncsbn.org/Delegation_joint_statement_NCSBN-ANA.pdf

Day, L., Turner, K., Anderson, R. A., Mueller, C., McConnell, E. S., & Corazzini, K. N. (2014). Teaching delegation to RN students. *Journal of Nursing Regulation, 5*(2), 10–15.

Mackoff, B. L. (2014). The practice of boundary clarity. *Nurse Leader, 8*(2), 23–27.

Mueller, C., & Vogelsmeier, A. (2013). Effective delegation: Understanding responsibility, authority, and accountability. *Journal of Nursing Regulation, 4*(3), 20–27.

Appendix A

Joint Statement on Delegation: American Nurses Association and National Council of State Boards of Nursing

In 2005, the American Nurses Association (ANA) and National Council of State Boards of Nursing (NCSBN) issued a joint statement on delegation, which can be accessed on the ANA and the NCSBN websites. The joint statement identifies nine principles of delegation:

1. The essence of professional responsibility and accountability
2. Care coordination and the use of assistants in providing patient care
3. Not delegating the nursing process but rather only parts of the process to assistive personnel
4. The significance of nursing judgment
5. Delegation to competent individuals
6. The components of effective communication between the RN and the delegate
7. The importance of two-way communication in the delegation process between the delegator and the delegate
8. The importance of critical thinking, professional judgment, and the five rights of delegation:
   - The right task
   - Under the right circumstances
   - To the right person
   - With the right directions and communication
   - Under the right supervision and evaluation
9. The role of the chief nursing officer is ensuring adequate infrastructure for delegation and supervision

Data from American Nurses Association (ANA) and National Council of State Boards of Nursing (NCSBN). (2006). Joint statement on delegation. Retrieved from www.ncsbn.org /Delegation_joint_statement_NCSBN-ANA.pdf and nursingworld.org/MainMenuCategories /Policy-Advocacy/Positions-and-Resolutions/ANAPositionStatements

Appendix B

Delegation Assessment: Why Don't I Willingly Delegate or Accept Delegated Tasks?

In groups of three, develop your response(s) to each situation. Which principles of delegation were followed, and which principles were not followed?

1. Overdelegation
   - Would you pass my medications for me and sign off my orders? I'm really busy.
2. Underdelegation
   - I'll do it myself. The nursing assistant argues with me when I ask her to do something.
   - I'll do it myself. I always have to do it over.
3. Refusal to accept assignment—legitimate delegation
   - I don't have enough experience to perform that task.
   - I don't know how to do that very well [fear of criticism for mistakes—lack of self-confidence].
   - I'd rather not risk the patient's life.
   - I have too much work already.
   - It's always me that gets the work; ask someone else.
   - I'm too busy, I won't be able to do a very good job, but if that's what you want. . . .

Appendix C

Process of Delegation

1. Select a competent and capable person; consciously assess that person's skill, experience, and attitude.
2. Assign the task/duties to immediate subordinates.
3. Clearly and realistically define the goals, priorities, and outcomes for both the delegator and the delegate; give complete information.
4. Confer authority and the means to do the job; grant permission (authority) to take all the actions necessary to perform these duties.
5. Create an obligation (responsibility) on the part of each employee to perform the duties satisfactorily.
6. Keep in contact and give feedback during and after the completion of tasks.

> The great question about power is who should have it. —John Locke

CHAPTER OBJECTIVES

Upon completion of this chapter, the reader will be able to do the following:

» Understand basic elements and characteristics of professional negotiation.

» Define the unique characteristics and obligation of the clinical leader in facilitating and coordinating negotiation and its processes.

» Delineate the elements and characteristics of dynamic negotiation and the stages necessary for successful negotiation processes.

» Outline the principles and characteristics of negotiation and problem solving as a part of the clinical leadership experience.

» List at least six components of negotiation and the characteristics of each.

» State at least three reasons why the clinical leader must use negotiation processes every day as a part of leadership expression.

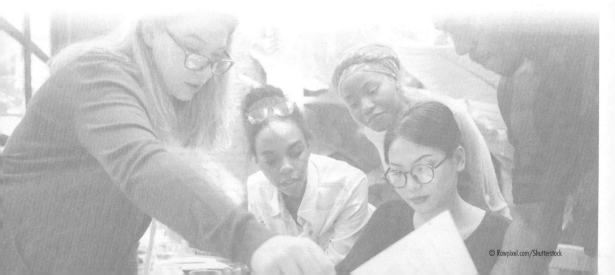

Overcoming the Uneven Table: Negotiating the White Waters of the Profession

Negotiating skills are not optional for the clinical professional. At all levels of professional practice, the elements of negotiation are continually used in the role of agent and while acting in the best interests of persons and the public. The nursing professional continually negotiates with peers and patients, administrators and assistants, and a host of other professionals representing a wide variety of constituents having an influence on the work of the nurse.

Effective **negotiation** is entirely a learned skill. Although some people may be born with particular talents that enhance their ability to negotiate, effective negotiation is more typically learned through the process of discipline and application. In fact, much of the skill and talent necessary to negotiate well can be improved through continuous and effective use and refinement of skill development and learning. People who are less naturally gifted with the basic negotiating skills can easily learn and adapt to the process of working with others to find common ground, to reach agreement, or to move collectively within a diverse set of circumstances (Deleuran & Jarner, 2011).

Becoming an effective negotiator requires learning some basic skills to help refine understanding and clarify the factual foundations for decision making and collective action. In all negotiations, it is important to be able to apply good listening techniques, effective questioning methodologies, useful verbal and nonverbal communication approaches, and creative mechanisms in advancing win–win solutions and shared values.

CRITICAL THOUGHT

Negotiation does not produce winners or losers. Rather, it leads to a mutually beneficial solution to a common issue in a way that engages the stakeholders and invests them in the deliberation process.

Principles and Basic Skills of Negotiating

Working toward achieving universally recognized and acceptable solutions is a discipline just as much as it is a process. Each party to a negotiation recognizes that the other parties have something that is important to each individual sufficient to require their interaction, communication, and some level of argument. Basic processes of negotiation occur every day over things as small as deciding between items on a lunch menu to resolving the complex vagaries of a multinational contract. Despite the difference in scale, the principles that drive these negotiations are generally consistent.

Negotiating is not about winning or losing. In fact, if winning and losing are a part of the negotiation or the result of the negotiation, the dialogue can be considered as having failed. A win–win outcome is an essential characteristic of negotiation and forms one of its foundational principles. Negotiation is undertaken to identify and engage in a process that clearly establishes needs and wants, with all parties working to reconcile their interests in a way that results in mutual advantage or value. In short, all parties must win something meaningful to them for positive negotiation to be satisfied. Because of the nature of win–win approaches to negotiation, developing effective skills and high levels of preparation are critical to successes between the parties to a negotiation (Heller & Hindle, 2008; Kozina, 2014).

Because negotiation is a skill, recognizing the principles and foundations that guide it is the first step to developing the essential insights and skills that ultimately make negotiation successful. The following principles are applied to ensure a positive exchange:

- Understand your own position.
- Collect data on the other's position.
- Concession is a strategy, not a loss.
- The solution must be mutual.
- Expect to be surprised by what emerges.
- The solution may be other than expected.
- The exchange must be thought fair by stakeholders.

In addition, a set of core skills must be developed and refined to ensure successful negotiation:

- The individual must be able to discern, identify, and declare specific goals for which the risk of negotiation is worth undertaking. These goals establish an entry position but also support flexibility, which indicates a willingness to engage in dialogue and negotiation.

- The parties must maintain a certain level of flexibility and fluidity with their wants and needs. Insisting on a firm and unyielding attachment to positions, demands, or needs eliminates the grounds for meaningful negotiation and polarizes the process before it even begins.

- Both parties must demonstrate a willingness to be open and available, and they must be willing to entertain a wide range of potential options and considerations that can provide creative and unique ways of satisfying needs and finding common ground.

- Good negotiators are well informed, are clearly prepared, and understand as much about the matter under negotiation as possible. It is important to know as much as possible about all points of view and positions on the issue. A good negotiator knows how to argue on behalf of the other positions at the table almost as well as the parties who make those arguments do.

- Negotiation essentially relies on the use of good communication skills and positive interaction. Some level of competence in communication is sound preparation for the meaningful dialogue of negotiation. All negotiation reflects the use of words and language combined with the communication capacity of body language, gestures, and tone. The better prepared and disciplined the individual is in these negotiation skill sets, the more positively positioned he or she is for effective negotiation.

- Listening is perhaps one of the most essential foundational skills in effective negotiation. Strong negotiators carefully listen to messages being delivered by others and take note of the context as well as the content of the message. Here again, body language, gestures, tone, use of language, and the ability to discern supporting information or communication in a way that helps clarify true meaning all contribute to the effectiveness of the interaction.

- A good negotiator knows how to sort the extraneous from the valuable, and the high priority from the unimportant. He or she continually remembers the purposes and principles that bring individuals to the negotiation table, and the negotiator recognizes the needs and wants that reflect how those purposes might be fulfilled. When negotiators

CRITICAL THOUGHT

The ability to listen carefully is one of the most important leadership skills associated with good negotiation. Hearing the real messages that are the basis for negotiation is critical to obtaining the right outcome.

are more aware of their negotiating partners' personal needs and wants, they are better able to satisfy them with a wider range of options. Problems can usually be solved in a number of ways, so being open to alternative options that can address needs and wants provides a wider range of choices for getting issues appropriately addressed.

Practicing negotiating skills in noncritical situations can help an individual develop his or her negotiating talent in a risk-free developmental environment. Negotiation is such an important skill that formally including it in the continuing education developmental program for nursing staff should be considered; such an approach would signal that this skill is part of the tool set necessary for good clinical care. Refining negotiation skills in the common and ordinary activities of daily life helps hone them for more specific and directed circumstances. The professional must know that just as negotiation occurs in personal life (e.g., negotiating who takes the children to school and who picks them up, choosing a favorite restaurant, resolving a difference on child rearing), so this same process occurs—and uses the same principles and skills—in the work arena.

Give and Take: The Principles of Exchange

Important to negotiation is the understanding that every party needs to gain from the interaction. That is, something of value must be exchanged. For individuals to feel as though they have accomplished something by participating in the negotiation, they must feel that they are taking something meaningful away from the process. In negotiation, if one side wins and the other loses, the negotiation has essentially failed.

REFLECTIVE QUESTION

The most important issue for an individual involved in negotiating is what his or her precise bottom line is. When you think of a recent conflict with a coworker or family member, what was your essential bottom line beyond which you were not willing to go?

People must first be clear about what it is they most need or want from the negotiation process. This notion of an individual's bottom line helps establish the ground upon which the individual will negotiate. At the same time, individuals in the negotiation need to know that to obtain a satisfactory outcome for themselves, there must be a fair exchange that results in a satisfactory outcome for other stakeholders to the negotiation. Individuals engaged in negotiation must recognize that flexibility is a vital element to ensure that the process is successful. The give-and-take, balance of power, and back-and-forth of the negotiation process provide a continual recalibration of the dynamic between the parties as each moves to meet his or her needs and the chosen methods and mechanisms satisfy each stakeholder.

Stages of Negotiation

Like any formal process, negotiation involves several phases or stages that participants move through as they advance to mutual solutions and satisfaction. Typically, an equitable negotiation moves through the following stages: (1) readying for negotiation; (2) establishing the framework for the negotiation; (3) intensive interaction; (4) bargaining; and (5) closing the interaction, which sometimes includes another step: (6) implementing the agreement.

Readying for Negotiation

Detailed *and* intense preparation for negotiation is a hallmark of truly successful interaction. Information is always the source of power in the negotiation process. Those who are best prepared for negotiation will best benefit from it. As part of this preparation, it is important not only to become fully aware of one's own arguments and justifications in the negotiation process but also to be able to argue the views of other participants with equal adeptness. Identifying the issues at the table and appreciating all of their nuances will help the individual better understand his or her own position and its relationship to the other potential positions at the table.

Achieving such a thorough understanding of the issues at hand requires some level of objectivity and broad-based assessment. Although emotion is clearly a legitimate element of the interaction process, preparation for the negotiation should be as free of the emotional component as is possible, so that the individual will be open to all the information and data that are influencing his or her position and informing the negotiation process.

An honest interaction and confrontation with the data informing the negotiation provides an analytical perspective that helps participants avoid surprises that might directly affect the success of the negotiation. Here again, the individual bottom line—that is, the essential nonnegotiable point below which the participant cannot go—needs to be clear and specific. The individual establishes this so-called best alternative to a negotiated agreement (BATNA) as the absolute point of reference and the essential "get" that is necessary to make the negotiation successful for him or her. A "badly" negotiated agreement, from the perspective of any party, is generally worse than no agreement at all.

Establishing a personal bottom line raises the question about what happens when the parties to the negotiation cannot reach a satisfactory agreement. Each negotiator must place himself or herself in the context of the other negotiators and consider what might happen if an agreement is not reached. Remember, each participant in the negotiation has his or her own bottom line. Developing an awareness of that bottom line and the individual's relationship to it advances a deeper understanding of the negotiation process by facilitating mutual understanding of the variety of bottom lines held by the parties to the negotiation.

After establishing a bottom line and selecting the approach to be used to support it, the negotiator should practice his or her approach to the interaction. By doing so, individual participants essentially choreograph their interaction in the negotiation and step through all the points at issue, arguments and counterarguments, positions, and interactions that might come up during the negotiation. Much like a game of chess, the steps and stages in the approach to negotiation require that participants think through as many of the moves and positions in the interaction as possible. Each participant should recognize that other participants are likely as prepared and will have also done their homework for the negotiation.

In summary, preparing for the negotiation involves the following activities:

- Be fully aware of one's own position.
- Know the arguments that support and oppose the position.
- Understand all the issues at the table.
- Study the other parties' positions and issues.
- Be clear about personal, emotional hooks.
- Establish the beginning, personal bottom line.
- Determine the best personal approach.

Establishing the Framework for the Negotiation

Although preparation for the negotiation is an important first step, it is also important to establish the terms of engagement for the negotiation encounter. Preparations for the negotiation are almost as important as the negotiation itself. Because of the anxieties that arise owing to the nature of confrontation and the stresses associated with opposing points of view, the negotiation leader must seek to establish the rules of the negotiation and the terms of the engagement. The goal here is to provide a structured and positive environment for the negotiation. Such a milieu allows the parties to clarify their expectations with regard to the process and to operate within the context of fairly formal rules of dialogue. Major elements of those roles of dialogue are as follows:

- Establish a rule that allows participants to speak without interruption.
- Identify each other by first names, leaving titles and roles outside the negotiating room.
- Establish agreement with the behavioral parameters, refrain from attacking, eliminate put-down behavior, and ask clearly structured questions that can advance understanding and clarity.
- Refrain from coarse, crude, profane responses or negative use of language.
- Listen with respect and sincerity, attempting to fully understand the other party's communication and generation of interests.
- Respect differences and understand that each participant is entitled to his or her own perspective.
- Let go of failures and nonsolutions generated from past interactions; focus instead on decisions made from the current negotiated point forward.
- Agree to make an intentional effort to refrain from arguing, belaboring points, venting, or making comments of long duration. Each participant should agree to use the negotiating time in a fair and equitable manner.
- Establish and respect needs for break time and time away from the negotiation.
- Establish regular times for rest and recuperation and breaks from the negotiation as a way of supporting individual needs and maintaining sufficient energy for the long-term negotiation process.

Much of the preliminary work in establishing the terms of engagement provides a positive environment within which a generative, solution-seeking approach to negotiation can unfold. Eliminating as many of the sources of negative energy and a negative negotiating environment helps accelerate the likelihood of a successful negotiating process.

CRITICAL THOUGHT

Confrontation often creates anxiety. It is wise for the negotiator to understand which issues create anxiety, practice with a friend or colleague in objectively making an argument, and work with them in dealing with the emotional aspects of the negotiation process. Practice diffuses emotional intensity and strengthens presentation skills.

Intensive Interaction

Interaction with others during the negotiating process reflects the understanding that each participant has of the process as well as the role of each participant in the negotiation. Guidelines for such intensive interaction include the following points:

- Keep in mind that negotiation is a process, not an event.
- Remember your emotional hooks.
- Keep in mind that each session builds on previous sessions.
- Recalibrate your position after gaining more data.
- Better articulate others' real positions at the table.
- Identify emerging points of convergence/agreement.
- Discern the best personal approach.
- Keep the intensity of negotiations level and consistent.
- Take breaks after tough issues or during lull moments.

Assessing the characteristics of the other parties helps the individual participant characterize his or her own approach and the conditions influencing the interaction. While preparing for the negotiation, the individual comes to more fully understand both his or her own position as well as the positions of the other participants. Each argument should be objectively reviewed in depth and in detail to develop a specific counter to that argument. In addition, participants should assess the strength of the other parties' positions in an effort to find points of convergence or emergent elements of agreement. Sorting through others' basic arguments and starting points can give participants a clue as to the other predominant positions and the other participants' bottom lines. Besides assessing the argument of the negotiation, participants should be reviewing others' skill in advocating for their position, capacity for negotiation, and clarity with regard to presenting facts and expectations.

At the same time as the participants are assessing one another's arguments, elements related to lack of specificity, weaknesses of the argument, lack of clarity, or factors with which the other participants are unaware may also serve to inform other participants about a particular argument or point of view. Ultimately, the goal of such preparation is to provide points of comparison with one's own argument, utilizing this information to help strengthen, clarify, or reformat a particular position. Remember, the issue here is not to be right but rather to be factual, clear, precise, and understood.

Because negotiation is generally continued over a series of sessions, previous sessions provide exposure, background, prior information, and new data that inform subsequent sessions. Even so, previous sessions may not be a strong indicator of the action and interaction of the current round of negotiation. Each negotiation session stands on its own merits and reflects only the activities that occur within that session, even though they may be an aggregate of the work of previous sessions. While subsequent sessions always build on previous sessions, each session brings forth its own dynamics and generates conclusions that may not have been as easily reached in previous sessions.

An important aspect of the ongoing negotiation process is the opportunity for individuals to note and identify points of convergence or common ground. As the negotiation sessions unfold, emerging areas of common ground may become apparent. Early agreements on particular issues of conflict can provide the floor for subsequent clarity and agreement on more difficult issues—a process called **chunking**. Instead of reaching a point of broad generalized agreement, the final agreement may actually represent an aggregation of smaller agreements that, when looked at comprehensively, satisfies the needs of the participants (Boulle, Colatrella, & Picchioni, 2008; Kobayashi & Viswat, 2014).

If you are the leader of the negotiation process, it is important that you create a safe space where the negotiation can unfold with a sense of balance and equity. Certainly, a neutral location that is comfortable, easy to access, and as informal as the negotiation requires is an important consideration. Comfort and attention to the supporting details related to the location itself will be important. The leader provides a good sense of control and an environment supportive of the negotiation situation. To do so, the leader orchestrates and manages the atmosphere, space, structure, and processes associated with the negotiation. Supplying supporting materials and information, as well as paper, pens, and other practical items that facilitate the process, is helpful. Attention to detail also means ensuring that bathroom facilities are nearby, lighting is soft yet supportive, the room temperature is appropriate, and required audiovisual supports are available and work properly. It is also important to have a clock available so that everyone is aware of the time—managing time is critical for various elements of the negotiation process. It may also be important for the leader to ensure that there are alternative places where individuals or groups can gather to do individual work in a private and uninterrupted environment. Following are some guidelines for creating an environment supportive of negotiation:

- The environment of negotiation is as important as the negotiation.
- Soft balanced lighting reduces emotional intensity.
- The room temperature should be neutral, between 68 and 72 degrees Fahrenheit.
- Water should be available at each position at the table.
- There should be alternative locations for party breaks or caucuses.
- Pens, papers, and flip charts should be available for the process.
- A box of tissues should be available at each position.

- The restrooms should be noted and should be nearby.
- The space should allow for parties to mingle informally.

Leaders will frequently be conducting negotiations between two or more parties and must be aware of the dynamics related to the intensity of the interaction. They should be able to assess the tone and mood of the participants by reading body language, which reflects levels of stress through nonverbal signals such as gestures, facial expressions, and body movements. The leader's preparation helps the individuals both anticipate and determine the best approach for initiating the negotiation. The levels of stress, the intensity of the issue, and the relatedness of the participants, in turn, help the leader predetermine which particular approaches may best break through the stress, create comfort, and reduce the intensity at the beginning of interaction. In particular, the leader's skills in reading nonverbal signs and body language (e.g., gestures, eye movements, and facial expressions) can be applied to determine which particular approaches may be necessary to initiate the dialogue and sustain it. The leader should pay attention to even small gestures and movements, such as fidgeting, wringing of hands, raised eyebrows, crossed arms, sitting back in the chair, and eye contact; these are indicators of the mood and emotional intensity of the participants.

Participants of the negotiation should realize that negotiation is both an art and a science. The structural part of negotiation reflects more of the science of negotiation; the flow, dialogue, and interaction of the participants reflect more of the art of negotiation. Some dos and don'ts related to the intensity of interaction at critical points in negotiation might be as follows:

- Do listen carefully to all parties.
- Don't make lots of concessions at the earliest stages of negotiation.
- Do allow plenty of room for self-maneuvering in suggesting or proposing positions.
- Don't make opening statements or offers so polarized or extreme that the position is lost.
- Do emphasize conditional offers that reflect what you will give based on what someone else offers.
- Never say "never."
- Do probe participants with regard to their feelings, insights, and attitudes.
- Do avoid closed-ended questions that can be answered with yes or no; instead, expand on open-ended questions to seek explanation or understanding.
- Stay away from demeaning, diminishing, alienating, and angering other parties.

In a negotiation, it is important that all parties remain open to options and opportunities that may arise in the process of communicating and interacting in the negotiation. Avoid making thoughtless, quick, or brash statements that might polarize the negotiation or rule out any movement by the other parties. Make sure that proposals are broad based, open ended, and exploratory, allowing all parties to expand on and consider options and opportunities for consensus, convergence, or identification of common ground. Parties to negotiation should avoid forcing other parties into a corner, as this merely narrows the opportunities for movement and reduces the chance that further negotiation might lead to concessions or consensus that would help move the parties toward resolution.

Seeking clarification of other participants' points or contributions is a critical element for ensuring clarity and specificity. The leader and participants to the negotiation want as much as possible to be clear about what is actually being negotiated and where participants are in relationship to the information and elements on the table for discussion. Remaining in a questioning mode helps create a context for clarification and understanding and promotes an environment that supports an open negotiation process. Although not all parties to the negotiation may be positively disposed toward this process, it is important to be able to pursue the factual elements embedded in all responses to keep the negotiation balanced.

At times in the negotiation, the leader will recognize tactics that seek to delay, offset, stall, or send a negotiation off course. The leader has to manage threats, insults, intimidation, bluffing, dividing, emotional intensity, and boundary testing. Awareness of the potential of these behaviors in any human interaction is critical for facilitating the negotiation process. In each of these situations, the leader must be willing to implement strategies to offset the imbalance created by negative behaviors:

- If participants make threats, the parties must be reminded that negotiation cannot occur under conditions of duress, and that compromise and concession can be found only if the behavior that drives the threats is offset by sound principles of communication.
- If insults occur, diffuse them with a balanced and calm reaction and a restatement of the principles that guide the dialogue and the

CRITICAL THOUGHT

The leader periodically translates for the parties, enumerating points of convergence, issues, understanding, and opportunities for agreement. This restatement provides clarity and helps participants form language that clearly communicates their understanding.

interaction. Allow the participants to restate their position within the appropriate context and proceed with a more constructive dialogue.

- When participants use intimidating language, identify and recognize it and its impact in reducing the positive context for negotiation and the negative connotation it implies. Restate the original contribution to the dialogue and ask for clarification and response with regard to its accuracy free of emotional intensity.

- When a party makes obtuse, nonspecific, dubious assertions (lying, for example) that represent bluffing, restate the individual's original position in clear terms and wait for a factual response. Use question statements to clarify the issue and counteract the obfuscation or bluff.

- When a participant tries to exploit disagreements (using disagreement for personal advantage), restate the area of disagreement for clarification and enumerate the particular positions of participants as a mechanism for confirming those positions.

- When leading questions are used to confuse, identify weakness, or force concessions, delay answering a series of questions, break down the questions into single units, and seek specific answers to each individual question as it relates to the originating issue. Any question that is not topically specific should be eliminated from the clarification.

- When an individual's response includes emotional extremes, such as anger and accusations, blaming and pointing fingers, reactions, and polarization, affirm the commitment to fairness, equity, and balance. Refocus the conversation on specific issues and remind the participants of the terms of engagement. If necessary, taking a break from the process can provide an opportunity for emotions to be addressed and balance to be reestablished.

- When participants infringe on the terms of engagement, clearly enumerate and restate the terms to reemphasize their role in the negotiation process and to remind participants of the value they play in balancing negotiation. Here again, ensure that clarity is established, language is precise, and process is followed consistently.

Leading a negotiation process is a challenging and sometimes difficult experience, especially when a wide variety of personalities are involved and must be dealt with in the effort to maintain balance at the negotiating table. Each participant brings his or her own cultural, social, and personal behavioral set of values that can facilitate and sometimes constrain a positive negotiating environment. Negative behaviors will invariably arise, and sometimes negative personalities will be present. Rather than ignore or minimize these conditions, it is important that the leader

CRITICAL THOUGHT

The leader should be fully aware of the emotional content embedded in each participant's position. The leader should anticipate the potential for emotional reactions and outbursts and respond with a strategy that honors the legitimacy of the emotional feelings, yet places them in context with the process at the table. The leader never stifles emotions. Instead, the leader ensures that their expressions are appropriate and that they do not direct the negotiation.

of the negotiation identify patterns of response to negative negotiation behaviors. Some examples of common behaviors and recommended responses to them follow:

- The perennially unclear negotiator: It may be helpful to be more visual with regard to establishing a higher level of clarity for this kind of negotiation. Putting thoughts in writing, using visual presentations, placing submissions in a bullet-point format, or restating the participant's contribution as a way of clarifying it is helpful to supporting this kind of negotiator.

- The indecisive or uncertain negotiator: Careful and structured conversations are central to affirming positions and points. Periodically restating and reviewing the elements of the dialogue will help clarify and confirm the parties' positions. Staying focused on the question and exploring specific issues with the indecisive negotiator using new wording or language helps advance clarity and facilitate movement.

- The overly aggressive negotiator: Keep the discussion fact based and free of emotional content. Make sure language is clear and intent is clarified. Reinforce the terms of engagement and make it clear that threatening or repressive behavior will not be accepted at the table. When emotions are running high, allow for their expression and use breaks as opportunities to spend time with personal, negative emotions and to diffuse their intensity.

- The overly emotional negotiator: Recognize and accept the feelings and expressions of the negotiator. Help the negotiator translate his or her emotions into a language that clarifies and specifies their expression. Patiently allow for emotional moments but provide a context for them to prevent them from limiting the dialogue. Allow time for emotional expression during breaks and away from the negotiating table to ensure less emotional intensity at the table. Balance emotional feelings with factual affirmations and translation of feelings into positions (Heller & Hindle, 2008).

SCENARIO

You have two colleagues, Nancy and Jane, who express significantly different views on delegating patient care activities to nursing assistants. Each feels strongly about her position. Nancy believes that any activities where nursing assistants demonstrate competence should be delegated to them. Jane, however, believes that delegation should be selective, ensuring that particular skills are reserved for the registered nurse. Nancy and Jane have maintained these conflicting positions for some time now, and it is becoming an issue with regard to the appropriate delegation standard on the unit.

You are a clinical leader on the unit and currently chair the unit's Practice Council. You would like to resolve this issue the most effective way possible and have set a meeting date with Nancy and Jane to address their differences.

Discussion Questions

1. How might you prepare Nancy and Jane for this dialogue?

2. How will you prepare yourself as leader to facilitate their interaction?

3. Which key data will you need to inform the discussion at the table?

4. Who else will need to be present at the table and what will their role be?

5. Which conflicts do you anticipate and how will you prepare yourself for them?

Bargaining

Bargaining is the phase of negotiation that emphasizes the give-and-take related to the variety of positions at the table. As the work of exchange, it includes the following elements:

- Bargaining involves give and take.
- Positions often shift during the bargaining phase.
- Trade-offs are suggested and made during bargaining.
- At this time, the legitimate positions are determined.
- Points of convergence and agreement emerge in this phase.

- The potential for conflict and shutdown accelerates.
- The potential for movement and agreement also accelerates.
- The essential skill of the leader is to keep bargaining on track.
- Positional restatement is frequently made to validate understanding.

A number of different bargaining approaches exist, most of which reflect positional bargaining. With this approach, the negotiator attempts to bargain in a way that supports his or her position as the most correct of the various positions at the table. Positioned bargaining has some value in that it requires the development and support of a rationale for a particular position. A stated position indicates the appropriateness and logic of the position and helps clarify and justify its validity. Imbalanced or polarized positioned bargaining can provide a baseline for the consideration of additional approaches or positions that may spin off from an originally fixed position.

In open and balanced negotiation, the bargaining process initiates the serious give-and-take necessary to identify legitimate positions and gauge the degree of support for any particular position or view. If bargaining is open and equitable, and a positive goal is sought for the resolution of the negotiation, bargaining can begin to reveal points of convergence, areas of common ground, or particular positions that appear more legitimate and appropriate for resolution. In an absolute winner-take-all approach to negotiation, positions can become polarizing and limiting, providing a set of absolutes from which the position holder will not deviate. In such a case, the true bargaining process never unfolds; instead, people hold to their positions regardless of the nature of the dialogue or the potential for a mutual solution or satisfaction. This hardening of positions has the potential to, at worst, shut down the negotiation or, at least, limit its effectiveness. If such intransigence holds strong from the outset, the negotiator may need to remind the parties very early that negotiation and mediation as a resolution process may not be appropriate for them. Instead, arbitration—a process in which a decision is made by a neutral "judge" rather than reached through dialogue between the participants—may be a more suitable option.

When clarifying positions and contributions to the bargaining process, it is important to compare proposals, positions, and suggestions from the negotiating parties to the original positions. The leader in the negotiation will often want to restate positions in light of subsequent information or discussion to illuminate movement, new information, the potential for new positions, or new decisions made about original positions (Lewicki, Saunders, & Barry, 2009). In doing so, the leader tries to ensure the discussion and dialogue have a firm foundation in fact. In this process, particular bargaining positions may be strengthened, refined, or altered, creating a new floor for further dialogue and bargaining.

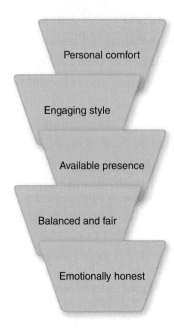

Figure 13-1 Negotiation facilitation

The most important skill of the facilitator/leader of negotiation is keeping the bargaining on track, ensuring that it does not move far afield into ever-widening issues that do not relate more specifically to the positions and issues at hand. Bargaining should be focused, be detailed, and move inexorably in a direction that suggests positive progress and some level of satisfaction from the participants. To achieve this end, the facilitator/leader will have to keep a level head and bring all personal skills to the fore (**Figure 13-1**). Although positive bargaining should not necessarily reflect a win–lose scenario or positioning, the leader should be prepared to see particular positions or emergent positions grow in intensity and viability as more data and dialogue reveal a particular direction and more relevant choice making.

Because bargaining is the predominant centerpiece of the negotiation process, the leader should ensure that good notes are taken, records are provided, and movement is recorded. As particular and seminal points of reference, decisions, or new positions emerge, they should be documented, restated, and validated, and the general determination of support for the decision should be obtained from the parties to the negotiation (Garner & Lovering, 2004).

Because bargaining lies at the heart of the negotiation process, it demands the most skill and takes the most significant time commitment and attention to detail of all the phases. In this stage of negotiation, all of the skills associated with understanding dialogue, body language, language of expression, communication, styles of negotiation, and points of convergence will be very important to the leader/facilitator. As with any significant skill, time and experience are the greatest moderators of competence and success. When first tackling this challenge, novice leaders may want to consult with negotiating mentors or have such people present in their own negotiating process to support their own negotiation learning and development.

Critical elements of the bargaining process that the negotiating leader may need to keep in mind throughout the interaction include the following items:

- Help the participants at the table separate relationship concerns and issues from the substance of the issue being negotiated. It is not that relationships and feelings are not important and should not be considered; rather, it is that the negotiation has a purpose and, ultimately, that purpose must be fulfilled.

- Constantly look for shared vision, issues, terms of reference, language, and goals. Ultimately, values will define the solution, and parties to the negotiation must essentially value the solution they participated in obtaining.

- As a leader, use objective criteria, data, decisions, and progress as a basis for subsequent decision making. Decisions should be based on principles, not made under pressure, and reaffirming those principles is critical to the successful process of negotiation.

- Sort through the issues one at a time so that the table does not become crowded with a competing or complex array of issues and processes such that the key point gets lost in the complexity.

- Avoid terms and language that are grounded in finality during the process of negotiating. As much as possible during the earlier stages of dialogue and interacting, emphasize open-ended approaches. Decisions should emerge, not be forced.

- Summarize the process to date frequently. This step helps the parties remain clear about the progress, current positions, and issues presently at hand.

- Help the participants avoid ultimatums, terminal language, and polarized positioning. Negotiation is a process, not a terminal event, and all of its elements should be used liberally.

- Take regular, if not frequent, breaks in a format that allows the participants to interact in an informal and friendly environment. Strengthening relationships always diminishes polarization.

CRITICAL THOUGHT

Bargaining is one of the more critical moments in the negotiation process. It is during this phase that the role of the leader/facilitator is critical to ensuring success. Participants are balancing on the edge of dissolution–resolution and need help in specifically refining understanding, potential for agreement, convergent and divergent positions, and renewed focus on real issues.

Closing the Interaction and Implementing the Agreement

As a process of negotiation unfolds successfully, a number of things should have occurred. New positions should be clarified and well defined, trade-offs noted, bargaining trades clearly articulated, specific consensus achieved, particular documented agreements made available, and final understandings affirmed. These essential elements ensure the final stages of the negotiation process are reached and indicate its point of closure. At this moment in the negotiation process, it is important for the negotiation leader to confirm the terms of the agreement and ascertain whether full understanding on the part of all parties has been obtained. The final form and language are important to the specificity and clarity of the agreement and must be sanctioned by all parties to the negotiation. All terms of agreement must be restated and documented in language clear enough for all parties to understand and to validate. All parties should have an opportunity to review, question, and clarify the agreement and to be satisfied before final language is created that will bring the negotiation process to closure.

After agreement has been achieved, documented, and signed off by the parties, the process moves from closure to implementation. Therefore, it is important to address the following elements prior to expecting the agreement to be put into action:

- All the facts of the agreement should be in place. Documentation should be specific, clear, and focused, and all the participants should indicate they agree with the final documents.
- An action plan for implementing the agreements should be identified by each of the participants in a way that demonstrates a consensus of understanding regarding role and action related to the agreement and commitment to implementing subsequent action.
- The parties should clearly understand the contribution of each participant to the implementation of the agreement; that is, all parties should understand their particular and specific roles and the activities associated with those roles in implementation.

- Specific mechanisms for verifying and validating action and performance in fulfillment of the agreement should be included in the action plan in a way that clearly demonstrates support for the agreement and the performance of its elements and expectations.
- Opportunities for regathering the negotiating parties to evaluate commitment, performance, progress, and further considerations relative to the agreement should be provided at regular intervals as a way of ensuring both progress and performance.
- A specific timeline for satisfaction and completion of the work of the negotiation should be clearly established as well as the individuals most accountable for determining performance and progress. A timeline and accountability provide definitive criteria against which to measure the success of the negotiation and its application and performance.

SCENARIO

Building on the previous scenario in this chapter, assume that agreement has been reached and Nancy and Jane have converged to the point of resolution. As a nursing leader on the unit and chair of the Practice Council, you are now interested in establishing a standard for delegation. Form a small team of colleagues to respond to the following questions.

Discussion Questions

1. Because you are attempting to establish a standard of delegation for practice on the unit, which critical elements of delegation are required to inform that standard?

2. Now that Nancy and Jane have agreed, who needs to be involved in the standards development process that reflects their agreement?

3. How will you obtain consensus around the standard once it is established as a protocol for practice?

4. What is the role of the Practice Council? How will the Council establish the expectations for performance with regard to the new standard on delegation?

5. What is the role of the unit manager in relationship to the established new standard for delegation?

CRITICAL THOUGHT

In recent years, collective bargaining has shifted from an exclusive and more positional-based strategy to a format that represents stronger ownership of common interests and mutual advantage. Traditional, conflict-based collective bargaining often results in negative processes and long-term bargaining. Bargaining from the perspective of mutual interest establishes a stronger foundation for seeking common ground and helps to share responsibilities for problem resolution.

For more information check out www.lmpartnership.org to see how Kaiser Permanente uses **"interest-based bargaining"** to grow the organization and the unions it employs.

Negotiation is a fundamental element of all human interaction. It reflects the uniqueness and differences that each person and group brings to relationships, interactions, performance, and the satisfaction of wants and needs. The clinical leader will continuously confront situations that demand some level of negotiation and agreement. The elements of negotiation outlined in this chapter form a basic foundation upon which the skills of negotiation can be built. However, the clinical leader should be encouraged to read and study further the particulars of negotiation, especially those related to individual skills and needs as a part of the learning dynamic associated with developing and growing personal negotiation competence. Through learning, practice, and the wisdom of time, the clinical leader can develop excellent skills and become a powerful resource in problem solving, relationship building, and effective decision making (Lewicki & Barry, 2010).

The Clinical Leader and the Unique Characteristics of Collective Bargaining

Collective bargaining is a formal process of negotiation defined and protected by the National Labor Relations Board (NLRB) in fulfillment of the National Labor Relations Act (NLRA) (Taft-Hartley Act) and the subsequent adaptations to health care in Public Law 93-360. These laws govern collective bargaining activities specifically in unionized hospitals, but they also have implications for supervisory roles in non-unionized environments, providing opportunities for professional workers to file unfair labor practices in any healthcare environment. The details of labor–management relationships that operate under the auspices of these various labor laws can be found in management texts or union information resources. The clinical leader—the focus of this text—must be aware of the specific characteristics and processes associated with collective bargaining in hospitals and healthcare settings that are unionized and have collective bargaining agreements (Carrell & Heavrin, 2009).

Unionized healthcare institutions operate under formally negotiated agreements between staff and management known as collective bargaining agreements. These agreements predominantly address salaries, benefits, and working conditions, all of which are specifically negotiated between employers and their employees' union. Usually these agreements are renegotiated over defined periods of time and cover a specific number of years. In addition, such negotiated union agreements clearly define the rights of management as distinct from those of employees. Historically, these agreements have operated as an outflow of positional bargaining, as the collective bargaining process often demonstrates. This model of negotiation has often resulted in contentious, polarized, and negative relationships between the parties. In recent years, broader and more engaging collective bargaining negotiating processes have been unfolded in a way that facilitates and strengthens the relationship between healthcare organizations and their staff. These negotiations focus more on principles and relationships than on simply the facts or factors around which a negotiation is often based. Such more principled approaches help the parties to the negotiation focus on mutual challenges, problems, issues, interests, values, and finding common ground. Many of the principles of negotiation discussed in this chapter apply to the formal process of collective bargaining (Blanpain, Bamber, & Pochet, 2010).

For the clinical leader, it is important to understand the fundamentals associated with leading in a unionized environment and operating within a collective bargaining agreement. If the staff seek union representation, sections of the NLRA are triggered when a formal petition for representation is filed, initiating a complex series of events. In particular, aggressive campaigns are launched seeking the signed and dated authorization cards from employees that must accompany the petition for representation within a specified time frame. During this time, the employer cannot interfere with or impede upon the rights of the employees to take advantage of the opportunity for collective bargaining. Although at least 30% of employees must authorize their representation by the union for the collective bargaining process to move forward, union members typically seek majorities of 50% to 60% to ensure that the highest level of support is demonstrated to the NLRB and the employer. If the 30% minimum level of interest is met, staff members vote in a formal NLRB-supervised union election. Prior to the election, the employees, the union, and the employer all have a chance to indicate their desired positions with regard to the forthcoming election. Through a secret ballot, nonmanagerial staff vote under the observation and supervision of the NLRB. A simple majority of votes cast determines the outcome. If the NLRB decides that the vote was valid, it supports the outcome, the union is certified, and the formal process of collective bargaining between the union and the organization is established (Carrell & Heavrin, 2012).

Critical elements of collective bargaining include the following points:

- Employees are represented by a union.
- All employees covered by the union agreement must abide by its requirements.
- Union members elect representatives to negotiate on their behalf.
- After negotiation, a collective agreement is arrived at by employer and union.
- Union contracts set out the obligations and requirements of both the employer and the union.
- Time limits exist for the union contract, after which the agreement must be renegotiated.
- Union members must pay dues to their union.

In the United States, petitioning for union representation and collective bargaining is essentially considered an employee right. Under the NLRA, employees have a right to self-organization and to become members of labor organizations; subsequently, they have the right to bargain collectively through representatives of their own choosing for the purpose of advancing their own mutual interests. These rights are protected by law, and both union and employer must uphold the agreed-upon contents of the formal bargaining agreement between them.

As a clinical leader, the individual's bargaining environment will be shaped by the agreement between the union and the employer, and the leader will often be required to address its elements, represent its principles in his or her own behavior, and advance the interests of the agreement when potential and real conflicts arise between the agreement and the behavior of staff and management. To meet this responsibility, the clinical leader must be aware of the requirements of the collective bargaining agreement and his or her role as a staff leader in adhering to its requirements and in resolving issues and concerns related to the agreement. For example, the collective bargaining agreement may affect staff relationships and negotiation in the following ways:

- The collective bargaining agreement may limit the possibility of either management or staff changing any component of the agreement in a way that compromises the agreement or places people at threat in relationship to it.

- The collective bargaining agreement may effectively minimize asking staff about their union activities or collective bargaining–related activities if such questioning constrains or coerces them in ways not permitted by the NLRA or the specific collective bargaining agreement.
- The collective bargaining agreement may limit the employer's, management's, or clinical leader's ability to suggest benefits or favors that are not contained within the agreement and have not been formally agreed to by the employer or the union.
- The clinical leader should not act as an agent of either the employer or the union in issues or content related specifically to the collective bargaining agreement in a way that would jeopardize the agreement or marginalize behavior covered by the agreement.
- Clinical leaders should avoid rumor, gossip, unsubstantiated dialogue, or inappropriate discussion regarding the employer, the union, or the collective bargaining agreement in a way that diminishes, polarizes, or in any manner subverts the agreement or the relationship between the employer and the union.
- Clinical leaders must avoid personal discussion of opinions and feelings about the employer, union, or collective bargaining agreement in any way that is not consistent with the content of the collective bargaining agreement.
- Just as the clinical leader expresses support for the management and organizational leadership of the institution, so the leader should also extend respect and support to union leadership, especially as it relates to the elements of the union obligations in fulfilling the requisites of the collective bargaining agreement.

Collective bargaining creates equity in the workplace by giving workers a stronger voice through collective action and serves as a counterforce to the equally

CRITICAL THOUGHT

Usually, when management adheres to sound principles of professional shared governance, demonstrates contemporary leadership principles and practices, and relates to professional knowledge workers as partners in the workplace, and when equity is the driving force of relationships between them, unionization is frequently deemed unnecessary.

powerful collective voice of organizational management. Generally, the desire to unionize in an organization indicates the employees' sense that their collective self-interest and benefits have been challenged or that organizational management does not directly and positively support employees. Usually, when management adheres to sound principles of professional shared governance, demonstrates contemporary leadership principles and practices, and relates to professional knowledge workers as partners in the workplace, and when equity is the driving force of relationships between them, unionization is frequently deemed unnecessary. In contrast, failure to adhere to strong evidence-based principles of leadership, shared governance, empowerment, equity, and engagement creates the landscape that advances the potential for employee interest in unionization.

Collective Action, Collective Bargaining, and Employee Strikes

Every collective bargaining agreement has a particular life span. When the agreement nears its end, the parties go back to the negotiating table to renegotiate a new contract and timeline. This is generally a tenuous period of time where issuing of positions and counter-positions by the employer and the union determines the subsequent content of the collective bargaining negotiation. Representatives from the union and the employer establish a process and time frame for negotiating their positions, interests, and proposals in pursuit of mutual agreement, which will result in a contract supported by both management and union membership.

Negotiations can continue for an extended period of time depending on the distance separating the various parties' positions, the intensity of the negotiations, and the number of items to be addressed. If much work has been done by the employer and the union ahead of time, the collective bargaining process can often be simple and straightforward. Conversely, if the parties' positions require a great deal of negotiation, dialogue, and member contribution, the negotiation process can be quite extended. If the parties can reach a satisfactory agreement and both employer and union membership certify that agreement (the union has its members vote their support), the contract is completed and signed. However, if a solution to disputes and disagreements cannot be satisfactorily reached at the bargaining table, the union may exercise its right to strike if its members vote to do so.

A strike is a mass refusal of employees to work. It is associated with the following characteristics:

- Picketing occurs to discourage employees from working or others from conducting business with the employer.

- A strike occurs in response to employee grievance or lack of agreement on a contract.
- Strikes are used to pressure employers to reach an agreement with the union.
- Accommodations to the strike regarding patient care must be made by the employer.
- Union or non-union workers may cross strike lines to provide patient care on behalf of the employer.
- Strikes stop when they are settled by agreement by the union and employer or by court action.

In health care, strike preparations usually involve altering the workload of management to ensure patient care is not threatened and to address the critical needs of the healthcare facility. While union member employees are on strike, other staff and management usually fulfill the limited obligations of patient service. For the clinical leader, it is important to keep in touch with the human resources department for guidance on acceptable professional behavior, action priorities, personal roles, and approved conversations during an employee strike period.

Negotiations usually continue during the strike. The pressure of the strike process and the slowdown of normal healthcare organization work and patient-care activities usually create additional pressure on the employer and the union to settle their dispute. Often emotions run high during the strike process and can create challenges for the clinical leader both inside and outside the organization. Traditional liaisons and friendships between the clinical leader and other members of the staff can frequently be challenged and stretched thin during emotionally turbulent times, especially over the strike period. At these times, the leader must stay faithful to the principles of the contract, good leadership expression, and personal emotional balance. The clinical leader must remember that collective bargaining is an exercise of basic American rights but is also fraught with

CRITICAL THOUGHT

The clinical leader must ensure a safe environment for temporary staff, patients, and those who cross the picket line. Bullying, shaming, and toxic behavior may reveal itself in this environment. The clinical nurse leader has an ethical duty to support care and the nursing profession by addressing issues quickly and appropriately.

all the human emotional vagaries that intensive and complex interaction frequently entails. Patience, consistency, and adherence to the letter of the law and the collective bargaining agreement should positively guide the clinical leader in maintaining a balanced work environment and positive relationships with peers and managers.

Negotiating in the Profession of Nursing

To a large extent, any professional relationship is a continuous and dynamic negotiation. Consequently, negotiating skills and capacity are essential characteristics of the clinical leader. Developing and enhancing negotiation skills will expand the capacity and enhance the viability of the leader in a wide variety of leadership scenarios and circumstances.

Negotiation is not simply a formal process. Rather, it is an element of human communication and interaction that deals with values, exchanges, and problem solving. Critical thinking and problem-solving skills serve as a fundamental part of the negotiation process and shape this process so that it yields positive results and advances the interests of those involved. Negotiation is simply disciplined communication. Furthermore, it comprises communication that reflects purpose, value, and outcome. None of these elements takes precedence over the others, and all essentially work in concert to advance relationships, improve conditions, and have an impact on people and work.

For the clinical leader, certain critical elements of communication and negotiation drive the role and relationships in all processes of interaction and engagement:

- The clinical leader applies his or her translational capacity to deliver messages and communicate with others. The leader always uses language and images that can be understood and effectively repeated by the listener.
- Listening for tone and context is as important as listening for message. The clinical leader always "reads between the lines" of the message by observing other indicators (e.g., body language, gestures, movements, attitudes, facial expressions) that accompany the language and often signal the existence of additional matters of significance to the communication.
- The clinical leader recognizes that every individual deserves respect and should be heard and have a voice. Sometimes this voice needs to be clarified and focused, and the clinical leader provides the tools to

ensure an accurate and correct representation of the message and its meaning.

- Messages must have focus, specificity, and clarity to have value. The clinical leader establishes a high standard of clarity and works to support individuals and teams in achieving it.

- Knowing when it is time to move the message forward is a central communication skill for the clinical leader. Often points get stuck in the morass of repetition at a time when people are eager for clarification, agreement, and forward movement. The leader knows when a point has been made and is ready to move the message forward at this time.

- Keeping the discussion focused and iterative (dealing with one issue at a time) helps people resolve problems and keeps the discussion from dissolving into confusion, confabulation, obfuscation, and too much complexity. Trying to address too many issues at a time actually facilitates conflict; staging and singling out issues helps sort and align them in a format so that they can be accurately addressed.

- The clinical leader needs to be aware that issues have personal meaning and are accompanied by feelings of ownership and emotional attachment. Although the leader must separate fact from emotion, it is important to support people's feelings and provide opportunities for their expression as a part of the exploration and problem-solving process.

- Solution, resolution, and achievement are all products of good negotiation, communication, and problem solving. The clinical leader knows that there are processes and solutions for dealing with all human activity, interactions, and relationships. Patience, consideration, the discipline of good process, and the effective use of collective wisdom all act in concert to solve problems with integrity, equity, honesty, and effectiveness.

The professional knowledge worker continually deals with the translation of knowledge into action directed toward a positive impact. This discipline guides the action of the professional and informs the strategies and interactions necessary to advance the work of the profession. Because of the intensity of the professional work, the centrality of human relationships to professional action, and the profession's social obligation to positively impact society, complex interactions and relationships must be negotiated. The clinical leader is charged with facilitating and coordinating these interactions; through the use of good communication and negotiation skills, he or she seeks to refine and advance the essential interactions and intersections necessary to translate knowledge and collective wisdom into meaningful action and purposeful impact.

Leaders cannot lead if they do not have the capacity to negotiate. However, negotiation is a learned skill; it is also a journey more than a single event. This continuously unfolding dynamic matures and develops as the skills of the negotiators are advanced and refined and can be directed toward meaningful purpose and a positive outcome. It is not always easy to keep the focus of negotiation and the intent of the negotiators aligned with the desired outcome. During the path toward resolution, the skill, discipline, and attributes of the leader and the processes associated with negotiation become critical to the efficacy and effectiveness of knowledge work and the knowledge worker. Ultimately, consistency and faithfulness to the principles and practices of good negotiation will yield the benefits of a positive context for knowledge work. The result is sound and purposeful relationships and interactions and effective deliberation and decision making that serve the interests and values of the community.

SCENARIO

Aaron James, RN, BSN, clinical leader for the neurology unit, was confronted by a staff member who was angry with a colleague. According to this nurse, the colleague "was consistently abusive to her" and she was "at the end of her rope with her." The angry nurse wanted her colleague to be disciplined and fired for the manner in which she had been treated. The nurse stated that this behavior had been going on for several months. Although she tried to avoid crossing paths with the colleague, she felt as though the offending nurse deliberately sought her out to "berate and demean her."

Aaron noted that the colleague of whom this nurse was speaking had also been on the unit for more than 20 years and had not been the subject of this kind of behavioral complaint before. Nevertheless, something was clearly missing in the two nurses' relationship. While he had heard snippets of information from others about potential bad feelings between the nurses, this occasion was the first time he had actually seen an emotional response and received a specific complaint. Aaron knew he would have to explore this incident further to assure it did not go further and to provide an opportunity for the nurses to confront and address their issues surrounding this conflict.

Discussion Questions

1. Having seen the emotional reaction and heard the response from one of the nurses in this conflict, what is the first thing that Aaron should do in proceeding to address this issue?

2. After clarifying the elements involved in the issue and recognizing that the two nurses had legitimate concerns, Aaron has decided to mediate a conversation between them. What are some of the things that Aaron should consider as he prepares for this conversation?

3. Aaron is aware that these two nurses need to find common ground and negotiate their differences so that they can continue to work together as colleagues. What are some of the things Aaron will need to do to create a "safe space" for these conversations?

4. The negotiation will need to go through a series of steps or stages as it proceeds toward agreement and resolution. With your learning team, outline the elements of this process of negotiation and identify some of the issues related to each element that Aaron will need to be aware of as he facilitates the dialogue and helps the participants negotiate their relationship.

5. After agreement has been reached between these two nurses, what timeline should Aaron establish for evaluating progress and performance relative to their agreement? Which elements of the evaluation might Aaron seek to address?

SCENARIO

The medical unit practice council had just recently received the new LEAD (lower-extremity arterial disease) guidelines and had reviewed them as a part of assessing how they informed changes in nursing practice. Elaine Ray, RN, BSN, was chair of the Practice Council and had noticed that these new LEAD standards would affect clinical protocols for wound care and nursing practice standards for patients with compromised arterial blood flow. During the discussion held by the Council, a number of conflicting issues arose with regard to appropriate application of the standards of practice and their implication for changing existing protocols and routines of the nursing staff.

(continues)

(continued)

Elaine knew that there were a number of challenges involved in the discussion and decision making around appropriate clinical standards for management of arterial wounds, as well as the need for staff engagement in practice changes. In the initial dialogue in the Practice Council, she noticed widely differing points of view on how the LEAD standards were to be translated and applied to practice and how the protocols and procedures would be constructed to guide effective practice. The Council was eager to undertake its work in developing protocols and procedures but was challenged by the diversity of insights, views, and recommendations from its members about what those new practices might be and how they might be implemented on the unit.

Discussion Questions

1. Clearly, there is strong opportunity for using negotiation and communication skills as Elaine facilitates dialogue and decision making around the adaptation and application of the new LEAD practices. Assume Elaine's role as Practice Council chair and, with your learning team, plan out a strategy for negotiating the variety of views regarding a standard and reaching a consensus on an acceptable standard.

2. As Elaine leads this process and moves it toward defining particular standards, there will be times when the group members become entrenched in their positions. What are some of the strategies that Elaine might consider to help move people off their positions and into a place of acceptable agreement around a practice standard?

3. Strong emotions often come to the fore when people are attached to beliefs and practices. What are some techniques or processes that can help Elaine deal with these emotions and attachments to positions by addressing them yet moving participants forward in the decision-making process?

4. Is there a role for testing and experimentation of approaches when absolute agreement cannot be reached for a single approach? How might that response be structured?

5. When a decision has been reached by the Practice Council for a particular protocol or standard of practice, what are some of the characteristics and elements of a valuation that need to be incorporated into its implementation as a way of validating the usefulness and effectiveness of the protocol/standard?

CHAPTER TEST QUESTIONS

Licensure exam categories: Management of care: advocacy, concepts of management

Nurse leader exam categories: Knowledge of the healthcare environment: governance; Leadership: systems thinking, change management; Communication and relationship building: influencing behaviors

1. Working toward achieving universally recognized and acceptable solutions is a discipline just as much as it is a process. True or false?

2. The negotiator must always be firm and resolute with his or her bottom line throughout the negotiation to make sure personal objectives are met. True or false?

3. A willingness to be open, available, and have a wide range of potential options and considerations can provide creative and unique ways of satisfying needs and finding common ground. True or false?

4. When gathering data for negotiation, the individual should focus on his or her own position, strengthening it with evidence strong enough to counter the other parties' positions. True or false?

5. Positions should be broad based and open ended to provide room for alternative solutions. True or false?

6. Threats and challenges always arise during a negotiation. Each negotiator must be prepared to counter these with stronger challenges to point out the evidence and veracity of his or her own position. True or false?

7. When leading questions are used to confuse, identify weaknesses, or force concessions, the leader should delay answering the series of questions, break down the questions into single units, and seek a specific answer for each individual question as it relates to the originating issue. True or false?

8. Employees seek union membership when management fails to listen to them and employees cannot get what they want from the system. True or false?

9. Collective bargaining is governed by laws that prescribe how employees can form a union, collectively organize, negotiate, and strike. True or false?

10. Negotiation is not a leadership skill but rather a learned skill that anyone can apply to any situation that demands negotiation. True or false?

References

Blanpain, R., Bamber, G., & Pochet, P. (2010). *Regulating employment relations, work and labour laws.* Frederick, MD: Kluwer Law International.

Boulle, L., Colatrella, M. T., & Picchioni, A. P. (2008). *Mediation: Skills and techniques.* Newark, NJ: LexisNexis Matthew Bender.

Carrell, M., & Heavrin, C. (2009). *Labor relations and collective bargaining.* New York, NY: McGraw-Hill.

Carrell, M., & Heavrin, C. (2012). *Labor relations and collective bargaining: Private and public sectors.* New York, NY: Prentice Hall.

Deleuran, P., & Jarner, S. (2011). *Conflict management in the family field and in other close relationships: Mediation as a way forward.* Portland, OR: DJØF International Specialized Book Services.

Garner, S., & Lovering, M. (2004). *Conflict resolution.* Princeton, NJ: Films for the Humanities and Sciences.

Heller, R., & Hindle, T. (2008). *Essential manager's manual.* New York, NY: DK.

Kobayashi, J., & Viswat, L. (2014). 3-D negotiation in a business context. *Journal of Intercultural Communication Academic Librarianship, 34*(1), 1.

Kozina, A. (2014). Managerial roles and functions in negotiation process. *Business Management & Education, 12*(1), 94–108.

Lewicki, R., & Barry, B. (2010). *The essentials of negotiation.* New York, NY: McGraw-Hill.

Lewicki, R., Saunders, D., & Barry, B. (2009). *Negotiation.* New York, NY: McGraw-Hill.

Appendix A

Negotiation Skills Assessment

To ensure successful negotiation, the leader must have specific skills. This is a simple and basic inventory of negotiation skills. For each of the points made, select the appropriate answer. The higher your score, the greater your negotiation skills' value. This assessment should be looked at as a developmental tool, not a test.

1. Almost never
2. Sometimes
3. Often
4. Regularly

I collect relevant data in preparation for a negotiation.				I work to understand the other parties' positions.			
1	2	3	4	1	2	3	4
I understand my own position in the negotiation.				I am able to state my position in clear and precise language.			
1	2	3	4	1	2	3	4
I understand and use an appropriate range of negotiation strategies.				I know what my bottom line is, and I negotiate to support it.			
1	2	3	4	1	2	3	4
I recognize that all parties must take something of value from the negotiation.				My body language is consistent with my meaning and message.			
1	2	3	4	1	2	3	4
I remain positive and persistent in the negotiation process.				I recognize opportunities for compromise and consensus when I see them.			
1	2	3	4	1	2	3	4
I am determined to reach a mutually satisfying agreement.				I respect and honor all differences and seek to learn from them.			
1	2	3	4	1	2	3	4
I find I consistently negotiate win–win situations.				Scoring: 1–13 Need more learning/skills 14–27 Learning and growing 28–40 Building skills well 41–52 Growing into a negotiator			
1	2	3	4				

> If we want unity, we must all be unifiers. If we want accountability, each of us must be accountable for everything we do. —Christine Gregoire

CHAPTER OBJECTIVES

Upon completion of this chapter, the reader will be able to do the following:

» Understand the basic elements and characteristics of professional accountability.

» Define the unique characteristics of an obligation of ownership and its relationship to accountability.

» Delineate team and interdisciplinary characteristics of accountability and the need for discipline-specific clarity in directing purposeful teamwork.

» Outline the unique characteristics of professional accountability and its role in fulfilling a profession's social mandate.

» List at least five elements of the role and relationship of accountability and undertaking risk in clinical practice.

» State the essential relationship between performance and accountability, and describe the impact of the leadership role in the clinical service environment.

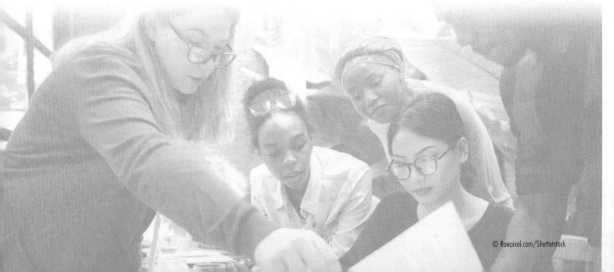

Accountability and Ownership: The Centerpiece of Professional Practice

All professions are grounded in principles of accountability (Tilley, 2008). Professions have a social obligation to the society that empowers them. That accountability is invested in the profession as a whole and incorporated in the individual practices of each member of the profession. This obligation for social accountability informs the social contract between the society that licenses the professional and the professional who acts in the best interests of the society that empowers her or him. In turn, this social contract forms the centerpiece of the profession's role in society and sets the framework for the role and performance obligations of the profession and each of its members.

Each individual brings to her or his role a specific accountability representing the individual's full commitment to the characteristics, skills, competencies, and capacities that will contribute to and advance the interests of the society that the individual's profession serves. Vital to undertaking professional work is a precise and clear understanding of the nature of the profession, its accountability for performance, the contribution that it makes in fulfilling its work, and the relationships among the profession's members and between its members and the people the profession serves. This chapter serves to discuss the role of the individual in relation to professional accountability and ownership; it builds on the work of Chapter 9, which addresses the role of professional governance and guides teams to collective accountability within organizational structures.

There has been extensive historical debate about whether the structural, functional, and behavioral characteristics of nursing and nurses truly represent the character of professional practice (Moanojovich, 2005). On a superficial level, many of the elements that characterize professional practice are present in

CRITICAL THOUGHT

Perhaps one of the most challenging aspects of accountability is the lack of clarity regarding what it means in the context of work. Furthermore, there are many challenges in terms of how accountability is evidenced in the work of the team and how it influences the outcomes of work. There is no other concept in work that is cited as much as accountability, yet is so little understood.

At its simplest level, *accountability* reflects the sustainable achievement of definitive outcomes. *Responsibility*, by comparison, entails meeting expectations and effectively performing actions in the exercise of doing work. Thus one concept—accountability—is about the achievement of results and the other—responsibility—is about the quality of the work effort. An individual, therefore, can be responsible without being accountable. In fact, responsibility without accountability is one of the work crises of the current age. Many people do good work and work very hard on processes or activities that have a questionable relationship to the achievement of sustainable outcomes.

Because of the traditional business fixation on process and action, short-term and interactive products are often perceived as signs of performance effectiveness and progress. In reality, sustainable results can be achieved only over much longer periods of time. To achieve them requires better tying the actions of work to their products. Much research has been devoted to exploring the goodness of fit between the effort of work and its results (Simon & Canacari, 2012). Effectiveness is best indicated by the tightness of this fit—that is, the match between the expectations for results and the actual results. The better this relationship, the more sustainable the outcome is and the more valuable the relationship between the two is. Ultimately, this set of circumstances creates the ideal work relationship by directly connecting responsibility and accountability.

To achieve such a direct connection between responsibility and accountability, a clear understanding of the elements of accountability and the expectations for performance of each of the parties is required. Without it, there exists no foundation for defining or delivering accountability.

nursing—a foundation in a specific body of knowledge, a disciplined educational pathway, a rigorous code of ethics, clearly articulated standards of practice, and the licensing body that ensures the appropriate rigors of regulation. If these were the only arbiters of the character and content of a profession, then nursing would clearly meet those conditions. However, much of the debate with regard to the professional character of nursing relates to the educational level of the majority of its practitioners, its dependent role in relation to other disciplines, lack of clarity about its specific contribution to the health of society, and an ongoing lack of a disciplined, professional self-governance structure, evidenced by the many other broad constituencies that claim to represent nursing's interests. In addition, nursing continues to lack political clout, a locus of power, policy influence, and presence at the decision-making tables where health policy is set, strategic decisions are made, and health resources are allocated.

Many in health leadership would assume that the lack of a place at the decision-making table would be a problem in key roles related to policy, politics, strategy, and decisional power. This factor may be a clear indicator of the limited role that nursing plays in critical health decision making and is reflected in the limited independent parameters that the nursing role represents in the broader social landscape. This subordinating social condition and lack of primary ascendancy of the nursing role on the broader societal stage indicate to some observers that nursing is a subsequent or dependent work group that fails to meet critical indices of truly professional behavior.

The challenge faced by nursing in gaining recognition as a true profession seems generally to be supported by the evidence. While nurses represent the single largest professional healthcare group in the United States, their minimal role in those forums that set direction and make decisions for the healthcare system suggests that nursing is not a key player at the healthcare decision table nationally, regionally, locally, and in health organizations. While this level of representation is now undergoing significant changes, in the past it has provided the clearest testament to nursing's lack of place, position, power, and role in societal decision making related to health policy, strategy, resource allocation, and provider roles (Jameson, 2009; Patton, Zalon, & Ludwick, 2015).

CRITICAL THOUGHT

Expectations are the foundation for performance. Every worker has the right to know what is expected and which skills are necessary to meet those expectations; otherwise, the worker should not be in the role.

CRITICAL THOUGHT

Accountability for excellence rests with those who do the work!

The Professionalization of Nursing in the 20th Century: The Path to Accountability

Nursing's journey to professional equity has been long and somewhat torturous. The history of the maturation of the nursing profession closely matches the tenure and circumstances of the journey of women to social and political equity (Buhler-Wilkerson, 2001; Goodnow, 1938; Hein, 2001; Kahn, 2014; Lagemann & Rockefeller Archive Center, 1983). Much of the character, content, and role of the nurse mirrors the unfolding role of women over the centuries. Women's long presence in subsequent, subordinating, passive, and secondary roles in a historically paternalistic equation serves as the contextual framework for their same subsequent, subordinating, passive, and secondary roles within the context of nursing. Finding legitimacy, obtaining a voice, establishing theoretical and practice foundations, building a legitimate body of knowledge, and claiming "space" for the value and roles of nursing practice in health care are all challenges that have characterized the long and arduous journey to establish legitimacy, value, impact, and equity for the professional practice of nursing (Group & Roberts, 2001). A number of historical texts detail the account of this journey and serve to exemplify and validate the content and character of this long process (Bonvillain, 2007; Nicholson & Fisher, 2014).

During the 20th century, the profession of nursing evolved significantly as leaders sought to formalize and give structure to this field. Nursing is clearly one of the oldest practices in history, yet it is one of history's youngest professions. It is only since the time of Florence Nightingale that nursing as a profession and practice has been codified and formalized in a manner that provides a disciplined framework and content, grounded in science, evidence, precedence, standards, and ethics (Dossey, 2005; Fitzpatrick & Whall, 2005; McDonald, 2010).

Many of the social characteristics of traditionally masculine professions (e.g., law, medicine, architecture, engineering) served as the exemplar that nurses used to translate and shape the parameters of the emerging nursing discipline (Cope, 1958). Because nearly 100% of nurses in the past were women, many "feminine" modifications and adaptations of practice were created to accommodate the contemporary reality, which served to set the limits on nursing's role, position, authority, and power structure (Pollard, 1911). Much of the regimented, formalized, hierarchical, militaristic, and religious overlay to the structuring of the nursing profession in the 20th century strongly reflected the social requisite of establishing limited parameters and containing the nursing function within prevailing perceptions of what was appropriate for women during this era (D'Antonio, 2010; Group & Roberts, 2001; Mason & Leavitt, 2011).

The emerging equity in nursing during the latter half of the 20th century changed the parameters and patterns of nursing roles and relationships from regulation to practice, in parallel with the changing roles and characteristics of women in the rest of contemporary society. As equity has become more apparent in women's broader role expectations, education, opportunities, performance factors, pay, and position in society, these changes have likewise been reflected in the nurse's role (Cowen & Moorhead, 2011).

The role of the contemporary nurse reflects the steps taken on this journey to equity by women in society; it also demonstrates the impact of these changes on nursing as a whole. Today, the world of nursing includes a large number of graduate-educated nurses at the master's and doctoral levels, researchers and practice leaders, and advanced practitioners who practice both independently and interdependently to provide value-based health services to specific populations (Cowen & Moorhead, 2011). While the noise of the products of equity has not yet subsided, the relevance and value can no longer be legitimately contested.

SCENARIO

Florence Nightingale was the original accountability-based nurse leader. In her time, she confronted many of the vagaries of transformation and change as society moved out of the Victorian age and into the industrial age. Nightingale confronted many challenges related to beliefs, social attitudes, gender, science and technology, women's roles, and a host of other cultural and contextual barriers.

In our time, many new challenges have arisen and created a landscape for transformation and change. In small groups of four or five colleagues, discuss the parallels between the changes confronted by Florence Nightingale and the challenges of contemporary change. Focus your discussion on the similarities between what Florence Nightingale encountered on the cusp of a new age and what you as clinical leaders will encounter on the cusp of this new sociotechnical age and era of health transformation and reform. Enumerate how Nightingale addressed those challenges and indicate how her actions may serve as an exemplar for confronting leadership challenges in the contemporary age.

CRITICAL THOUGHT

Much of the history of nursing parallels the history of the women's movement. Many of the experiences that nurses have in the workplace reflect the same experiences that women share in a wide variety of work settings. The challenges associated with achieving equity in nursing match challenges in realizing equity for women in our larger society, and many of the requisites to do so are precisely the same.

Nevertheless, nurses have not reached the end of the road to professional clarity and social equity. While much has been done and the foundations of the profession have been established beyond question, many of the historical insights, notions, and attitudes about the nursing role and its legitimacy and equity remain subject to debate. Resolving these issues will require concerted action on the part of nursing professionals and their partners in asserting the legitimacy, value, and contribution of nursing to advancing social health. In turn, equity and the obligations and demands of equity-based accountability will become important cornerstones of the role of the profession and are now the requisites of the behavior and practices of every professional.

Maturing the Profession: The Age of Accountability

For professionals, responsibility is not the definitive foundation for work—accountability is. Historically, the nurse was judged to be an acceptable worker if he or she simply did what was required and characteristic of the function of the role. For this employed worker to be evaluated as competent, the individual needed simply to focus on the work and do it well.

This focus on the function of work and how well it is done forms the foundation for demonstrating the exercise of effective responsibility (Oliver, 2004). One can be responsible without being accountable; responsibility and accountability are fundamentally different concepts. Responsibility is embedded in the work and its processes, encompassing how well they were done and how effectively they were completed. This focus on responsibility characterizes the individual's performance as a reflection of process, action, task, function, and job. Responsibility sees the individual from the perspective of the work and values that individual as a reflection of what work was done and how well it was completed.

Such a focus on responsibility creates a task frame—a "job" orientation. In fact, it describes job-driven work and creates the conditions that enumerate the characteristics of jobs and job categorization of work. In most historical work-places, this perspective is evidenced in a number of ways. Notably, job descriptions are often laundry lists of functions and activities ascribed to a role. These functions and activities zero in on the elements of work rather than the results that demonstrate the impact of work. In addition, performance evaluations review the worker within the context of the capacity to function and the ability of the individual to do or perform the work. The responsible person's behavior and ability to do the work, get the job done, and get along with others who are also doing their jobs are all included in the list of functional competencies that represent responsible behavior. These characteristics reflect how well a person does the work, how much of that work gets done, and how effective the person is in doing that work. Such an evaluation of work tends to concentrate more on the quality of the work processes, the character of the effort, and the content of the functions of work (issues of responsibility), and less on the value of the work, the meaning of the work, and the impact the work has on making a difference.

This focus has largely resulted from a slavish attachment to process and function and the heavy emphasis on job orientation. Even as the nursing profession is fundamentally driven by value and meaning, much of the character of the profession's work remains delineated by job functionalism, process, activity, and task focus. It is not unusual to hear a nursing professional speaking of his or her work essentially as a job—that is, a laundry list of tasks, functions, actions, processes, and effort. As a result, a stronger *employee work group syndrome* operates to frame the work of nursing as perceived from the position of *job*.

The job characterization of the work of the nurse leads to an entirely different assumption than can be obtained through the lens of professional practice and behavior. The (inaccurate) assumption is that nurses can do jobs responsibly but cannot act accountably. When this frame of reference is adopted, nurses can be perceived only in the context of job performance. Regardless of how much

CRITICAL THOUGHT

The primary focus of accountability is the achievement of results and the effect of those results over the long term. Sustainable organizations do not simply look for sustainability in the next increment of time. Instead, they establish a long-term vision and tie their work processes to all the efforts necessary to achieve this vision. Ultimately, individuals and teams must define their accountabilities as reflection of this long-term viability. Embracing this focus on accountability instead of process responsibility calls for rethinking of a unilateral focus on job elements and processes.

activity is identified as "professional" in most job categories, every profession should certainly be able to demonstrate professional behavior and create a frame of reference within which particular work activities can be characterized. In short, if the nurse wishes or seeks to be treated as a professional, he or she must be able to demonstrate behaviors consistent with professional delineations.

Accountability and Ownership

There can be no accountability without ownership. Accountability assumes some level of intensity of the individual and an investment in and ownership of the role, tasks, and activities as they represent the characteristics and demands of the profession (Malloch & Porter-O'Grady, 2009a). In a profession, preparation for work occurs in the academic setting and incorporates prerequisites, examinations, regulation, and often licensure as requirements for entry into the profession (Gebbie, Rosenstock, & Hernandez, 2003).

Professions are knowledge dependent. Professional knowledge workers operate in the workplace with the assumption that they have been adequately prepared in the principles and practices of the profession sufficient to generate trust in their efforts and to ensure competence in the application of their work. Membership in the profession is a requisite to role performance at work. However, in many organizations, the notion of membership as a part of the script and relationship between the organization and the professional worker is not fully or adequately addressed. In fact, participation in job categorization (being an employee) overcomes recognition of membership in the profession (being a professional). As a result, the relationship between the individual and the workplace unfolds through the lens of job categorization, with the individual being seen as an employee rather than as a professional. The job then becomes the contextual framework for the relationship between the individual and the workplace, with job parameters being established that favor functionalism, task focus, process orientation, action

CRITICAL THOUGHT

Ownership is commitment to the following:

- Fully applying one's own skills
- Growing and learning to enhance talents
- Development of others
- Evaluating effectiveness of contribution
- Continual lifelong learning

over reflection, and measures of productivity embedded in action rather than in impact (Werhane, 2007). Ultimately, the professional worker becomes divorced from the drivers embedded in professional membership and, instead, becomes more strongly attached to job requisites and the action- and function-based drivers embedded in job performance.

For the nursing leader, it should be clear that creating a job context for work cannot produce professional outcomes. When the job predominates, the obligations of professional membership and its accountability dissipate, and the expectations for performance at the professional level simply never come to fruition.

To navigate this scenario successfully, the leader must be able to revise and recalibrate the professional worker's relationship to the organization. Leadership, therefore, is charged with creating an organizational context that does not impede membership and ownership of the work (as job categorization of the work does); instead, the structural context for professional work becomes a framework within which work expectations unfold (a professional structure). For that to happen, the following circumstances and conditions are required in terms of the role of the leader and the structure of the organization:

- Professional ownership implies that the ownership of the work belongs to the profession, not to the workplace. The relationship of the workplace to the profession is one of partnership, not dependency, creating a strong framework for horizontal rather than vertical interaction.
- Contemporary research on the orientation of professional/knowledge workers suggests that the traditional incentives often seen in employee-driven models will not motivate the action of this worker. In fact, the use of such traditional incentives actually impedes or diminishes the commitment and motivation of the professional/ knowledge worker to the work and the workplace.
- Clear indicators of performance expectations and deliverables must be established within the professional role charter or contract of nursing. From the very outset, their selection must be done in a way that clarifies the expectations of professional membership, enumerates specifics regarding obligations of ownership, sets peer-based expectations, and forges an agreement to participate fully in the life of the profession in the workplace.
- Employee work group models, job descriptions, job performance, job measures, job satisfaction, and job orientation—indeed, all job categorizations—must be separated from the identification of professional characteristics, roles, expectations, and performance

factors if professional behaviors are to be exemplified as normative factors in the workplace.

- Contemporary leaders should onboard new professionals through the use of well-identified professional processes, such as granting privileges instead of hiring, peer-based selection of incoming members instead of management hiring practices, credentialing processes, peer-based protocols, clinical/career advancement mechanisms, and continuous professional development as foundational to the onboarding process.

- As with most professional bodies, the development of terms of behavior, operating rules and regulations for professional members, professional bylaws, and professional decision-making councils should increasingly become the framework within which the nursing discipline makes decisions about its character, content, ethics, contribution, and mechanisms for advancing the interests of the organization and its users.

- Normative shared leadership practices and professional governance structures create the behavioral and operating frame of reference for the nursing profession and establish a milieu where both the organization and the profession can work collaboratively, collaterally, and seamlessly to advance the health interests of the community and the particular health needs of people.

The critical element of understanding and valuing the effectiveness of the profession of nursing in the healthcare workplace is the recognition that professional outcomes cannot be advanced, demanded, strategized, or expected in the presence of an organizational structure and operational arrangement that is based on an employee work group. Professional behaviors are simply unachievable when the prevailing infrastructure of the organization is designed to support job behaviors. Congruence between professional structure and professional ownership is an essential correlate to sustaining professional behaviors (**Figure 14-1**). In the absence of a structure that reflects commitment to professional membership, ownership, and partnership, expecting performance that reflects such a commitment becomes an effort in futility.

At the same time, the individual professional must come into the professional organization with a clear understanding of the obligations of membership in the professional community and ownership of the profession's work. A strong part of the preparation of the professional entails deepening that individual's understanding of the terms of membership in the profession and the obligations that membership incurs. Often, new members of the nursing profession share an equal burden of responsibility for accepting job categorization; fixed,

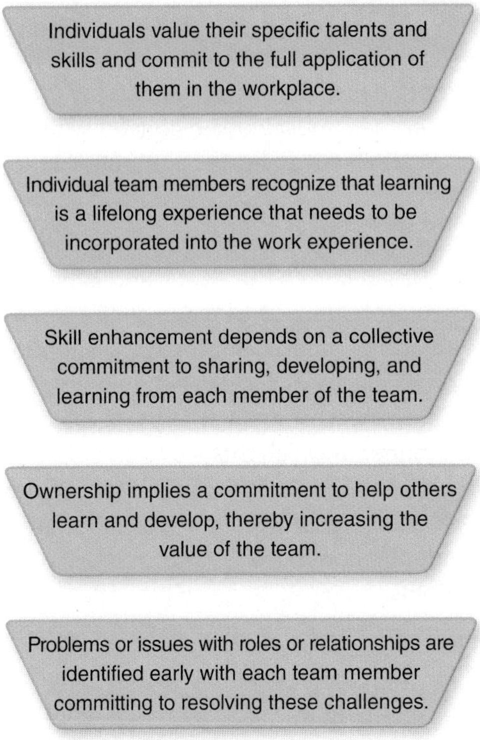

Individuals value their specific talents and skills and commit to the full application of them in the workplace.

Individual team members recognize that learning is a lifelong experience that needs to be incorporated into the work experience.

Skill enhancement depends on a collective commitment to sharing, developing, and learning from each member of the team.

Ownership implies a commitment to help others learn and develop, thereby increasing the value of the team.

Problems or issues with roles or relationships are identified early with each team member committing to resolving these challenges.

Figure 14-1 The critical elements of ownership

finite, and functional work patterns; and an addiction to the safety of ritual and routine. If individuals have an attachment to these patterns of behaviors, they should not consider membership in a profession. Professional membership is a significant obligation—it demands full engagement, ownership, and investment in the life of the profession. Embracing roles that advance the ethics, standards, evidence, and best practices of a profession is equally, if not more, important to the profession and the quality of patient care than is the functional action of the nurse. Frequently, nurses can be heard saying, "I'm too busy with my patients" to participate in deliberations and decisions about standards of care, protocols, evidentiary dynamics, and best practices. One is simply left to wonder if the nurse is truly too busy to participate in those processes that define the foundations of his or her practice and inform its action, what the justification for that busyness is, and how legitimately it represents best practices and the state of the art and science of nursing. For the professional nurse, accountability and ownership are not options.

CRITICAL THOUGHT

Every team member has a specific accountability for achieving the team's goals. All team members must work in concert with others to ensure that both individual and collective efforts contribute to the achievement of team goals.

There are basically two kinds of team goals to which individuals contribute. First, some goals relate to the needs and activities of the team that fulfill the purposes and direction of the organization of which the team is a part. These goals and objectives are the work priorities of teams and provide the framework within which team action unfolds. Second, the team has its own specific service or functional goals that relate to the work that it does and the manner in which that work is completed. Here the team focuses on the application of standards, protocols, processes, pathways, and plans. These goals identify the framework for individual and team action and provide the context within which individual and collective performance unfolds.

Team members recognize that if effectiveness is to be achieved, the efforts of individual team members must converge around team goals. All activities related to the function of the team should coalesce in a way that advances performance against the anticipated goal achievement. It is in failing to recognize this fundamental reality for all teams that infrastructure and relationship begin to break down. When any one member's performance operates out of synch with the team's goals, the integrity of the team begins to disintegrate. It is important for team members to recognize that although individual work is unique and important, it must ultimately advance the team's work effort as well as fulfill the organization purposes for that work. Good teams assess the relationship between the work of individuals and the collective work of the team and its effect on achieving outcomes.

CRITICAL THOUGHT

In the professions, the identity of the person and the professional are one. The work (practice) of a professional is not a separate part of his or her life. In the professional, the practice and the person are so tightly linked that they are one and the same thing.

The Cycle of Personal Accountability

At a personal level, the individual professional must draw specific conclusions and certain references to his or her personal ownership of membership in the profession, contribute to its work, and fulfill the obligations of the social trust that membership in the profession implies. This means that at a personal level the individual understands the nature of the relationship of the person to the profession.

One notable characteristic of a professional is his or her recognition of the intensity of the fit between the person as individual and the person as professional. In the professions, these elements converge to create in the person a unity between professional identity and personal identity. The individual must continually reflect on the value of that connection, explore how that connection is best represented in the life and action of the person, and consider what that convergence between person and professional means in terms of sense of self, values, self-expression, and the broader role of the person in society.

This personal deliberation on accountability is a fundamental part of role identification with a profession. Its calls upon the professional to assess who and where the individual is in relationship to his or her profession and how that match is expressed as a part of personal commitment.

Some of the issues and elements that relate to this self-assessment are as follows:

- Action is driven by principle. The question for the professional is whether action and principle in personal expression are coherent and consistently linked in such a way that the expression of the work of the discipline represents the principles that drive it.

- Personal action is informed by commitment to learning and knowing. The professional seeks to ensure that clinical action is informed by knowledge and evidence that the choices made are the most rational and best fit with the needs to which they are directed. In so doing, the professional affirms personal commitment to continuous learning, growing, and adapting as a part of ensuring that practices are meaningful and relevant.

- In the interests of reflective practice, the professional engages in personal self-reflection as part of his or her personal assessment of the goodness of fit among values, decisions, actions, and outcomes. This personal reflection seeks to more deeply assess the intensity and effectiveness of the personal work of the professional and the difference that work makes in the lives touched by the professional.

- The accountable professional is able to identify incongruence, brokenness, or inadequacies and make effective judgments about how best to change his or her role and practice to become more effective. As a result of this corrective and adaptive capacity, the individual has a professional opportunity to be flexible, to be innovative, and to better align work with the evidence that both justifies and validates it.
- In the interests of personal ownership of the profession, the individual recognizes his or her role in relationship to other members and works to join with them in the collective effort to advance and improve the profession and its work. The individual professional recognizes that the profession is not an objective entity but rather the sum of the collective wisdom of each member within the profession. The profession can do nothing for the individual if the individual is not acting on behalf of the profession. The profession has no life except that of the collective energies of the members who constitute it. It can do nothing without the concerted action of its individual members. Members move a profession; a profession cannot move its members without their engagement.

Accountability in Action

Certain critical elements of ownership should be evident in the practice of each professional nurse. In nursing, as in all professions, this ownership accompanies membership as a part of the set of individual obligations that each nurse must bring to his or her practice. These obligations inform the contributions the nurse makes to the profession, to the organization, and to the patients. Critical elements of professional ownership include the following:

- The individual nurse values his or her specific gifts, talents, and skills and agrees to fully apply them in the work of the profession in a way that positively impacts the patient's experience.
- The individual professional member of the staff recognizes that his or her competence depends on continuous and dynamic lifelong learning and practice. This fundamental commitment to membership is evidenced by continuous advancement of the nurse's learning experience.
- Competency and skill enhancement depend on the individual's commitment to membership and contributions to the collective activity of deliberating, sharing, developing, learning, and deciding on standards and protocols of practice that are required as a part of a collegial agreement.
- Individual ownership implies a commitment to engage with others in their learning and development and in mentoring and sharing in the

learning process in a way that advances the value of the profession's work and its impact on the patient's health experience.

- Each professional member recognizes the inherent challenges and issues in professional relationships and collegial action. The individual acknowledges and accepts the obligation to fully engage those differences and to find common ground with others in a way that demonstrates the profession's capacity to problem solve in concert with other professions.

Each individual member of the professional community recognizes that he or she has an inherent obligation to make a contribution to that community in a way that will benefit both the individual and the community (Porter-O'Grady, 2004). Put simply, the life of the individual professional cannot be advanced or improved if the life of the discipline is not addressed as a whole. Team performance, in fact,

REFLECTIVE QUESTIONS

- Does the work I do relate well to the purposes of the team?
- Do my work efforts integrate well with the efforts of others on the team?
- Am I clear on the essential value of each element of my work?
- Do the efforts of all team members link to and integrate well with expectations?
- Do I reassess my functions and activities regularly to determine their relevance?
- Do I join with the team in evaluating effectiveness of work effort?
- Is there clear evidence that my work and the outcomes directly relate well?
- Am I willing to adjust my work activity when a change is clearly indicated?
- Do I actively problem solve with team members to resolve critical issues?
- Am I flexible in adjusting my work activities when the team needs to change?
- Do I actively join with team members in identifying specific work changes?
- Do I initiate discussions and dialogue when problems in work processes emerge?
- Is there a willingness on the part of all team members to confront one another?
- Do I join with the team in celebrating successes and accomplishments?

is just the aggregation and synthesis of individual performance. The success of this performance reflects agreement on and understanding of the principles and standards of practice and the common action that represents the consensus of professional members. In complex responsive processes (the positive interplay between the organization, work teams, and individuals), there exists a deep understanding of the goodness of fit between the action of each individual member of the profession and the collective impact the profession has on the lives of the individuals served by the profession. The more unilateral and nonaligned the action of the individual is, the less significance or value the impact has on advancing the work of the profession. Conversely, the more aligned, collaborative, and integrated the actions of individual members are, the more impact these actions have on the profession as a whole and the more likely the profession can sustain its promise of quality and effectiveness.

Individual Role Accountability and Team Performance

Clearly identifying the elements and characteristics of the individual professional's role is a critical first step in relating it to the collective work of the profession. Each individual must know the unique contribution he or she makes as a member of the profession and clearly recognize that his or her individual contribution has a direct impact on team effectiveness. Teams are effective only to the extent that their members coalesce their unique and individual contributions

CRITICAL THOUGHT

Focusing on team goals includes the following:

- Incorporating team goals and individual work
- Defining the fit between individual and team
- Clarifying organizational work expectations
- Identifying team performance factors
- Specifying individual needs related to work
- Supporting each other in the collective work
- Removing impediments to team effectiveness
- Ending incongruent individual performance
- Evaluating progress regularly and often

around a common aggregated contribution that cannot be achieved unless synthesis emerges between all members' efforts (Stacey, 2009). Before team effectiveness can be delineated, the basic foundations of individual contributions and the unique character of those contributions as they integrate with team effort must be established to ensure a lasting positive impact.

Several elements of individual accountability affect the collective or team effort of any discipline. Each individual professional member must realize that one of the primary arenas of accountability is the extent to which he or she supports the professional colleagues on the team. Here again, the individual member of the team contributes to the team to the extent of his or her unique gifts and role. Each of the critical elements of ownership previously identified has a specific and direct impact on the life of the team, its viability, and, ultimately, its clinical outcomes. Some of those relationships can be best described as follows:

- Individual member skills, when connected to the unique skill set of every other member, create the framework for the collective team contribution. It is the aggregate of the individual skills that evidences the value of the collective work of the clinical team. Diversity of contributions (from the team efforts) and clarity regarding the unique character of those contributions (based on the effort of each member of the team) are critical to ascertaining the value of the team and the impact of its collective efforts.

- Teams cannot be constructed simply because people want to meet or work together; instead, teams are purposeful in their origin. Given this fact, the construction of the team is a critical first step in team performance. There must be a goodness of fit between members of the team and the work of the team. This goodness of fit is not an accidental achievement. The leader must do intentional work in assessing the unique and specific characteristics of team members to ensure that their fit coalesces across the team to make the contribution to which the team is directed.

- Accountable teams are relational bodies. Members must be able to act synergistically, reflecting an agreement on their contributions and the activities of their collective effort. In short, they must be able to work well together. This relationship competence and integrity of team members is a critical element of team effectiveness and should be considered a fundamental part of the work.

- Individual and collective accountability requires both the person and the team to understand that the relationships in the team and the functions of the team demand a continuous openness and availability to learning. Therefore, learning is embedded in the individual and collective action of the team as the team continues to unfold its work. In doing so, the team members discover new facets, insights, and approaches refining the work that make a difference in the team's outcomes.

- Purpose-driven teams are formulated as a primary mechanism for fulfilling that purpose. Teams do not exist just to exist. In turn, leaders must realize that a constant reference back to purpose, meaning, and goals serves as a critical reminder to the team of its reason for being and the driver for its work. Achieving outcomes means fulfilling the team's purpose and staying focused on this connection. This is critical to the sustainable effectiveness of the team.

Individual accountability is represented in the person's commitment to the team effort, which represents the profession's collective obligation to have an impact on the health of those served and to make a difference through that collective effort. It is important, however, for each individual professional to remember that the team cannot be effective if the questions of individual accountability and ownership are not addressed and resolved by each member as a part of understanding his or her own unique contribution to the efforts of the team. In fact, accountability is the centerpiece of every meaningful professional action.

Delineating Professional Work and Accountability

Historically, job descriptions have been used as a vehicle for delineating the role functions, tasks, and activities of the nurse (Zedeck & American Psychological Association, 2011). Organizations have historically placed a great deal of stock in these job descriptions as a justifiable and legitimate framework for defining functional performance expectations. The problem with this approach is that the dynamic nature of professional work, the significant dependence on individual relationships and critical judgments, and the highly variable nature of the user (the patient) seriously belie the validity and value of work defined as a fixed, finite, functional, and incremental set of activities (Malloch & Porter-O'Grady, 2009b). The only product of this framework or approach to defining work is a continual fixed notion that results in static ritual and routine. In fact, standardized, static, ritual, and routine mechanisms become the product of these environments. Job descriptions simply codify this pattern of behaviors and produce the incorrect assumption that work elements for the professional can be codified and

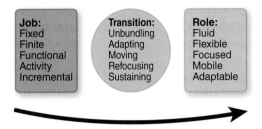

Figure 14-2 From job descriptions to accountability

fixed in a set of activities that are essentially nonvariable and rarely change. Of course, this is simply not true.

For the professional to be effective, professional performance must be tied to role (**Figure 14-2**). This connection is a reflection of the relationship between action and outcome, moderated by the needs of the user (the patient), in a dynamic interaction that is fluid, flexible, focused, portable, and mobile. The professional must be intuitive, incisive, responsive, and adaptive to the needs of the patient (the user). Although standards form the floor of practice and lay the groundwork for good judgment, they do not encompass the full expression of judgment and the adaptability necessary to accommodate the specific and unique needs of each person served. Principles, standards, and practices must be adapted and adjusted to reflect the very real and powerful influences of the user's resources, experience, behaviors, circumstances, culture, and responsive capacity. Established and fixed functional delineations of this work simply do not adequately address or appropriately codify personal demand in a way that legitimately meets patient needs. The more firmly the role is embedded in ritual and routine and fixed practice, the less capability the individual nurse has for rendering the kind of critical judgment necessary to be appropriately adaptive and responsive in a way that advances quality and outcome and adequately addresses the unique needs of the user. When such critical adaptability is lacking in practice, any vehicles or measures of quality, impact, and outcome suffer from diminishing returns and ultimately cease to exist. Describing and characterizing the role of the professional requires a different configuration than job descriptions can provide.

This does not, however, abrogate the responsibility of the professions to codify and frame practice in such a way that it can be effectively delineated and delivered with excellence, demonstrating positive impact. Evidence-based practice and the evidentiary dynamics of applying it call for the professions to establish a true cause-and-effect relationship between the principles of practice and their application. An evidence-based approach to defining practice requires real-time, just-in-time, and readily accessible information resources that serve to inform practice-in-process, thereby creating the conditions to immediately alter, adjust, or change practice in a way that demonstrates congruence with the evidence. Thus the following information factors affect accountable performance:

- The ability to generate the right information
- The quality of the information gathered
- The willingness and ability to share the right information
- The technology and hardware supporting the use of information
- The accuracy with which the information is translated
- The applicability of the information to the work
- The competence of the worker in using information
- The ability to evaluate the effectiveness of information

This new demand for asserting the foundations of practice indicates how professional roles and functions must adjust to the use of more high-tech tools and approaches to defining, delivering, and evaluating care-in-process. Because of the just-in-time nature of digitally related clinical delivery and of user-driven service structures, professional work must be fluid and flexible and respond to the evidence in a way that indicates how and when it needs to change. Role descriptions, performance charters, and professional accountability call for the individual to be accountable for transitioning to higher standards of practice as they are applied, including using digital tools of practice and documentation. Clinicians have no choice but to reconfigure practice to address the emerging evidence for changing it, make effective use of the technical tools that provide real-time data informing practice, make immediate changes within the process of practice, and demonstrate a highly refined willingness to own the outcomes of practice rather than simply manage the tools of practice. The tools of practice—technology hardware, data, information, evidence, and past practice—are continuously changing, of course. Specifically, they are moving clinical work in the direction of a high-level sociotechnical clinical environment. Rigorously defining and codifying these tools does nothing to advance the meaning and work of the profession. In contrast, molding and shaping these tools to better match user needs and demands is clearly part of the work of the professional. Doing so requires defining and advancing an adaptive and predictive capacity and establishing role protocols that state the requisites for these skill sets rather than provide a laundry list of tasks and actions. Clinical leaders should be aware of the need to transition away from traditional job descriptions and toward these more accurate professional role delineations in a way that more effectively supports the professional role, defines the requisite capacities for effective professional judgment, and better identifies the interface between the technology that supports just-in-time clinical practice and the viability of the professional nurse.

In summary, the following work factors affect accountable performance:

- The competence of the individual to do the work
- Staffing and scheduling arrangements supporting the work
- The goodness of fit of the individual's work effort with the team's collective effort
- The team's ability to understand the contribution of each member
- The work tools affecting the ability to do the work
- The utility of managing and applying information
- The clarity of expectations with regard to performance
- Time or workload affecting the ability to accomplish the work

From Process to Outcome Focus

The primary point of accountability is to be able to demonstrate impact, results, and effects in the service relationship, all of which are sustained over the longer-term continuum of health (Kleinpell, 2009). Effective and sustainable organizations and the professions that practice in them do not always simply look at incremental and action steps in isolation to determine their impact and effect. Instead, in the interest of sustainability, they work to establish a longer-term vision of the clinical role and its impact on patients and populations and tie work processes to the collective effort to make a difference in the lives of the individuals they serve. Ultimately, the professional individuals and the teams within which they work must define their unique and collective accountabilities as a reflection of their commitment to achieving long-term impact and viability. This focus on accountability—instead of simply process responsibility—calls for rethinking the unilateral, compartmental, late-stage engagement of work; it requires developing a much more integrated, collective, interdisciplinary team framework for those elements of the process that produce meaningful impact on patients and populations.

In the contemporary healthcare environment where value is the driver, it is imperative that clinical organizations and their professionals focus their work on advancing sustainable and meaningful health for populations and communities. Individual providers serve the population one patient at a time. However, that service should reflect the providers' understanding that each patient represents the whole of his or her population, and these populations in turn represent the larger community. Through their service, nurses demonstrate that the individual and collective actions of the professional and their clinical teams can result in

CRITICAL THOUGHT

Accountability points to remember:

- Accountability must always be experienced within the role.
- Accountability cannot be externally directed or controlled.
- Accountability must be owned by those who do the work.
- Accountability must be directed to outcome, not process.
- Accountability is represented by team commitment to goals.

SCENARIO

Michael Cullen, RN, BSN, the clinical nurse leader on the medical-surgical unit, has been experiencing significant staffing problems for the past year. Michael has found it difficult to match the needs of patients with the availability of professional nursing staff. The problem has not been so much a shortage of nursing resources but rather a wide variability in patient acuity and census that has created difficulty in scheduling and staffing.

Michael has recognized the need to blend financial, administrative, and clinical realities and create a framework for appropriate staffing at a level that would meet the needs of the patients yet still operate within the unit's specified financial constraints. Furthermore, he wants to engage the professional staff in a way that would help bring ownership to the processes developed and to the standards created while designing and organizing an evidence-based approach to resource use.

Michael has discussed these issues with Nancy Mays, RN, MSN, the manager for the unit. They have laid out a grid that accounts for labor productivity, clinical nursing work, productivity measures, workload issues, patient and staff variances, and value and quality issues related to the delivery of nursing care. They realize that all these elements will need to be included in a systematic plan directed toward meeting patients' needs and defining specific nurse staffing and patient care delivery relationships.

Michael and Nancy have been challenged with clarifying the next steps in initiating an evidence-based approach to nurse-driven patient care. They both recognize that each of the elements will need to be explored with regard to existing information, best practices, research-based information resources, and experiential data generated out of the practice environment.

They have called on you as their practice consultant to help them organize a systematic process for patient care using evidence-based approaches. To initiate this process, they have formulated the following questions.

Discussion Questions

1. How does the unit create a model that integrates the elements identified in the scenario and establishes a framework for planning evidence-driven care?

2. How can we engage the staff in the process of planning and implementing an evidence-based model so that there are higher levels of ownership from each of the practitioners?

3. Can we link patient needs, workload measurement, staffing skills and competencies, acuity needs, and resource parameters in an ongoing dynamic application that can adjust to the reality of a highly variable census?

4. As the consultant to this process, your obligation is to help gather the information necessary to answer these questions and assist management and clinical staff in developing a partnership around an evidence-based format to address practice, resource, and quality issues on the nursing unit. Where might you begin, and how can you help them through these initial steps based on the information in this chapter?

positive health impacts on populations and communities. This principle drives and informs individual accountability and collective action in a way that represents the value, sustainability, and continuing viability of clinical practice. The following elements, therefore, are critical to understanding accountability within the context of impact:

- Accountable organizations and the professionals within them clearly identify who they serve and how they serve them in a way that demonstrates a meaningful positive impact on the health of that population or community. These professionals commit to redefining, refining, and advancing their processes and mechanisms as necessary to ensure this impact is positive and sustainable.

- Professionals who fully understand personal accountability continually join their efforts with one another to recalibrate, redefine, and accelerate the value of their work effort as a reflection of the goal of achieving population and community health. All clinical work adjusts its goals as service effectiveness advances in light of the mission of continuing the positive impact on the health of populations and advancing the health status of communities.

- Professional organizations that are committed to impacting the health of the individuals whom they serve understand the essential character and needs of accountability and create structures and infrastructures that support both individual and collective autonomy. They define accountability and action in a way that takes best advantage of economic utilization of resources and effective application of evidence and knowledge in positively impacting populations and communities.

- Emphasis on effective clinical systems does not just address processes or outcomes. The focus of effectiveness is on establishing a tight goodness of fit between processes and outcomes that demonstrates effective interactions, actions, relationships, and interfaces between the work of the professions, the needs of the user, and the health of the community.

REFLECTIVE QUESTION

How many of the following characteristics, which demonstrate accountable self-management, do you possess?

- Personal sense of ownership
- Role self-confidence
- Good role fit with others
- Willingness to clarify ambiguity
- Good problem-solving skills
- Relating well with others
- Strong communication skills
- Not seeking permission
- Tolerating differences
- Easily exploring alternatives
- Questioning rituals for relevance
- Good self-evaluation skills

- Accountable partnerships do not simply exist among professionals, their disciplines, and their organizations. Individual members of the community also share in the accountability for advancing the health of that community. The contract for effective health is between the provider and the user, the organization, and the community. Such a contract is forged through a convergence of accountability and action that exhibits a mutual commitment and effort to advancing the conditions, circumstances, and actions that lead to healthy patterns of behavior.

Accountability Is About Adding Value

Accountability is not simply about doing a job well. In fact, accountability has little to do with job orientation. For this reason, job models should be minimized when dealing with professional workers. In the past, leaders would often acknowledge individuals for having done a good job. Nevertheless, simply doing a good job does not necessarily mean that the right job was done (Bowles & Candela, 2005; Ulrich, 2014). Value is derived from doing the *right work* rather than doing a *good job*. Creating a strong connection between the activities of the professional and the right work is a critical and fundamental part of the contemporary leadership role. Today, the value of one's work depends on how strong a goodness of fit exists between the work of the professional and the impact that work has in making a difference in those to whom the work is directed.

Work is not inherently valuable. Simply doing work and keeping busy is not a source of value. Work is valuable only to the extent that it is informed by purpose; if its purposes are not fulfilled, the work does not demonstrate real value. Value is evidence of how directly the work connects to its contribution, to the intentional fulfillment of its purposes, to the achievement of its ends, and to its sustainability. This value notion of work is critical to a deeper understanding of its application and the professional's willingness to validate the sustainable value of the outcomes of the work and the dynamic processes that produce those outcomes.

Ultimately, value is the product of a measured and defined relationship between an effective process (cause) and a meaningful outcome (effect). It represents the convergence of the full range of variables that make up the complex elements of good decisions and actions necessary to good practice. As an outgrowth of purpose, meaning, expectation, performance, and outcome, the visible expression of value indicates how these dynamic factors operate in concert to ultimately shape patient outcomes. For their efforts to yield value, both individual professionals and their teams must fully apply their energies and talents to configure work in a way that will lead to the desired impact and outcome.

Although work and action may be highly variable, their dynamic nature does not diminish the importance of the fit between selected clinical actions and the particular health impacts achieved through those actions. For the professional, the ongoing challenge of creating this "fit" is the central constituent of clinical work. The role of the clinical leader is to create the conditions that support assessment of the evidence, adjustment of clinical action, management of clinical information (documentation), and evaluation of impact. For the professional, these attributes and behaviors require a stronger set of skills and performance factors for their realization than the historical, functional, or task-based delineation of the nursing role would support. The never-ending dance among the individual professional, the clinical team, the user, and these care attributes and behaviors creates the essential conditions for a living expression of value in a way that drives toward positive health impacts and outcomes.

The Individual, Creativity, and Accountability

Professional practice implies that the individual pursues innovation and creativity as part of his or her practice. Clinical leaders should encourage and advance the creativity and innovation embedded in practice as a part of supporting the adaptive capacity of each nurse; adaptation is necessary to ensure that the most relevant and appropriate practices and behaviors unfold in such a way as to make the most difference in the lives of the individuals the healthcare organization serves (**Figure 14-3**). Everyone is born creative, but life's circumstances may either bring out or diminish creative efforts and expression over time. Often, in job-based organizational arrangements, the need for uniformity, similarity, and standardized performance mediates against the action of innovation and creativity. Life experiences, challenges to personal growth, continuous threats to dynamic self-image, and social structural limitations that create rigid parameters that impede creativity all work in concert to limit innovative expression.

Although organizations must carefully manage the creative effort and carefully construct the infrastructure for innovation, they can ensure that both thrive in

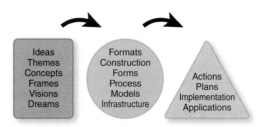

Figure 14-3 Generating the creative urge

the system. This means, of course, that the system design must value and generate the conditions amenable to innovation and creativity. Such a continuously active and dynamic process requires good leaders to be both aware of the requisites of innovation and creativity and clear about the discipline necessary to focus innovation and creativity on the purpose and values of the system.

Innovation and creativity demand infrastructure and leadership behaviors characterized by openness, trust, free expression, and availability to ideas in a way that moves the organization beyond habit, rote, ritual, and routine. Creative leadership and organization reflect the leader's capacity to embrace the different and the creative, to challenge existing patterns and practices, to push the walls, and to reflect in new ways, generating new patterns of response. All too often, the most significant leadership deficit is failure to create an effective and safe environment where creative and innovative practitioners can emerge and positively change patterns and practices to advance the science and art of practice, the experience of the user, and the impacts and outcomes of patient care.

True accountability assumes that openness and availability to creativity and innovation are fundamental parts of a meaningful and appropriate clinical environment. Out of this clinical context, the impulse to create, to improve, and to advance—an urge that is present in each nurse—is continually expected and supported. Professionals have a right to expect that practice will respond to changes in the evidence, new technology, environmental shifts, and new insights; indeed, nurses are accountable for adjusting their work to such shifts.

Leaders who create an environment that supports creativity and innovation in their practitioners provide a context for excitement, generativity, and a high level of engagement that enthuses the team, converges positive forces, and generates a deeper accountability as well as a broader desire for involvement. This challenge clearly calls upon leaders to embrace their own self-creativity and to recognize, even in their own leadership, the urge to innovate. The leader who is limited in his or her leadership of clinical creativity ultimately fails to recognize in others the creative urge and the value of tapping that innovation in a collective effort to make positive change and to personally embrace the intentional construction of the future.

There is no doubt that in most workplaces it is often difficult to live in a creative and innovative way. Certainly, the normative expectations of work that emerge as part of the day-to-day effort can bury the creative urge in ritual and routine. Nevertheless, the leader must recognize that the effort for innovation and creativity involves systematically addressing risk. This effort must be intentional, not accidental. Unless it is well served and purposeful, the creative and innovative urge will be sublimated in a way that guarantees its nonexpression. Although some regulatory, procedural, policy, or performance requisite might

SCENARIO

Stephen was the newly elected chair of his unit-based Practice Council. He was not familiar with the demands of this role but wanted to respond with his best effort. He looked at the rules of engagement for the Council and reviewed the terms of reference for its actions on the unit. Stephen was a little concerned when he saw the following statement: "The Practice Council has the accountability for the practice decisions on the unit; because the Council represents the clinical staff and reflects its accountability for practice decisions, its deliberations and decisional processes always lead to action and therefore require staff compliance." He was unaware of this level of authority and sought to clarify it with his manager.

During this discussion, Stephen learned that his role was seen as a clinical leader who fully participated in decisions that affected the work of others. His manager explained that her role was to support the Practice Council's decisions and to help Stephen in the processes associated with dialogue, discussion, negotiation, and making and implementing decisions. She also encouraged him with her personal commitment to help him develop leadership skills and facilitation processes.

Stephen welcomed this support but remained a little intimidated that he would be responsible for the staff making decisions that could affect practice and patient care in a direct way. This policy was a powerful break from the past, when the manager was the prime mover and controller of decisions. Here accountability meant that clinical decisions were placed with the staff, where those decisions had the best chance of being implemented and evaluated. This clearly increased staff engagement and extended their role in having an effect on the work of the organization.

Discussion Questions

1. Given your knowledge of accountability, what advice would you give Stephen to help him get started in building and expanding the notion of accountability for all of the staff?

2. How do you change the staff participation terms of engagement from invitation to expectation?

3. What might be one of the first arenas for building the expectation of accountability?

CRITICAL THOUGHT

The leader is the role model for safe risk taking and appropriately engaging the innovative or different. Colleagues will not take risks if the leader does not make it safe to do so.

always be cited to block an expressive or experimental response, it is the leader's obligation to place these parameters in context and define mechanisms that raise the standard of practice and impact patients in a way that belies the limitations of past practice, policy, and regulation. This is accountability in action (**Figure 14-4**).

Regulatory socialization has historically been well entrenched in the healthcare organization, resulting in an emphasis on sameness, consistency, policy, and

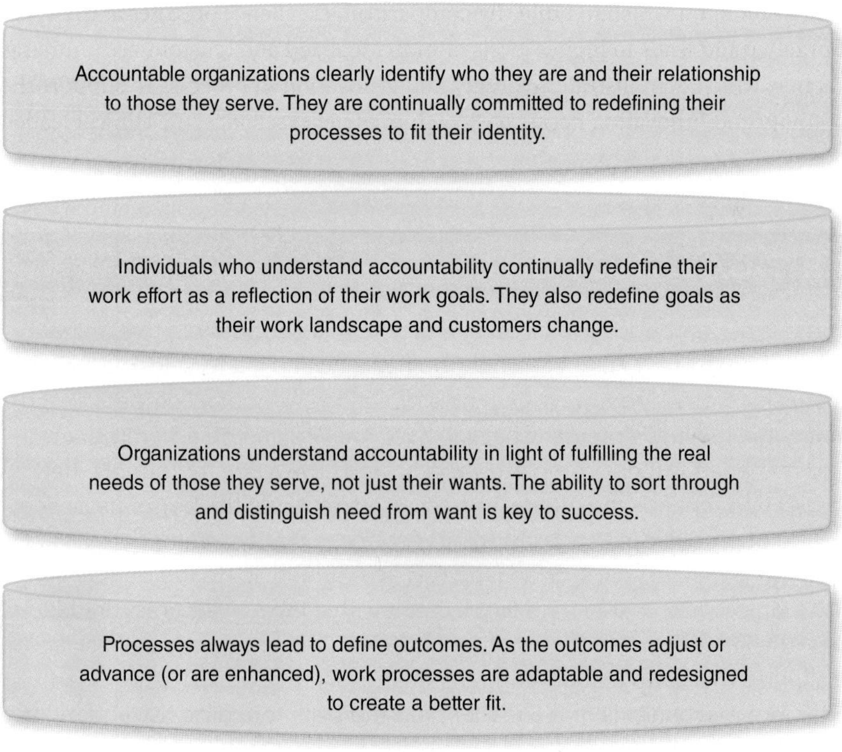

Accountable organizations clearly identify who they are and their relationship to those they serve. They are continually committed to redefining their processes to fit their identity.

Individuals who understand accountability continually redefine their work effort as a reflection of their work goals. They also redefine goals as their work landscape and customers change.

Organizations understand accountability in light of fulfilling the real needs of those they serve, not just their wants. The ability to sort through and distinguish need from want is key to success.

Processes always lead to define outcomes. As the outcomes adjust or advance (or are enhanced), work processes are adaptable and redesigned to create a better fit.

Figure 14-4 Accountability in action

routine at the expense of the potential of innovation. The presence of these perceived constraints often reflects uncertainty about applying the innovative practices needed to stimulate creativity and transformation. Also, the vast amounts of time spent in meeting the sometimes mindless requisites of regulation, policy, ritual, and routine limit the leader's ability to explore outside the box within the work environment—that is, to find opportunities to move above and beyond the regulatory "floor" of organizational life. Missing from the leader's role is the capacity that creates an opportunity to explore differently and provide unique incentives for innovation and contribution.

In reality, the leader's focus on creativity and innovation in a highly changing social construct is absolutely essential to advance sustainability, life, and meaningful impact on the work of the organization and the life of the community. The wise and effective leader acknowledges that creativity is not an option but rather a necessary condition for growth and adaptation. This leader recognizes that standardization sets the "floor" of practice, whereas innovation and creativity operate effectively at the "ceiling" of practice. Standardization creates a platform that expresses the principles and foundations of practice; it constitutes the essential foundation upon which to build. By comparison, excellence operates at the apex of practice and leads to higher levels of individualized and "customized" nursing practice, which demonstrate creativity and innovation in process. To support the creativity and innovation necessary to achieve true excellence, the clinical leader

CRITICAL THOUGHT

There is risk embedded in all human action. It is not possible to eliminate risk. If there were no risk, life would be flat—indeed, lifeless. Risk is a sign of reaching out in new ways or in new directions without a compass or the ability to absolutely predict what will happen. Risk can be accommodated and managed but not completely eradicated. The more thoroughly the leader understands the nature and occurrence of risk, the better he or she will be at predicting it and designing responses that accommodate risk or manage it well. In fact, a good leader is able to anticipate the degree of risk inherent in a change and to predict it with a level of accuracy. In this way, the leader can help the staff grapple with the implications of risk and maximize their own responses to the changes in the work. The risk management mechanisms of the leader help the staff normalize risk and more easily engage it.

continuously seeks opportunities in his or her own self-expression to validate and value the innovative and creative and to create a context that provides a safe space for that same urge to be expressed and fulfilled by every member of the professional community. This is not an addendum to leader accountability but rather its centerpiece.

Accountability and the Engagement of Risk

The only truly effective work that leaders do is to create an enabling context for the successful efforts of others. Leaders become ineffective when they ignore the obligations associated with creating the context for work and become deeply involved in the machinations related to the content of work. In professional organizations, the content of work is the obligation of the profession, not the manager. In every professional organization that operates consistently with professional values, the discipline protects its right and obligation to own the activities of its practice and to put control over those activities in the hands of those who do the profession's work. When leaders fail to create a context that supports the professional practitioners in owning and managing the content of their work, effectiveness and accountability diminish and, over time, dissipate.

The leader creates a safe space for the professional to identify the work, define it, undertake it, and evaluate it. In addition, the leader enables the professional to engage with the risk and take on the effort necessary to advance successful work. To do so, the clinical leader must always be prepared to create context, conditions, and organizational circumstances that will facilitate ownership of work and delivery of work at the point of service by owners. In short, leaders do not ask others to behave and perform in a manner in which the leader himself or herself does not behave and perform.

All effective leaders are comfortable with ambiguity and can lead within the context of "the potential." This potential occupies the space between what is and what will be. The leader is called upon to observe, assess the environment, predict the trajectory, and identify the adaptive characteristics necessary to thrive in the context of what is coming next that will both change work and impact performance (Porter-O'Grady & Malloch, 2010). This ability to live in the potential is a critical skill for contemporary leaders; this adaptive and predictive capacity must be incorporated into the role and expression of leadership. In turn, it informs the creation of context and becomes the primary work of the contemporary leader.

Context frames action. As a leader more clearly articulates the appropriate contextual framework for responding to shifts in the environment and necessary changes in the organization, this leader creates positive conditions for staff investment and engagement. Such efforts lay the groundwork for the actions of the professional staff as they begin to move into new, enhanced, transformative experiences associated with the content and quality of their work and the impact of their work on the individuals they serve. The dynamic changes, adjustments, shifts, and challenges to the current work of the professional staff should be anticipated by the leader, who uses his or her predictive and adaptive capacity to discern the impact of the changing context on the character and content of professional work. Based on this role and the perspective that it brings, this leader can prepare the staff for the demand for change, shifts in the environment, changes in the system that will ultimately impact their work, and calls for deeper investment in those changes.

All this requires assuming a certain level of risk. In taking on this burden, the clinical leader must demonstrate a personal willingness to confront the vagaries of change and work transformation. The leader, as part of this strategy, models the behaviors that must ultimately be exemplified by the professional staff in their practices. In the leader's effort to make it safe for staff to reach out and embrace risk, the leader makes engagement with risk the normative behavior and reassures the staff that their own willingness to take on risk will not result in punitive, negative, or constraining behaviors on the part of the organization (Malloch, 2010).

In dynamic organizations, there is a deeper understanding that it is neither possible nor appropriate to eliminate risk. However, because of the nature of health care and the fear of negative impact on patients, risk in this industry has been given a contextual framework that represents danger, fear, and limitations. Like all leadership capacities, risk is an essential constituent of human effort. While negative risk must undoubtedly be limited in terms of its impact on patients, the risks inherent in creating the conditions of safety, appropriateness, innovation, and creativity on behalf of patients in a way that advances their interests should not be limited or diminished (Hueth & Melkonyan, 2009). Indeed, if risk is fully eliminated, the life of the organization would end.

Risk is a sign of the continuous and dynamic reach of the human experience in new directions and in new ways. Exploring new territory, often without a compass, advances human experience and improves it in important ways. Risk cannot be eliminated, but it can be well managed (**Figure 14-5**).

The better the leader understands and manages the nature and incidence of risk, the better the professional staff in the organization will become in predicting

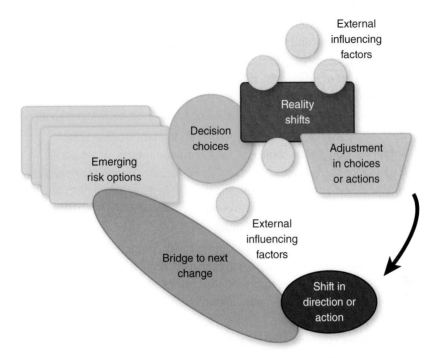

Figure 14-5 Cyclical engagement of risk and acting on it

risk, using its energy, and designing appropriate strategies for adapting it and making the necessary changes it demands. The good clinical leader is able to dissipate the potential for risk, decrease the degree of risk inherent in change, and predict the appropriate level of response with a high degree of accuracy. By creating a safe space for staff to deal with risk, the leader actually helps the staff develop a positive affiliation with the elements and character of risk and, in turn, grapple with its implications, maximize the potential for meaningful change, and adapt their own practice responses to its demands in a creative and role-enhancing way. For the leader, then, particular terms of engagement are essential for selecting the appropriate risk response and creating the conditions for managing risk well:

- Effective risk relates directly to current practice, and it must influence either positive work processes or clinical work outcomes to ensure that it is both legitimate and useful.
- All meaningful change encompasses some level of risk. This risk can often be found in the uncertainty embedded in change and in confrontations with past rituals and routines, often upsetting them and challenging their validity and continuance.

- Risk and error can often feel synonymous. Mistaking risk for error can create uncertainty and fear in the staff. Recalibrating error as a positive mechanism for learning, rather than as a negative cause for punitive action, is part of making the risk experience safer and more positive. This recalibration changes the context for risk and prevents the potential for error from becoming an excuse for failing to confront meaningful change.

- Risk calls leaders to live in the question and to push staff to raise appropriate questions about the work of the profession. The wise leader stops the trajectory of practice periodically to spend time with emergent and apparent risk, placing the risk in an appropriate change context and asking the staff to explore its potential in driving them to meaningful and appropriate changes.

- The leader works to manage risk appropriately, not to eliminate it. Risk can be anticipated and can be well managed. It is essential content that accompanies all change processes. Risk brings attention to the notable variables in the change dynamic that require thought, consideration, and careful response.

- Through her or his own relationship to risk, the leader demonstrates the value, contribution, and impact of risk on deliberation, action, and evaluation. The leader attempts to make risk a normative part of all intentional action and ensures that the team addresses the elements of risk as carefully as they address the components of the change process.

Accountability is always represented in the ownership of action, but not just any action. Action related to work reflects the professional's need to have a meaningful impact on or make a difference for the individuals the profession serves. Accountability always causes the professional to ask questions about meaning and impact, prompting the worker to think of personal action in light of its value and the effect it has on the service provided by the person and the profession. This tight fit between action and value is the clearest and strongest indicator of the presence of accountability embedded in the role of the professional. The effective leader consistently addresses issues of accountability and sets time aside with professional staff to help them reconnect with questions of meaning and value in their professional work. In this way, the leader keeps team members focused on purpose and value as the drivers of their work, ensuring that they do not become bogged down by the functions and activities of work.

Failure to adopt this focus and to be reminded of it on a regular basis may result in the loss of meaning reflected in the work of the professional. All too often, the vagaries and demands of day-to-day activity threaten to overwhelm issues of

CRITICAL THOUGHT

Ambiguity is the enemy of accountability. It is essential that performance expectations are clear and understandable at the outset, or performance will always be negatively affected. Some basic elements for role clarity are as follows:

- Precise language states the role in clear terms.
- Performance factors relate well to role tasks and functions.
- Terms of reference are precise and expressed as single items.
- Competence factors are clearly enumerated as the role's foundation.
- Factors included in the evaluation of the role are clearly stated.
- Individual performance is tied together with team performance.

meaning and value and cause individuals to be narrowly focused on the activities of the work rather than the purpose and the impact of that work. Such a perspective can lead to burnout—and it is the leader's obligation to prevent this potential from becoming reality. Burnout is often buried under the rituals and routines of daily activity and is evident in the failure to represent and access the meaning and value that drives the work and informs its content. In contrast, when the leader and the professional staff focus on value, they embrace accountability and acknowledge its centrality in driving the effectiveness of the work and its impact on the health of the community.

Accountability and Performance

Although accountability is not complicated, it is demanding. It requires of the clinical leader a deep commitment to its expression and an understanding of its meaning for the individual professional and for the profession as a whole. Accountability reminds the leader of the central component that differentiates professional work from other kinds of work. The sum of accountability of the individual and team is about making a difference and producing meaningful outcomes (**Figure 14-6**). Accountability serves as the cornerstone of the profession's commitment to the individuals and the communities they serve. It connects the social trust of the people for advancing health with the profession's responsibility to act as the agent of that trust.

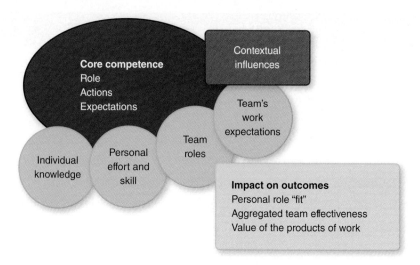

Figure 14-6 Factors impacting outcome

The central characteristics of accountability that are nonnegotiable for the profession represent the following principles:

- Accountability generally reflects the individual professional's commitment to performance and to action. It is this individual ownership of the profession's work that is necessary for action to be accountable.
- Personal accountability is the prerequisite to collective team effort and its ability to achieve and sustain desirable outcomes. Individual accountability and team action are one, and the effectiveness of the convergence of their effort is measured against the level of sustainable health for the individuals they serve.
- Accountability demands a dynamic convergence between ownership, action, impact, and outcome. The individual professional and the clinical team must link all of these factors to create sustainability in the service they collectively provide.
- Individual accountability cannot be sustained if the system structure does not allow it to be legitimately expressed by those who own it and if the infrastructure does not include a framework enabling partnership, equity, ownership, and accountability.
- The clinical team has a right to expect that each professional member will understand his or her unique contribution, make that contribution to the fullest extent of his or her competence, and demonstrate that the collective skills of the team members link and integrate well to advance effective group processes and meaningful clinical impact.

Clinical excellence requires the engagement, accountability, and ownership of all stakeholders in the collective in a common effort tailored to the needs and demands of those they serve. Increasingly, nurse leaders are being asked to play a role in creating the conditions and circumstances that lead to the establishment of broader-based interdisciplinary teams around patient populations and the continuum of care. Nurses will certainly be expected to coordinate, integrate, and facilitate these interdisciplinary clinical teams in a way that assures their effective linkage around the needs and demands of particular episodes of care, patient populations, or care continua. The ability of the nurse leader to more cogently define the nursing contribution to these multifocal, multidisciplinary teams will be critical to those teams' success. As the primary care foundations become more sustainable and act as drivers for earlier-stage engagement in healthcare interventions, the role of the nurse will continually expand and deepen. This evolution will require a more deeply understood and critically expressed clarity regarding the nurse's contribution to the team's functioning. In turn, the nurse leader's capacity for professional articulation will be a foundational skill and an obligation of the future expression of the role.

Excellence cannot be attained or sustained by any profession without significant clarity regarding accountability and the contributions that clarity makes to the work of each discipline that makes up the collective work of the clinical team. Excellence is a demonstration of accountability in action. This level of performance is impossible to sustain without a clear understanding of accountability and what its full realization entails. Ultimately, accountability is the centerpiece of professional action and must be evidenced in the life and activity of every professional provider. Accountability demonstrates that professionals have coalesced their efforts in the clinical team in a way that results in a positive impact on the health of the individuals they serve.

SCENARIO

Susan Brown, RN, BSN, is a medical-surgical team leader and Practice Council chair on her unit. Susan has become increasingly aware of the disparity between the shifting and broadening role expectations for nurses and the limitations on the scope and practice of nursing driven by the current components of the job description. Indeed, Susan and many of her colleagues on the unit have discussed how inadequately the job descriptions are in addressing the critical elements of the professional role of the nurse.

(continues)

(continued)

Their general perception is that the job descriptions are limited, functional, prescriptive, and unclear in regard to accountability and outcomes.

The Practice Council has been discussing for some time how it might approach better defining and articulating the professional role of the nurse. The Council members want to move away from the prescriptive, functional task items enumerated in the job description in favor of a sort of "charter of accountability" for nurses. While this charter is as yet unfocused in terms of structure and design, the Practice Council perceives that it should focus predominantly on the role of the nurse with regard to impact, outcome, and making a difference in the life of the patient. Discussion has centered on the notion that accountability focuses on the products of work rather than the processes of work; that is, it focuses on the difference the nurse makes rather than the actions the nurse takes.

The Practice Council is now ready to formalize these efforts and begin the process of moving away from job descriptions as the definitive document for outlining and articulating nurses' roles. The Council has settled on the notion of "charter of accountability" as a means for characterizing the professional role of the nurse. Its members are unsure of their next steps but are looking forward to undertaking a new plan of action.

Discussion Points

With your learning colleagues, assume the role of the Practice Council at the point of decision making in this scenario. Consider the next steps to change from job descriptions to a new way of defining accountability for practice of the professional nurse. Consider some of the material learned in other chapters and apply it to this scenario. Explore issues related to role expectations, performance, patient outcomes, evidence-based practice, and accountability for outcomes. Lay out a "map" that outlines the trajectory that the Practice Council needs to take to conceive, design, and implement this new foundation for defining nursing practice accountability. If you are part of a large learning team, break into small learning groups and assume responsibility for a particular component of the redesign of these foundations for nursing practice. Share the products of your work with one another and create linkages between each of the elements of the work to bring together a picture of the whole project representing a vision of how nursing accountability might be defined differently.

SCENARIO

The nursing staff Practice Council on the surgical unit has been struggling with issues around variance in nursing practice in relation to principles and practice of surgery-site infection control. They have noticed that their postsurgical incisional infection rates are increasing, but they have not been able to identify the cause. They did note, however, that there was wide variance across the unit in individual nursing practice in managing surgical wounds and suture sites.

Sharon Mentor, RN, BSN, chair of the Practice Council, has recognized that this wide variation in clinical practice on the unit is an unacceptable foundation upon which to evaluate the challenges associated with the rising infection rates. She realizes that the Practice Council needs to develop clarity on standardized clinical practice related to infection control if the nursing staff is to make any progress in understanding the current challenges and directly addressing the problem. Sharon has already made this a priority for decision making for the next Practice Council meeting. She has just finished gathering clinical data and evidence on some of the issues related to practice consistencies in nursing management of incisional care and dressing change. Her desire is to challenge the Practice Council to develop an algorithm for this practice and to evaluate current nursing practices against the standard suggested by the Practice Council.

Discussion Questions

1. Based on principles of evidence-based practice, what should be the foundation for creating a measurement instrument to evaluate current nursing practices related to incisional care and dressing change on the unit?

2. In your learning team, how would you differentiate between the critical short-term objectives of addressing immediate challenges to infection control and the long-term obligation for developing a standard of practice that can serve as a protocol for infection control on the unit?

(continues)

(continued)

3. As nursing practice for incisional care and dressing changes appears to vary widely within this surgical unit, which type of learning and developmental plan to help change individual practices would be consistent with the standard the Practice Council develops for these procedures?

4. Work with your team to construct an algorithm grounded in infection control principles that can be applied to incisional care and dressing changes as identified as a concern for this unit.

5. Present your model algorithm to faculty or practicing nursing professionals for evaluation and feedback with regard to the viability, thoroughness, and applicability of this algorithm for addressing the infection control issue.

CHAPTER TEST QUESTIONS

Licensure exam categories: Management of care: ethical practice, professionalism, concepts of management

Nurse leader exam categories: Professionalism: personal and professional accountability, ethics, advocacy

1. How is the professional nurse accountable for designing clinical processes that demonstrate individual competence and a deep understanding of the work?

2. What is the professional nurse's Accountability in the delegation process?

3. Individual ownership implies a commitment to engage with others in their learning and development and in mentoring and sharing in the learning process. True or false?

4. One of the unique characteristics of a professional is the recognition of the intensity of the fit between the person as an individual and the person as a professional. True or false?

5. Onboarding interviews are not nearly as important as exit interviews because the staff and leadership get more accurate information from exit interviews about the work environment and staff members' level of satisfaction with their work experience. True or false?

6. Individual accountability cannot be sustained if the system structure allows it to be legitimately expressed only by those who own it. True or false?

7. How is the professional nurse accountable for designing clinical processes that demonstrate individual competence and a deep understanding of the work?

8. What are the elements of a profession? In the profession of nursing, which elements have room for continued growth?

9. What is the role of the nurse leader on a team?

10. What is the role of the leader in evidence-based shared leadership?

References

Bonvillain, N. (2007). *Women and men: Cultural constructs of gender.* Upper Saddle River, NJ: Pearson Prentice Hall.

Bowles, C., & Candela, L. (2005). First job experiences of recent RN graduates: Improving the work environment. *Journal of Nursing Administration, 35*(3), 130–137.

Buhler-Wilkerson, K. (2001). *No place like home: A history of nursing and home care in the United States.* Baltimore, MD: Johns Hopkins University Press.

Cope, Z. (1958). *Florence Nightingale and the doctors.* Philadelphia, PA: Lippincott.

Cowen, P. S., & Moorhead, S. (2011). *Current issues in nursing.* St. Louis, MO: Mosby Elsevier.

D'Antonio, P. (2010). *American nursing: A history of knowledge, authority, and the meaning of work.* Baltimore, MD: Johns Hopkins University Press.

Dossey, B. M. (2005). *Florence Nightingale today: Healing, leadership, global action.* Silver Spring, MD: American Nurses Association.

Fitzpatrick, J. J., & Whall, A. L. (2005). *Conceptual models of nursing: Analysis and application.* Upper Saddle River, NJ: Pearson Prentice Hall.

Gebbie, K. M., Rosenstock, L., & Hernandez, L. M. (Eds.). (2003). *Who will keep the public healthy? Educating public health professionals for the 21st century.* Washington, DC: National Academies Press.

Goodnow, M. (1938). *Nursing history in brief.* Philadelphia, PA/London, UK: Saunders.

Group, T., & Roberts, J. (2001). *Nursing, physician control, and the medical monopoly: Historical perspectives on gendered inequality in roles, rights, and range of practice.* Bloomington, IN: Indiana University Press.

Hein, E. C. (2001). *Nursing issues in the 21st century: Perspectives from the literature.* Philadelphia, PA: Lippincott.

Hueth, B., & Melkonyan, T. (2009). Standards and the regulation of environmental risk. *Journal of Regulatory Economics, 36*(3), 219.

Jameson, J. (2009). Nursing policy research: Turning evidence-based research and health policy. *Choice, 46*(10), 1973–1974.

Kahn, L. (2014). New evidence on gender and the labor market: A symposium. *Industrial & Labor Relations Review, 67*(2), 283–286.

Kleinpell, R. M. (2009). *Outcome assessment in advanced practice nursing.* New York, NY: Springer.

Lagemann, E. C., & Rockefeller Archive Center. (1983). *Nursing history: New perspectives, new possibilities.* New York, NY: Teachers College Press.

Malloch, K. (2010). Creating the organizational context for innovation. In T. Porter-O'Grady & K. Malloch (Eds.), *Innovation leadership: Creating the land-scape of health care* (pp. 33–56). Sudbury, MA: Jones and Bartlett Publishers.

Malloch, K., & Porter-O'Grady, T. (2009a). *Introduction to evidence-based practice in nursing and health care.* Sudbury, MA: Jones and Bartlett Publishers.

Malloch, K., & Porter-O'Grady, T. (2009b). *The quantum leader: Applications for the new world of work.* Sudbury, MA: Jones and Bartlett Publishers.

Mason, D., & Leavitt, J. (2011). *Policy and politics in nursing and health care.* Philadelphia, PA: Saunders.

McDonald, L. (2010). *Florence Nightingale at first hand.* Waterloo, Ontario: Wilfred Laurier University Press.

Moanojovich, M. (2005). Nurse–physician communication: An organizational accountability. *Journal of Nursing Scholarship, 23*(2), 72–78.

Nicholson, S., & Fisher, V. (2014). *Integral voices on sex, gender, and sexuality: Critical inquiries.* Albany, NY: State University of New York Press.

Oliver, R. W. (2004). *What is transparency?* New York, NY: McGraw-Hill.

Patton, R., Zalon, M., & Ludwick, R. (Eds.). (2015). *Nurses making policy from bedside to board room.* New York, NY: Springer.

Pollard, E. F. (1911). *Florence Nightingale, the wounded soldier's friend.* London, UK: Partridge.

Porter-O'Grady, T. (2004). Accountability and action. *Health Progress, 85*(1), 44–48.

Porter-O'Grady, T., & Malloch, K. (Eds.). (2010). *Innovation leadership.* Sudbury, MA: Jones and Bartlett Publishers.

Simon, R., & Canacari, E. (2012). A practical guide to applying lean tools and management principles to healthcare improvement projects. *AORN Journal, 95*(1), 85–103.

Stacey, M. (2009). *Teamwork and collaboration in early years settings.* Setauket, NY: Exeter.

Tilley, D. (2008). Competency in nursing: A concept analysis. *Journal of Continuing Education in Nursing, 39*(2), 58–65.

Ulrich, B. (2014). The responsibility and accountability of being a registered nurse. *Nephrology Nursing Journal, 41*(3), 241–254.

Werhane, P. H. (2007). *Women in business: The changing face of leadership.* Westport, CT: Praeger.

Zedeck, S., & American Psychological Association. (2011). *APA handbook of industrial and organizational psychology.* Washington, DC: American Psychological Association.

Appendix A

Individual Role Accountability and Team Performance

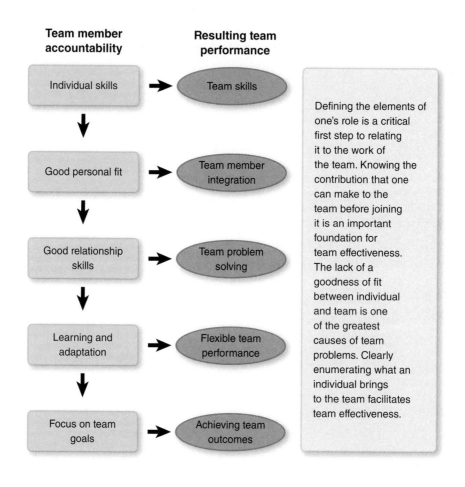

Team member accountability

Resulting team performance

Individual skills	Team skills
Good personal fit	Team member integration
Good relationship skills	Team problem solving
Learning and adaptation	Flexible team performance
Focus on team goals	Achieving team outcomes

Defining the elements of one's role is a critical first step to relating it to the work of the team. Knowing the contribution that one can make to the team before joining it is an important foundation for team effectiveness. The lack of a goodness of fit between individual and team is one of the greatest causes of team problems. Clearly enumerating what an individual brings to the team facilitates team effectiveness.

Appendix B

Fitting Individual and Team Goals Together

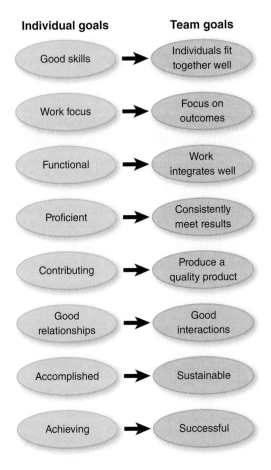

Individual goals → **Team goals**

Individual goals	Team goals
Good skills	Individuals fit together well
Work focus	Focus on outcomes
Functional	Work integrates well
Proficient	Consistently meet results
Contributing	Produce a quality product
Good relationships	Good interactions
Accomplished	Sustainable
Achieving	Successful

Appendix C

Creating a Culture of Accountability

- Bring people on board with the clear understanding of their roles and contributions as members of the team.
- Make sure everyone knows that participation is not optional and that every member of the work community must contribute.

- Include participation and ownership behaviors in the performance assessment process; review performance at least quarterly.
- Identify skill levels and developmental needs, and make sure they are addressed as a part of the individual's growth plan.
- Advise all members that accountability is about the achievement of outcomes, not just good work performance.
- Identify and resolve interpersonal conflicts early; the later they are engaged, the less likely they can be resolved satisfactorily.

Appendix D

Revisiting Invitation and Expectation

In a performance-driven organization, it should be clear to all participants that contribution, commitment, performance, and participation are expected. Team members should feel that they must be invited into ownership and participation in decisions and actions that represent the obligations of the team. Invitation indicates that accountability is optional. In effective team configurations, this is simply untrue. Membership implies ownership and accountability, and each team member must represent that in his or her role.

Invitation	Expectation
External orientation	Internal orientation
Passive engagement	Active engagement
Other-directed	Self-directed
Functionally driven	Purpose driven
Process oriented	Outcome oriented
Job mental model	Role mental model
Task fixed	Relationship based
Event based	Journey based
No ownership	Full ownership
Past active	Proactive

Appendix E

Responsibility Versus Accountability

Responsibility (20th century)	Accountability (21st century)
Process	Product
Action	Result
Work	Outcome
Do	Accomplish
Task	Difference
Function	Fit
Job	Role
Incremental	Sustainable
Externally generated	Internally generated
Quality effort	Quality impact

The terms *accountability* and *responsibility* are frequently used interchangeably. However, these terms and the dynamics to which they relate mean entirely different things. Perhaps the most important distinction between responsibility and accountability relates to their orientation. Responsibility focuses on the work, the competence of the worker, the effectiveness of the processes, the quality of the effort, and the excellence of its application.

Accountability, in contrast, focuses on the products of work rather than the processes of work. Accountability relates to issues regarding the impact of the work, the products or results of work, a difference the work makes, and whether the work mattered in relation to performance and expectations. Quite simply, accountability focuses on issues of outcome and calls attention to the effects of the work rather than the processes related to the work itself. Today, questions of accountability have become increasingly important as the relationships among work effectiveness, outcome, and work process become important.

Appendix F

Accountability and Impact

- Accountability always asks what difference the work effort makes.
- Accountability focuses the effort of the worker on the products of work rather than the processes of work.

- In accountability, the discipline is focused on creating a goodness of fit between work effort and results.
- Accountability suggests that evaluation and comparison occur between work and the products of work.
- Accountability implies that quality improvement focuses on work as a reflection of the value of its products/result.
- Accountability seeks to identify which specific elements of work make the key difference in its results.
- Accountability requires an internal generation or motive for excellence, not merely an external demand.

Appendix G

Role Clarity and Accountability Model

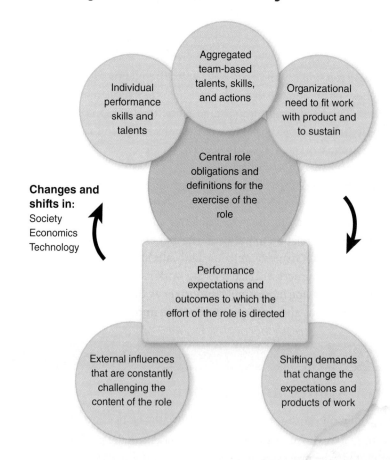

Appendix H

Accountability and Locus of Control

Accountability reflects the individual ownership of the decisions that attend to a particular role. A role holds decisional authority not so much because that authority is assigned to it but more because it is seen as legitimate to the role owing to the role's opportunity and obligation to directly affect outcome. The necessity to act in a certain way to affect a related, defined outcome is the authority basis for determining location and making decisions related to a particular work effort. A role is empowered to make specific decisions because of its direct relationship to the specific decisions and actions that result in the fulfillment of the purpose or products of the work. An accountability-driven organization has an infrastructure that supports and recognizes this approach to accountability and performance.

Role:
- Location
- Accountability
- Performance
- Competence

Accountable decisions flow from individual roles through the actions necessary to directly achieve outcomes and sustain an effective work–outcomes relationship.

Decisions:
Authority
Autonomy
Competence
Applicable

Actions:
Applied
Appropriate
Implemented
Good process

Outcomes:
Evaluated
Good fit
Effective
Sustainable

Accountability reflects the location of power in the hands of those who ultimately undertake the actions that produce results. Ownership of accountability is necessary to the achievement of sustainable outcomes. Without this dynamic interaction, all work is, at best, incremental and short term.

Appendix I

Ownership: The Center of Accountability

The central theme of accountability is the ownership of work. There is much controversy and disagreement about the locus of control for decisions and actions related to the work of organizations. In a private enterprise system, it is often assumed that the owner of the enterprise owns the means and processes associated with the organization. In truth, this is an incomplete view of the work relationship. Although the organization owns the products of work and influences the processes of work, unless a real partnership exists between those who do the work and those who own the means and products of work, there will be no sustainable, consistent, and accelerating outcome.

The challenge here is to incorporate the understanding that workers also have an ownership capacity. Because outcomes are generated from the efforts of the worker as well as the resources of the owner, a fundamental partnership exists between them. When this partnership is well described and shared, the processes and products of work have the potential to be continually effective and sustainable.

The wise leader understands this fundamental relationship and does everything to clarify its elements and to better describe the contribution that both people and resources make to the achievement and sustainability of the organization. This leader continually balances needs of workers with demands of the organization in a mosaic or dance of effort that ensures the energies of the worker (human capital) and the resources (financial capital) of the organization continue to contribute to success.

Balancing Ownership and Resources

Ownership of work	Resources
Internally generated	Externally generated
Skill based	Adequate
Continual improvement	Relate to need
Conscious contribution	Cost–benefit value
Full engagement	Shared with workers
Good processes	Gain shared
Effect on outcomes	Return on investment

Appendix J
Volume Versus Value

Many times, the professional worker will indicate that the amount of work done should be evidence of the importance of that work. Of course, nothing could be further from the truth. The amount of work one does has nothing to do with its meaning or value. Value is found in the effect of the work, or with its outcome. The inputs of work relate directly to the outcome and should advance or increase the value of the outcome at a faster rate than the cost associated with the input. There is no positive value if this exchange of the relationship between input and outcome is negative. Increasing one's work does not increase value; it just increases the effort.

Value is better represented when there is an expenditure of just the right amount of effort to maximize the products or outcomes of the work, and not an ounce more. In most effective workplaces, this relationship is important enough to be constantly defined and measured as a way of obtaining as much value as can be derived from the work effort.

Volume and Value Indicators

Volume of work	Value of work
Task focused	Results focused
Functional	Action based
Process oriented	Outcome oriented
Focus on the work	Effect of the work
Task completion	Achieving expectations
Many processes	Goodness of fit of effort
Worker centered	Making a difference
Immediate	Sustainable
Short term	Renewable

Appendix K

Some Risk-Dealing Rules of Engagement

- Risk must relate directly to the work being undertaken and have an influence either on positive work processes or work outcomes to be legitimate and useful.
- Risk usually accompanies all change and can be found in the noise or uncertainty of a change from past rituals and routines, upsetting them in ways that challenge their continuance.
- Risk often first appears as error, creating uncertainty or fear. Error is simply a form of risk that needs to be placed in context rather than become an excuse for not confronting change.
- Risk calls leaders and staff to question. It is wise to stop and spend time with the apparent risk, placing it in appropriate context and exploring what it is pointing out to all.
- Leaders cannot eliminate risk; risk can only be anticipated and managed. Risk accompanies all change processes and demands attention to the variables that affect the implementation of change.
- The leader creates the attitude that determines how staff will respond to risk. The more normative the leader can make the presence and experience of risk, the better staff will deal with it.

Appendix L

Path of Professionalism Engagement Through Your Career

Stage	Professionalism
Novice	• Engage in discussion about standards of care and best practices at the unit level. • Join a unit-level team in your organization. • Join professional organizations and network with peers within and beyond your organization. ▪ American Nurses Association ▪ Practice-specific nursing organizations

Advanced Beginner	• Initiate discussion about standards of care and best practices at the unit level. • Become an active member of a unit-level team in organization, participating on a project. • Engage resources and opportunities for continuing professional development at your organization or within your specialty.
Competent	• Enact change about standards of care and best practices at the organizational level. • Seek membership on an interdisciplinary or nursing department team in your organization. • Consider certification in a nursing specialty. • Become an active member of a professional organization at the local or state level. • Engage resources and opportunities for continuing professional development at your organization or within your specialty.
Proficient	• Engage in discussion about standards of care and best practices at the state or national level. • Seek a leadership position on a professional team in your organization. • Seek a leadership position at a professional organization at the local or state level. • Engage resources and opportunities for continuing professional development at your organization or within your specialty.
Expert	• Enact change in standards of care and best practices at the state or national level. • Engage resources and opportunities for continuing professional development at your organization or within your specialty. • Seek a leadership position. • Mentor others in their professional journey.

Data from Benner, P. (1984). *From novice to expert: Excellence and power in clinical practice.* Menlo Park, CA: Addison-Wesley.

Critical Thought, Leader Tip, and Scenario icons made by Freepik from www.flaticon.com; Callout icon made by Yannick from www.flaticon.com; Team Tip icon made by Chanut is Industries from www.flaticon.com

> What could be worse than being blind? That would be seeing and having no vision. —Helen Keller

CHAPTER OBJECTIVES

Upon completion of this chapter, the reader will be able to do the following:

» Understand the requirements of linking and integrating leader learning in a way that can be effectively applied.

» Define the basic elements of leadership and translate them into situations and scenarios that require leadership application.

» Enumerate the components of a leadership challenge or problem and the steps and processes associated with its resolution.

» Outline the approaches to issue identification and selection of appropriate strategies to reflect on the issue and to construct mechanisms for its resolution.

» List at least five major components of each chapter's leadership focus and explain the impact that focus has on the role of clinical leadership.

» State personal leadership growth and developmental needs that define the individual journey and trajectory of leadership and create a guide for personal leadership development.

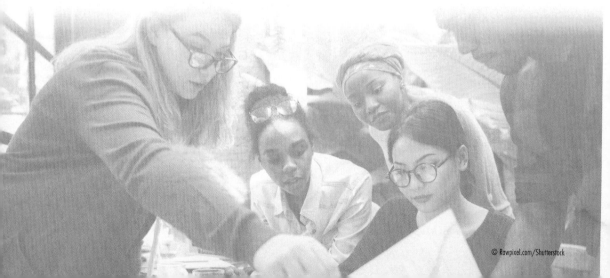

Integrating Learning: Applying the Practices of Leadership

This chapter serves as a comprehensive summary of the work of this text and as a tool for synthesizing the foundational leadership concepts that will inform the reader's leadership practices. The ability to use tools to express leadership capacity and to apply principles is the best indicator of leadership success. Keep in mind that this work is directed to the emerging clinical leader who does not intend to become a manager but who still needs the insights and tools necessary to express real leadership in the clinical environment. Fewer than 1% of all graduates with bachelor of science degrees in nursing will become managers, but most will aspire to excellence in practice and clinical leadership. How well the clinical leader achieves this goal is completely dependent on his or her ability to synthesize the capacities of leadership and apply them successfully to the practice problems and human relationships that serve as the foundation of clinical practice. Be sure to review the other chapters for key concepts and behaviors that can and should be integrated into your discussions and creation of new and better solutions for health care.

CRITICAL THOUGHT

The leader always stays in the question. The leader constantly recognizes that he or she does not own other people's problems and that the leader's role is to help others own their problems and develop the skills for resolving them.

In the Era of Health Transformation

Perhaps one of the most important roles of the leader is evidenced in the capacity to anticipate and predict future expectations and translate them for those persons whom he or she leads (Maxwell, 2010). Nothing is more important than helping the staff to anticipate change and translating that change into a language that colleagues can understand and, more importantly, actively engage in. These insights about the direction of the work journey are critical because they encompass people's hopes and desires to improve or make things better, and they demonstrate a capacity to make a difference that can be sustained over time.

At the same time, it is important for the leader to exemplify for the staff the ability to own the changes that lead to the realization of these opportunities in ways that will enhance both the work experience and the patient experience. Life is not static: If it is not positively pressed forward, it inevitably falls backward, diminishing opportunities and growth in ways that create conditions ripe for decline and contraction of the organization.

The leader essentially provides a beacon on the pathway to the future that illuminates the path itself and enlightens fellow travelers as to what they will find and what it will require of them to continue their own personal journey.

The Context of Healthcare Policy

There are a host of reasons why every nurse needs to be aware of the implications of healthcare policy. The demand for changes in our system has been long in coming (Phillips & Bazemore, 2010), and it requires leaders to be fully engaged in identifying and translating the particular changes embedded in the activities of reform to staff colleagues, regardless of their practice arenas. To be sure, we are in the midst of an unprecedented level of complex change that requires us to think differently and adopt a complex perspective. The good news is that this complexity is nothing new. The Affordable Care Act was seen as adding complexity; efforts to repeal and replace were as well. The constant for the leader is that healthcare policy will continue to shift the environment of the industry, and we must attempt to advocate, anticipate, and evolve our work and our profession to

REFLECTIVE QUESTION

Work cannot provide meaning; instead, it demonstrates how meaning is present. How, then, does the leader help others discern the meaning that drives their work so they do not lose touch with it? Remember, motivation is intrinsic not extrinsic.

maintain our high professional ethics and standards. The scenarios presented in this text are intended to challenge your thinking and sometimes even stump you until you can gather additional resources to assist you in your decision making—always knowing that it is who is at your table and how well you can work together that truly matters. We encourage you to enjoy this journey.

The most significant reality shift for providers is the radical move from a volume service framework to a value-driven model of both delivering and paying for healthcare service. Even today, years after the ACA became law, organizations struggle to find their way in value-based care. Some beacons have shown that a focus on outcomes and values is also good for business. For example, Kaiser Permanente, a large integrated health plan and provider system, has grown exponentially by focusing on affordability, access, and quality care.

For years, nurses have been objecting to the heavy dependence on the volume rubrics that are embedded in tasks, functions, procedures, and protocols, yet there is a lack of any real alignment with the values or outcomes to which they are intended or relate. In the emerging healthcare system, value drivers almost exclusively emerge as the sole frame of reference for health care. Unless the practice language changes to match the values perspective, our very practices will become the impediment to moving and engaging the systems and structures that could compete with them; in turn, we may be tempted to create fixes or superficial remedies that are inherently inadequate and not amenable to improving our practice.

The full script for American health care has being completely recalibrated and will continue to adjust as systems, organizations, leaders, and the population grapple with the changes. Even the most casual observer of the healthcare crisis can see that our traditional approach to service is unsustainable; even if a new

CRITICAL THOUGHT

What if nurses were paid for the impact they made, not the hours they worked? How would you quantify and qualify the impact of nursing on a given patient?

political administration does not like the prevailing place for changing health care, he or she will have to begin at point zero to transform a system that does not serve the country well. Eliminating the present does not return us to the past. Instead, it creates a new demand for making the system work effectively to fulfill the mandates to which it is directed.

A good leader recognizes the need for good policy and relevant direction (Hazy, Goldstein, & Lichtenstein, 2007). There must always be a good fit between the work of a system and its purpose. Indeed, when purpose is sacrificed on the altar of work, the work loses direction quickly and becomes devoid of the meaning that should be guiding it. The leader will constantly be bombarded with people who are addicted to the energy of activity—that is, who pursue activity just for the sake of activity—and will be unable to alter their vision or change their practice. Ritual and routine tend to inure people from both ownership and value, such that they descend into the morass of functionalism. Tasks and functions (job orientation) become their reason for being and subsume all their energy and creativity. We should not diminish the value of effort and work, but the leader does need to keep in mind that many who have entered into the ritual of work have surrendered their attachment to good judgment, critical reflection, and a search for real value. The leader must recognize these characteristics when he or she sees them and be prepared to identify and address them in ways that create sufficient change to make these traditional sanctuaries from accountability both untenable and unacceptable.

Several drivers in healthcare policy are changing the landscape of health care and require the leader to reconfigure both work and roles in the health system:

- Value drivers mean that impacts and outcomes are more important to good and sustainable healthcare service than are good processes and tasks. Process and task focus on the work; value focuses on outcome and impact. For the leader, much of the theory in this script addresses the challenge of helping colleagues deconstruct function and work as well as replace it with an understanding of what making a difference looks like and what it will take to get there.

- User-driven healthcare service means that the patient is the driver and that providers are respondents to that equation. In essence, providers must surrender ownership of health decisions to users; they must help users become competent in making the decisions they now own and guide them in making effective healthcare choices.

- Digital technology is now the predominant means of communicating and interacting with patients. It is no longer optional for a provider to claim technological incompetence in the course of her or his practice. It is simply impossible to practice and to prepare for the future of practice without sufficient technological competence to drive the digital clinical journey.

- In professional practice, collective wisdom is infinitely more valuable than unilateral action. If any practitioner sacrifices the products of collective wisdom on the altar of individuated practice, he or she is simply proclaiming to peers and patients that the practitioner's personal judgment about standards of practice and the protocols that express them is more valid and appropriate than those established through the collective mind of the profession as a whole.

- Anything effective in healthcare policy will be constructed and will be the product of the work that addresses an inadequacy or limitation in practice. Practice relevance will reflect the goodness of fit between what is considered normative behavior and what lies at the periphery of human behavior. Indeed, it may serve as a catalyst for changing the health priorities when a lack of goodness of fit becomes glaringly apparent.

- Any successful healthcare policy must address affordability, access to care, quality, and the patient experience. Not addressing one of these aims will leave the system vulnerable to failure and fragmentation.

Healthcare policy change, it should be apparent, serves as a stimulus for re-thinking and reconfiguring health care in a way that reflects real value for achieving objective measures of health and advancing the level of health of whole categories of health resource users (Berwick, Nolan, & Whittington, 2008).

The Management of Conflict

Principles of conflict management are essential to navigating the landscape of transformation and change, if only for confronting the divergent views among stakeholders that have a genuine and positive commitment to advancing health care. These differences must be managed in a way that moves individuals and groups toward consensus and agreement that will inform and guide subsequent action. As indicated in this text, conflict is a normative dynamic, and one that serves as a centerpiece in the leadership armamentarium. At every corner of the system and in almost every work process, the leader confronts differences that must be addressed and conflicting notions and processes that must be resolved. Applying the principles of good conflict management will be an essential skill set that will often make the difference between positive movement and stagnating immobility.

A few principles of sound conflict management to keep in mind are as follows:

- A good conflict management process identifies conflict in its earliest stages. The sooner conflicts can be addressed, the easier they will be to resolve. Conflicts ignored or left unattended too long can become intransigent and waste untold resources in their negative effect and in the work required to mitigate them.

- Conflict resolution is a dynamic process that has methods and techniques attached to it that must be addressed and utilized in a systematic and progressive manner. Through many years of application and research, the critical stages of conflict resolution and the activities associated with its success have been developed. Faithfulness to this process and consistency with its application will promote positive results and help the mediator ensure successful resolution.

- Human behavior can vary widely and sometimes be unpredictable, especially under conditions of duress or stress. The conflict leader must always be prepared for the potential of behavioral extremes and emotional drama in the mediation of conflicts. Emotion is a legitimate component of real problems; when ignored, it can have a devastating effect on progress and resolution. The mediator must develop both comfort and skill with addressing emotional expression as a part of the resolution process so that the positive work of mediation can bear the fruit of resolution.

- Resolution means the achievement of a mutual solution that meets the needs of all the parties to a conflict. It is no accident that the mediator role is often referred to as "neutral." The mediator has no agenda other than meeting the participants' needs and discovering a mutually derived solution. As soon as the mediator takes a position, he or she becomes a part of the conflict, in which case the effectiveness of this role dissipates and the conflict never really gets resolved.

- Conflict resolution and mediation are learned and developed skills that evolve with practice and application. A good mediator deals honestly with his or her own uncertainty and difficulty with conflict, working to resolve whatever personal barriers might exist in effectively handling other people's conflicts. Good mentorship and practice can improve the comfort and skills of the mediator in ways that ensure a meaningful and valuable experience for those experiencing conflict and who are working to resolve issues that keep them from mutually meeting their own needs and the needs of the patient.

A facility that embraces conflict demonstrates the strength and character of good leadership (Boulle, Colatrella, & Picchioni, 2008). In no other area of leadership are the skills of problem solving so critical. The vast majority of organizational problems are relational or interactional in nature. A leader who is able to confidently confront these issues with a high level of skill is an asset to people and organizations beyond ordinary value. Furthermore, the effectiveness in managing conflict translates into so many other leadership skills that its utility is invaluable. Remember: Conflict is a lucrative source of innovation.

The Centrality of Accountability

Perhaps there is no greater challenge to professional performance and impact than the personal expression of accountability. Accountability is the cornerstone of professional expression (Tilley, 2008). Some scholars suggest that it is the essential foundation of professional practice, such that one cannot be a professional without it. There is little doubt that accountability is the best indicator of whether professional behaviors are at work in the clinical environment.

Accountability is not as amorphous and ambiguous a notion as many are led to believe. In fact, accountability is a very precise notion with particular characteristics that mark it as a unique expression of human action (Connors, Smith, & Hickman, 2004). Three essential characteristics dictate the content of accountability and are essential to its definition—autonomy, authority, and competence.

Autonomy comprises the right to make decisions and take action. A person cannot be accountable for something over which he or she has no right to decide and to act. Having a right to decide and to act is critical to accountability: No matter where a decision might be made, if accountability does not exist in that place, the right to decide and to act does not exist either, and any decisions and actions that occur there cannot be fully realized and the outcome cannot be sustainably achieved.

Authority as related to accountability addresses the assurance that the necessary power to decide and to act is located in the place where the right (autonomy) to decide and to act is located. Accountability has no value if it has no power. Not only does it need expressive power, but that power must also be expressed by those who have the right to decide. In short, power must be located in the same place as the right to exercise it.

CRITICAL THOUGHT

There is no accountability if there is no autonomy to decide and to act, if there is no power to act, or if there is no competence to knowledgably exercise accountability.

CRITICAL THOUGHT

The further away a decision is made from the place it is exercised, the higher the cost, the greater the risk, and the lower the sustainability of the outcome related to it.

The third component in the definition of accountability is *competence* to decide and to act. While anyone can be given both the autonomy and the authority to act, there is no guarantee that an individual will do so competently. This notion of competent decision making and implementation of decisions is a critical component of successful decisions and actions. Having the capacity to make good decisions and to set the table where those decisions can be planned and acted upon is foundational to the action of accountability.

Some other elements of accountability are also essential to its exercise:

- Accountability cannot be delegated. It is internally generated and embedded in the professional role. While responsibility for tasks and functions can be delegated, the accountability for their fulfillment and the impact they create is held by the professional who is accountable for the results.

- Accountability is invested in individuals, not groups. It is a personal expression and attends to the action of the person, and it is in individuals that accountability is expressed and in those same individuals that its obligations are embedded.

- Accountability is about the products of work, not the processes of work. Accountability is demonstrated in what is achieved, not what is done. The action of work and how well it is accomplished demonstrate the fulfillment of responsibility. The impact of work and the difference it makes serve as the expression and evidence of accountability.

- Accountability implies change. Its positive impact suggests that a positive and desirable change has resulted and that the fulfillment of the goal to make change has been satisfied. There is no accountability if a change has not occurred, because a positive change is the only demonstration of the action of accountability.

- There is no accountability without consequence. Specifically, two consequences imply the action of accountability: negative and positive. Accountable professionals are continuously asking the questions of accountability. What happens with the expression of accountability and what difference is made? What happens if the accountability is not achieved?

Accountability is the cornerstone of professional action. It is the essential core of the expression of the role of the professional and is demonstrated by its positive performance and the achievement of desired outcomes. Without accountability, there is no promise to perform on the part of the profession and no commitment to advance the trust and interests of those served. It is essentially a part of the role of each professional and provides the best evidence of the value professionals have and the difference they make.

Structure, Organizations, and Professionals: Creating the Context for Practice

Professional practice is as strongly supported by sound organizational structure as it is by standards of excellence. A poor organization and supporting infrastructure for practice can create a negative framework for the practitioner and ultimately diminish the kind and quality of care he or she provides.

Professional knowledge workers need a very specific organizational context to facilitate good practice and positive outcomes (Porter-O'Grady, 2009). To date, organizational structure and professional practice models have not been extensively addressed in terms of the influence they have on creating a professional practice environment. The question as to whether nursing is a profession is best answered by the organizations that demonstrate their commitment to professional practice by providing a different way of doing business that best represents what both professional practice and professionals need.

Knowledge workers are intrinsically motivated. For them, their work is more than simply a job. Professional knowledge workers are generally licensed by the state and, therefore, are its agents in the performance of work that reflects a competency base and a particular kind of academic preparation. Society then entrusts these specially designated individuals with requisites for managing essential life processes in a way that acts in the best interests of society. Registered nurses are considered one of these groups.

REFLECTIVE QUESTION

What distinguishes knowledge workers from other employee work groups— that is, what requires the relationship between them and the organization to be structured differently? How does professional governance create the structure for framing this relationship between professionals and the system?

Being a professional does not guarantee that individuals will behave that way. Without an expressed code of ethics and standards of membership and performance, there would be no indicators related to the unique trust society has for these individuals. These codes of conduct and performance standards outline the particular expectations established for the professional. Members of a profession express mutual accountability for their membership and demonstrate that quality by adhering to the theory that underlies their discipline.

Professionals also govern themselves differently from other work groups. Professionals have a level of self-direction and shared governance that obligates them to manage the work of the profession, the relationships of professionals with one another, and their interactions with the people whom they serve (Styer, 2007). Because of the unique character of professional work and the charter bestowed upon professionals by society, they generally create a structure that affirms their unique obligation and empowers them with exclusive control over the work, its quality, and the competence necessary to do it to the level of satisfaction the peers would define and require of their members.

This structure, in turn, creates the context for sustaining a high level of competent professional practice. The historical context for the work of nursing did not have this enabling structure, and the advancement of the professional and professional practice suffered as a result. Research over the past two decades has revealed that both a context and standards reflecting staff ownership of professional practice work in concert to create the conditions that advance and sustain the work of the profession and lay the groundwork for performance excellence and high levels of provider and patient satisfaction.

Some well-validated essentials evidence a good fit between the supporting infrastructure and the capacity for sustainable professional practice:

- Professionals organize around decisions, not positions. Hierarchy means little to professions, and a structure that enables and supports horizontal relationships and interactions is an essential foundation for establishing professional practice. Decisions should always be generated by those who own them. Decisions should be made by the right person, in the right place, at the right time, for the right purpose.
- Decisions are driven from the point of service, such that 90% of decisions are made at the heart of the organization where professional services are provided. Thus most content-based decisions are made by the practicing staff, and the design of the structure indicates the locus of control for content decisions that are in their hands.
- A grid of accountability shows the locus of control for all decisions in the system and clearly identifies where decisions should be made

and by whom. This clear enumeration of decisions in the structure acknowledges the content of decisions and their legitimate owners, and provides a structural framework to ensure those decisions are made where they belong and by those who are accountable for their exercise.

- Clarification and distinction of decisions that are a priori management driven and owned and those that are staff owned are important distinctions of accountability in professional organizations. The professions own exclusive accountability for decisions regarding practice, quality, and the competencies required to do the work of the profession. Management accountabilities relate to the management of the human, fiscal, material, support, and systems resources that provide the context for the work of the profession. Each cannot do the work of the other, but both work in concert to support the mission of the organization, exercise stewardship over its resources, and fulfill the requirement and expectations of the professional service and care provided. This mutuality forges a bond between the profession and the organization and is the strongest demonstration of their partnership in meeting the healthcare needs of their community.

The integration of the social requirement to transform health care, resolve the conflicts that challenge this obligation in the day-to-day work of organizations and professionals, express the accountability to make a difference in the health and lives of the community, and advance the work of the profession is critical to building the profession and making a sustainable difference. Together, these conditions and activities demonstrate the potential and commitment of the professional nurse to ensuring the advancement of truly sustainable health (Institute of Medicine, 2010). The emerging leader must see them as the foundations of the work of the leader, work to advance them as a part of personal clinical leadership capacity, and demonstrate them within his or her own practice every day. Leadership is a dynamic work in progress and is a never-ending exemplar of the commitment to excellence and to making a difference in the world.

CRITICAL THOUGHT

The central principle of shared decision making is ensuring that the right decision is made by the right person, in the right place, at the right time, for the right purpose. Structuring for professionals is built around this centerpiece.

CRITICAL THOUGHT

America has the best doctors, the best nurses, the best hospitals, the best medical technology, the best medical breakthrough medicines in the world. There is absolutely no reason we should not have in this country the best health care in the world. —Bill Frist

CRITICAL THOUGHT

It is critical to synthesize all of the knowledge, skills, and abilities of nursing into an integrated whole that moves nurses from task completers to an overall demonstration of compassion and caring.

Thinking of nursing first as a job of caring and making a difference, as well as the work of giving medications on time, checking an X-ray to see if the doctor needs to be called, or taking an admission at 2:00 a.m. with a smile, reminds us of the synthesized whole of nursing work.

Resource Management in Health Care

Without people, physical settings, equipment, supplies, computers, and financial resources, the healthcare system would come to a halt. Ensuring that caregivers have the appropriate resources at the right time is complex and dynamic and requires proactive involvement from caregivers. Key issues specific to each of the categories of resources are highly interrelated within the system and are continually impacted by ethical challenges, professional role accountability, national and state legislation, and the evidence for increasing or decreasing resources. What is certain is that the allocation of resources is seldom a black-and-white decision; rather, it incorporates multiple considerations and exchanges of ideas to reach the best decision at a particular point in time.

Ethical Behaviors

The challenges of doing the right thing in health care cannot be overestimated. Multiple factors are continually interacting, changing, and impacting the processes of patient care. Perhaps the single most challenging issue is figuring out what the value of each participant in the discussion is and how the various participants will impact the decision. While it is believed that the values of the patient drive the decisions, this is not always the case. Further exploration is necessary whenever doubt arises about whether the patient's wishes and values are truly driving decisions. The importance of truth telling becomes paramount in getting to the best resolution of ethical dilemmas.

Also important are ethical issues specific to caregivers who are involved in errors. No longer is punishment following an error the expected action. Rather, the goal is to understand human fallibility and the influences of complex systems on practice breakdown. Remediation is always the goal when there is absence of intentional wrongdoing or a pattern of negligent behaviors. Ethical dilemmas create an emotional tool on individuals and teams. With more focus on caregiver burnout and suicide, the need to address ethical issues early has never been greater.

Moral courage is a critical professional competency that needs to be continually strengthened and modeled. The inherent risks in speaking up, challenging unethical decisions, and standing one's ground are significant and require collaboration and support for moral courage to be a reality.

Staffing Effectiveness

Achieving staffing effectiveness 100% of the time is the desired goal for all caregivers. Understanding staffing effectiveness measures and outcomes provides clear and objective guidelines for caregivers and leaders—but it also highlights the incredible challenges in achieving goals 100% of the time. Numerous strategies are available to inform staffing processes at various levels and times. Nurse–patient ratios, patient classification systems, legislative requirements, and different skill levels all enter into the equation for staffing effectiveness. Knowing

SCENARIO

As changes emerge based on healthcare policy changes, one must wonder if things will become better or worse: Will nursing be more humanitarian and respected as a profession, or will it become depersonalized in our attempts to provide healthcare access to all citizens and decrease costs?

Discussion Points

In a small group, think about a complex patient from your past. Describe the patient's complexity. Then create an ideal interprofessional team that might address the issues. List their professions, skill sets, and how you see them impacting outcomes. Also discuss how they might coordinate to build a seamless experience for the patient.

that many professionals are attempting to reduce the staffing process to mathematical algorithms to simplify the process should be cause for serious concern. Mathematical forecasting addresses only a small segment of the overall picture of patient care needs and nurse qualifications; the art and humanity of juggling staffing assignments in real time based on events of the moment are still essential for staffing effectiveness and nurse satisfaction. Both the art and science of staffing and scheduling are essential elements in ensuring staffing effectiveness. It is also clear that interprofessional teams are better equipped to manage complex cases. Nursing leaders should be at the forefront of coordinating teams that address the complexity of care.

Change and Innovation

Nothing ever stays the same! Learning how to thrive in the presence of continual change requires both art and science in the healthcare environment. Nurses need to understand their own attitudes, competencies, and values specific to change and innovation as a primary requisite for participating in change work. In an environment filled with both obstacles to and facilitators of change and innovation, there is no escaping the reality of change.

High performing organizations are competent in two types of change: innovation and performance improvement. Leaders must be competent in knowing how these two types of change create desired outcomes. Leaders must also understand that it is not a question of "either/or" but of "and." Innovation AND performance improvement are needed in high performing organizations. They create a dynamic that allows for novelty and refinement. In a value-based system, this dynamic is the engine by which organizations will become and remain sustainable.

As individuals become comfortable with the notion of embracing change and innovation, it is equally important to recognize that not all change is urgent or value laden. Some good ideas do not need to be implemented—unless there is evidence and rationale for making the change.

REFLECTIVE QUESTION

In the 1800s, nurses like Florence Nightingale and Clara Barton believed nurses no longer wanted to accept things the way they were; instead, they wanted to learn from past mistakes and improve the future of nursing. Do you think this is the overall feeling of nurses today? Why or why not? Describe facilitators and/or barriers to your rationale.

Policymaking

Policies are made at the national, state, and local levels; each impacts the direct caregiver in different ways. Policies are also the backbone of private organizations and agencies. Knowing the source of policies that govern patient processes is an essential first step in understanding the goals of the policies, the appropriate avenue for feedback, and supporting metrics to determine the value and impact of the policy.

In addition to knowing the source, content, and consequences of healthcare policies, it is important to recognize the role of the professional in providing feedback to policymakers when policies are no longer effective or do not achieve the desired goal. Too often, ineffective policies are maintained even when there is sufficient evidence to terminate them. Speaking up and providing input is consistent with ethical and professional practices.

Delegation

No individual can do everything for everyone. Complex patient care requires multiple levels of caregivers at different times to provide the necessary services, including surgical interventions, treatments, medications, therapy, nutrition, housekeeping, record management, and a host of other services. From the chief executive officer level to the patient, multiple caregivers interact with one another and oversee and direct different levels of care. Nurses, for example, collaborate with medical providers, therapists, pharmacists, and nutritionists and oversee licensed practical nurses, nurse assistants, clerical staff, and often housekeepers. The importance of effective delegation cannot be overestimated. Effective delegation ideally distributes the workload equitably and effectively.

Career Management

A career in nursing provides incredible opportunities to continually advance into numerous avenues and job roles. Proactively understanding and managing one's career requires not only a current license, but also continuing competence, participation in professional organizations, and mentoring nurse colleagues as they advance in their work. No individual should ever put his or her career on autopilot, expecting that little will change over time and that reentry into the workplace will not require updating and skill confirmation. A nursing career is both an incredible asset and an incredible obligation to the public.

Remember that nursing provides a wealth of opportunity to impact the world. Do not feel locked into a leadership trajectory when your passions lie in care. Do not take positions that do not bring out your best professional self. In many cases, the most successful and fulfilled nurses create their own paths. You can do the same.

CRITICAL THOUGHT

There is no medicine like hope, no incentive so great, and no tonic so powerful as expectation of something better tomorrow. —Orison Swett Marden

Concluding Thoughts

Learning and challenging our assumptions of the past is never-ending and sometimes overwhelming, but it is mostly energizing in that this work is a reflection of our vitality and abilities to create a better future and influence how that future evolves. The scenarios in the appendices of this chapter are intended to challenge your thinking, be outrageously creative, and push the walls of what we currently know and do in very special ways. The future will depend on nursing professionals continuing to learn creatively and take rational risks in pushing new ideas, projects, and initiatives forward quickly and effectively. The contemporary professional nurse is not afraid of failure—rather, when an idea or project or initiative does not work as intended, the work of course correction has already begun!

Best wishes on your journey. The healthcare world desperately needs your energy, wisdom, and passion for excellence in patient care.

References

Berwick, D., Nolan, T., & Whittington, J. (2008). The triple aim: Care, health, and cost. *Health Affairs, 27*(3), 759–769.

Boulle, L., Colatrella, M. T., & Picchioni, A. P. (2008). *Mediation: Skills and techniques.* Newark, NJ: LexisNexis Matthew Bender.

Connors, R., Smith, T., & Hickman, C. (2004). *The Oz Principle: Getting results through individual and organizational accountability.* New York, NY: Portfolio Hardcover.

Hazy, J., Goldstein, J., & Lichtenstein, B. (2007). *Complex systems leadership theory: New perspectives from complexity science on social and organizational effectiveness.* New York, NY: Vintage Press.

Institute of Medicine. (2010). *The future of nursing.* Washington, DC: IOM.

Maxwell, J. (2010). *The 21 irrefutable laws of leadership.* Nashville, TN: Thomas Nelson.

Phillips, R., & Bazemore, A. (2010). Primary care and why it matters for US health system reform. *Health Affairs, 29*(5), 806–810.

Porter-O'Grady, T. (2009). *Interdisciplinary shared governance: Integrating practice, transforming health care.* Sudbury, MA: Jones and Bartlett Publishers.

Styer, K. (2007). Development of a unit-based practice committee: A form of shared governance. *AORN Journal, 86*(1), 85.

Tilley, D. (2008). Competency in nursing: A concept analysis. *Journal of Continuing Education in Nursing, 39*(2), 58–65.

Appendix A

Exercise in Leadership: Advancing Evidence-Based Practice

This scenario exemplifies a situation that would draw on the learning and skills enumerated in a number of related chapters in this text. With a team of no more than five members, explore the issues presented in this scenario and use the principles and elements outlined in this text as your source for addressing Michele's leadership issues and resolving her questions and problems.

SCENARIO

Michele is chair of the Practice Council. There has been much discussion on the unit about implementing evidence-based practices in all of the nursing practice protocols. However, the staff know little about the foundations and principles of evidence-based practices and do not understand the implications of changing practice patterns to reflect the related principles and applications into every nurse's role.

A number of members of the Practice Council have expressed negative feelings about changing to incorporate evidence-grounded practices into their roles. One of them asked, "If what we are doing isn't broken, why fix it?" This person has managed to get a couple of the other members of the Council to support her opposition. The nursing manager is insisting that the Council seriously undertake this work because it is a "mandate" from the nurse executive, and the unit manager's "reputation is on the line."

Michele has some concerns about the process of implementing changes in response to a mandate from above. The organization has been operating within a shared governance structure for some time. To Michele, it appears that the move to evidence-based practice should be a staff initiative and come from the wider nursing division Practice Council rather than as a mandate from the nurse executive.

For Michele, evidence-based practice reflects a fundamental principle of accountability on the part of the staff. She feels that staff should want to validate their practice choices and application with data and demonstrate best practices in their clinical performance. She has noted that some questions have arisen regarding the level of understanding and commitment to personal accountability among all members of the staff. Michele knows that if evidence-based practice is to succeed, it will need the support of leadership and staff throughout its implementation.

The following are some questions designed to focus your deliberations and problem solving:

1. What preparation does Michele need to do in relation to her knowledge base about evidence-based practice before she brings the issue to the unit Practice Council? What information will she need to gather and provide for the Council members before they meet?

2. How will Michele present the concept to the Council, and what will she need to do to help them engage the concept and work to make it happen?

3. Michele has some conflict issues regarding evidence-based practice with Council members. How will she address the conflict? Which approaches should she use to persuade those who are opposed to the idea to embrace and work with the Council to make it happen?

4. Michele has some concerns about evidence-based practice being a response to a mandate. In keeping with the principles of shared governance, where does legitimate accountability lie for generating evidence-based practice? Where should the direction come from for requiring its implementation, and which shared governance mechanisms should drive it? What is the legitimate role of the manager in the requirement for and the process of implementing evidence-based practice on the unit?

5. Michele has expressed concerns about staff accountability. Because evidence-based practice depends strongly on staff's personal accountability for its successful implementation, what will Michele need to do to generate interest and accountability in the staff for practicing in a way that demonstrates evidentiary foundations for practice? How will she know when accountability is present?

6. Is there a point in time when the Practice Council should move ahead without full consensus? What are the criteria to do so? List the advantages and disadvantages of taking this step.

7. Create a mind map or visual graphic presentation of the problems and issues Michele must address and the ways in which she should deal with them as she leads implementation of evidence-based practice on the unit. Share your indicators of success for each element of the process that will demonstrate that you are making successful progress in making it work on the unit.

Appendix B

Exercise in Leadership: Increasing Capacity

The key concepts to be considered in this scenario are change, innovation, staffing effectiveness, policy, ethical issues, delegation, healthcare reform, and professional practice. The plan is to include the following items in a presentation to the leadership of the organization and interested community members:

1. John's assessment of his competence with change and innovation
2. The rationale for selection of team members
3. An assessment of other team members' competence with change and innovation
4. Identification of the who, what, when, and where of the change process
5. A list of supporters and nonsupporters of the change and the reasons for their positions
6. Ethical issues that could arise and how they will be managed
7. Changes in the staffing plan for days and nights
8. The addition of clinical and nonclinical roles and rationale for their addition
9. A list of rational risks that will be taken
10. Plans to address potential policy violations
11. A list of evaluation criteria and metrics to monitor the change
12. Completion of a performance demonstration document by each member of the team, identifying his or her contribution to the project and supporting patient care in the new model
13. A timeline for implementation and evaluation
14. Components of the expectation that cannot be met and what should be done instead to manage the new environment

SCENARIO

John is an experienced critical care nurse in a 12-bed unit. The facility is new and equipped with the latest technology. In general, the unit is well respected and attracts highly committed, professional nurses. Teamwork is above average, and nurse–physician relationships are quite good.

(continues)

(continued)

The strategic planning analysts for the organization have determined that the census for the critical care unit will triple in the next 12 months based on the anticipated increase in patients requiring care as a result of healthcare reform. There is neither enough time nor sufficient resources available to build more patient rooms.

The organization has indicated it plans to double nurse–patient assignments (from two patients per registered nurse to four patients per registered nurse), decrease the length of stay by 50%, and maintain quality outcomes at the 90th percentile. Currently, the outcomes are at the 95th percentile.

As a respected and competent clinical leader, John has been asked to lead a team of clinical caregivers to create a new delivery model that meets the identified needs for the future. John has also been encouraged to include any other stakeholders, including patients, to be on his team.

Appendix C

Exercise in Leadership: Clinical Technology Management

The key concepts to be considered in this scenario are technology management, change and innovation, ethical issues, healthcare policy, resource management, professional nursing practice role clarification, and the infrastructure for practice.

The team is asked to identify the following:

1. The change and innovation competence of each team member
2. The primary issues causing the dissatisfaction
3. Key stakeholders required to address the issues
4. Ethical issues specific to care of the oncology patient, reimbursement, and technology use
5. Issues related to professional nursing practice, use of technology, and compliance with regulatory mandates
6. Team dynamics including conflict, agreements, and challenges in addressing the issues
7. A plan to address the issues

8. A communication plan to inform key stakeholders of any changes
9. A list of evaluation criteria and timeline for evaluation
10. A timeline for implementation

SCENARIO

The use of clinical monitoring, documentation, and communication devices is at an all-time high in the oncology unit. Nurses have individual communication devices, portable tablets for documentation, badge locators for movements, and internal phones for special team assignments. Patients are linked to smart pumps, smart beds, cardiac monitoring, forehead stress monitors, and the communication system to call for assistance, order meals, and access television and movies.

Recently, feedback from patients has indicated a decrease in satisfaction and specific comments that more attention is being paid to electronic monitoring than to the patient. Given that the Hospital Consumer Assessment of Healthcare Provider Systems (HCAHPS) scores specific to patient satisfaction are now linked to reimbursement, there is an expectation that these issues will be addressed.

A request has been put forth for direct caregivers to volunteer to form a team, select a facilitator, and develop a strategy to effectively address this complex issue. The expectation is that the wisdom of an effective solution will come from experienced caregivers who are knowledgeable about the effective working of the systems and oncology care excellence. Participation on shared leadership committees is a preferred prerequisite.

Critical Thought, Leader Tip, and Scenario icons made by Freepik from www.flaticon.com; Callout icon made by Yannick from www.flaticon.com; Team Tip icon made by Chanut is Industries from www.flaticon.com

Glossary

Accountability   A demonstration that professionals have coalesced their efforts in the clinical team in a way that results in a positive impact on the health of those they serve; an obligation to account for or explain the events.

Accountable care organization   Networks of providers that are rewarded financially if they can slow the growth in their patients' healthcare spending while maintaining or improving the quality of the care they deliver. The accountable care model emphasizes population care, value-driven outcomes, the point of service at which patient care occurs, protocols for effective hand-offs, and inclusion of the family.

Analysis   Breaking down the components of a problem or issue into parts or elements.

Assignment   The distribution of work that each staff member is to accomplish in a given time period. Assignment occurs when the authority to do a task already exists.

Attitude   The manner, disposition, or inclination with which one approaches and reacts to situations.

Authority   The legal source of power; the right to act or to command the actions of others and have those orders be followed.

Autonomy   The right to self-determination; being one's own person without constraints by another's actions or psychological and physical limitations; the capacity of a rational individual to make an informed, uncoerced decision.

Balance sheet   A financial statement that includes assets, liabilities, and equity. It is a snapshot of the organization's financial position at a specific point in time.

Bargaining   The phase of negotiation that emphasizes the give-and-take related to the variety of positions at the table. Bargaining is the work of exchange. There are a number of different bargaining approaches.

Beneficence   The duty to do good. The term refers to actions that promote the well-being of others. In the medical context, this means taking actions that serve the best interests of patients.

Betrayal   A person's words or actions that indicate he or she lacks good intentions toward another; the breaking or violation of a presumptive contract, trust, or confidence that produces moral and psychological conflict within a relationship among individuals, between organizations, or between individuals and organizations.

Bioethics   A subdiscipline of applied ethics that studies questions surrounding biology, medicine, and the health professions.

Boundary crossing Brief excursions from an established boundary for a therapeutic purpose; for example, disclosure of bits of personal information or small gifts.

Boundary violation A deviation from the established boundary in the healthcare provider and client relationship where the healthcare provider's needs and the client's needs are confused.

Cash flow operating activities A financial report that shows the cash inflow and outflow activities or financial stability of the organization.

Chunking Instead of summarily reaching a point of broad generalized agreement, construction of a final agreement as an aggregation of smaller agreements that, when looked at comprehensively, satisfies the needs of the participants.

Classification The ordering of entities into groups or classes on the basis of their similarity, minimizing within-group variance and maximizing between-group variance.

Coach A person who assists others to develop viable solutions, to prioritize them, and then to act on them.

Code of ethics Guiding principles that enumerate the expectations of members of the profession and the personal and performance standards that represent what is best in the work of the profession.

Collective ethical wisdom The sum of individual and collective experience, knowledge, and good sense; know-how in which the individual and collective knowledge, experience, and good sense result in sound ethical decisions and judgment everywhere and every day.

Competence Application of knowledge, interpersonal decision making, and psychomotor skills expected for the practice role; having the knowledge, skills, and ability to practice safely and effectively; the potential ability and/or capability to function in a given situation.

Competency One's actual performance in a situation. Competence is required before one can expect to achieve competency.

Competent clinical practice Situation-specific performance requiring an integration of skills, including cognitive, psychomotor, interpersonal, and attitudinal skills.

Complex adaptive system A densely linked, intersecting, and interacting connection of agents, each making their own contribution and acting both independently in making that contribution and interdependently in linking that contribution to the independent but related contributions of other agents.

Conflict A metaphor for difference. It is more normal than it is exceptional.

Continued/continuing competence The ongoing synthesis of knowledge, skills, and abilities required to practice safely and effectively in accordance with the scope of nursing practice; the ongoing commitment of a registered nurse to integrate and apply the knowledge, skills, and judgment with the attitudes, values, and beliefs required to practice safely, effectively, and ethically in a designated role and setting.

Core schedule An aggregated, average staffing number and skill mix required for patient care, which includes caregivers, shift length, and calendar days.

Critical thinking Active, purposeful, organized thinking that takes into consideration focus, language, frame of reference, attitudes, assumptions, evidence, reasoning, conclusions, implications, and context when deciding what to believe or do.

Culture of nursing competence The shared beliefs, values, attitudes, and actions that promote lifelong learning and result in an environment of safe and effective patient care.

Dashboard A combination of graphics and numbers to quickly display important data elements.

Decision making A complex cognitive process that involves choosing a particular course of action from among alternatives. Decision making is an essential component of the problem-solving process.

Deep dive A tool to advance change and innovation in which a particular area is selected for observation in multiple ways. Workflows, photos, interviews, and observations are gathered by a team to analyze current processes and brainstorm new ways of doing the current work processes.

Delegate The individual staff person receiving the delegated task.

Delegation The transferring to a competent individual the authority to perform a selected nursing task in a selected situation.

Delegator The individual making the delegation.

Developmental stretch assignments Assignments to improve employee satisfaction and engagement through autonomy and leadership practices.

Directed creativity A tool to advance change and innovation in which a situation is proposed to encourage and advance new ideas.

DRG Diagnosis-related group. A system used to help clinicians and hospitals monitor quality of care and utilization of services. It has been used by Medicare to pay hospitals.

Emergent Conditions that are driven by new sociopolitical realities, economic changes, technological advances, evidence of best practices, and a host of related shifts that demonstrate that holding onto current practices is an impediment to better engaging work processes in the best interests of those they serve.

Employee recognition Acknowledgment of outstanding behaviors, communication, accountability, valuing diversity, delivering excellence, and teamwork.

Employee rounding Regular rounding in work areas to identify employees' most critical needs, safety issues, and clinical concerns.

Equality A measure of condition.

Equity A measure of value.

Ethical dilemma A problem that confronts one with a choice of solutions that seem, or are, equally unfavorable; a complex situation that often involves an apparent conflict of moral imperatives, in which to obey one would result in transgressing another.

Ethical erosion The subtle, even unnoticed, slippage of ethical standards; a pervasive, subtle negative dynamic resulting from a decreased focus on values in small and often unnoticed slippages; slight deviations from the normal course of events.

Ethical fading A process that obscures the ethical dimensions of a decision.

Ethics The philosophical study of right action and wrong action; also known as morality, ethics delineates the highest moral standards of behavior.

Ethics of care A recently developed moral theory based on the insights of Gilligan that rejects the traditional male-centered ethics that focused on rationality, individuality, and abstract principles in favor of emotion, caring relationships, and concrete situations.

Evidence-based practice Practice based on facts and truth; the integration of the best research evidence with clinical expertise and clinical values.

Evidentiary dynamics Nursing practices based on research conducted so that evidence may be presented.

Federal Register An unbiased source of information, the official daily publication for rules, proposed rules, and notices of the U.S. federal government.

Fidelity Duty to keep one's promise; the quality of being faithful.

Forecasting Projection of employee need based on census, patient acuity, and skill mix of available resources.

Health advocacy Supports and promotes patients' healthcare rights and enhances community health and policy initiatives that focus on the availability, safety, and quality of care.

Health policy Policy directed toward promoting the health of citizens; the aggregate of principles, stated or unstated, that characterize the distribution of resources, services, and political influences that impact the health of the population.

Healthcare economics A branch of economics focused on efficiency, effectiveness, and behavior in the production and consumption of healthcare goods and services.

Hearing (legislative) The principal formal method by which committees collect and analyze information in the early stages of legislative policymaking

Income statement A financial statement that includes information about revenue sources and expenses at a specific point in time.

Individual accountability Knowing the requirements and behaviors of effective delegation.

Innovation A product or process that redefines the social and economic potential of an organization or group.

Institutional policies Policies that refer to rules that govern the workplace.

Interest-based bargaining A negotiation strategy in which parties collaborate to find a "win-win" solution to their dispute. This strategy focuses on developing mutually beneficial agreements based on the interests of the disputants.

Justice The elimination of arbitrary distinctions and the establishment of a structure of practice with a proper share, balance, or equilibrium among competing claims.

Leader A person who coordinates, integrates, facilitates, and provides a context for the performance of the people in the organization.

Licensure The process by which an agency of a state government grants permission to an individual to engage in a given occupation.

Manager An organizational position and function. Managers have subordinates and a vertical relationship to those they manage.

Mediator A person who manages the conflict resolution process.

Medical futility Care at the end of life from which there is little hope of benefit; the belief that in cases where there is no hope for improvement of an incapacitating condition, no course of treatment is called for.

Mentor A wise and trusted advisor who guides others on a particular journey. A mentor provides support, challenge, and vision.

Mentoring The process of a more accomplished person assisting others to develop expertise and learn new skills based on the mentor's personal, untapped wisdom, reinforcing their self-confidence, supporting real-life situations, and sharing personal experiences when appropriate.

Mind mapping A tool to advance change and innovation in which software is used for collecting, organizing, and synthesizing large amounts of data in layers with complex relationships.

Moral reasoning The process in which an individual tries to determine the difference between what is right and what is wrong in a personal situation by using logic.

Morality Designates the conventional beliefs of a particular society; the degree of congruence between what one perceives as right and one's actual behavior.

Negotiation An attempt to identify, enumerate, and undertake a process that clearly establishes needs and wants and where all parties work to reconcile their interests in a way that results in mutual advantage or value.

Nonmaleficence Duty to do no harm.

Nursing certification The provision of tangible recognition of professional achievement in a defined functional or clinical area of nursing.

Onboarding The early processes of socializing nurses into the workplace to achieve optimal employee engagement.

Organizational accountability Providing sufficient resources, staffing, and appropriate staff mix; implementing policies and role descriptions; providing opportunities for continuing staff development; and creating an environment conducive to teamwork, collaboration, and client-centered care.

Organizational integrity The means of producing stronger, sustainable performance through ethical pathways consistent with the vision, mission, and values of the organization.

Organizational policies Policies that pertain to positions taken by organizations to govern the workplace and behavior.

Patient acuity The level of need or dependency of an individual patient.

Patient care delivery model A method or system of organizing and delivering nursing care, including the manner in which nursing care is organized to deliver the care necessary to meet the needs of the patients. The delivery system encompasses work delegation, resource utilization, communication methodologies, clinical decision-making processes, and management structure.

Patient classification system A tool to improve the clarity and objective identification of patient care needs. The goal of the system is to provide the most valid and reliable information specific to work that needs to be done for patients.

Performance improvement Measuring the output of a particular business process or procedure, then modifying the process or procedure to increase the output, increase efficiency, or increase the effectiveness of the process or procedure.

Personal integrity A state of wholeness and peace experienced when our goals, actions, and decisions are consistent with our most cherished values.

PICO approach A methodology used to form a clinical question, in which P is patient or problem, I is intervention, C is comparison intervention, and O is outcomes.

Policy The choices that a society, segment of society, or organization makes regarding its resources, involving setting goals and priorities, and deciding how and which resources should be used to achieve those goals. Policies reflect the values and beliefs of the leaders who make the policies in a society and/or organization.

Pragmatism An American school of philosophy that rejects the esoteric metaphysics of traditional European academic philosophy in favor of more down-to-earth, concrete questions and answers. A moral action is distinguished from an immoral action in that the person acts from a sense of duty, not from inclinations or feelings.

Principle A law or rule that has to be—or usually is to be—followed, or can be desirably followed, or is an inevitable consequence of something, such as the laws observed in nature or the way a system is constructed.

Profession An expression of a role and its relationship to the world, representing a social contract and reflecting high expectations for its exercise from those who will depend on it.

Professional boundary The limits of the professional relationship that allow for a safe, therapeutic connection between the healthcare provider and the client. These include, at a minimum, time, location of patient care money, exchange, favors or gifts, self-disclosure, and physical contact.

Professional governance   The accountability, professional obligation, collateral relationships, and decision-making of a professional, foundational to autonomous practice and achievement of exemplary empirical outcomes.

Public policy   An authoritative ruling relating to a decision made by government.

Rationalization   When a person knows what is right and doesn't want to do it; a term used in sociology to refer to a process in which an increasing number of social actions become based on considerations of teleological efficiency or calculation rather than on motivations derived from morality, emotion, custom, or tradition.

Remediation   The process whereby identified deficiencies in core competencies are corrected.

Research   The systematic examination of an idea using rigorous principles of experimentation and measurement.

Research utilization   The use of knowledge that is typically based on a single study.

Responsibility   Reliability, dependability, and obligation to accomplish work.

Right choices   Those choices that conform to ethical norms or principles, such that others can know whether one has made the appropriate choice.

Scheduling   The long-range plan that combines the organization's goals, legislation, regulation, and accreditation requirements and planned patient demand.

Setting the table   Knowing how all the decisions need to be served, which talent or expertise needs to be gathered, how large the team should be in relation to the issues it will be addressing, and which particular gifts and skills

will be present on the team as they deliberate the questions before them.

Shared governance   A structural format for nursing to implement a more horizontal locus of control in organizations. This framework provides support for the professions, their interaction, and their collective obligation to advance the interest of health care.

Social media   The use of web-based and mobile technologies to turn communication into an interactive dialogue; a group of Internet-based applications that build on the ideological and technological foundations of Web 2.0 and that allow the creation and exchange of user-generated content.

Social networking   Specific social activities to support team building, seasonal challenges, and common needs.

Social policy   Policy intended to enhance the public welfare.

Staffing   The real-time adjustment of the employee work schedule based on census, acuity, and the mix of available resources.

State Nurse Practice Act   An act that regulates nursing practice— including requirements to enter into practice—licensure maintenance, scope of practice parameters, and disciplinary action.

Statement of purpose   A statement that serves as an anchor for the work of a team and indicates the direction for team activities.

Statute   A law passed by the legislature.

Supervision   The provision of guidance or direction, evaluation, and follow-up by the delegator for accomplishment of a task delegated to another; watching over a particular activity or task being carried out by other people and ensuring that it is carried out correctly.

Synthesis   The act of combining and integrating numerous complex elements or components of the system to view the system as an integrated whole.

Terms of engagement   General rules of relationship and interaction that the team adheres to as a way of maintaining a positive communication and interaction environment within the context of the team as it completes its work.

Trust   One individual's willingness to be vulnerable to another based on the belief that the other is competent, open, concerned, and reliable, thus rendering risk taking more rational and realistic.

U.S. Department of Health and Human Services   The overarching federal administrative agency concerned with monitoring the quality of health care in the United States.

Utilitarianism   The principle of utility, or the greatest happiness principle; actions are chosen that will produce the greatest amount of happiness for the greatest number of people.

Veracity   Truth telling, or the duty to tell the truth.

Whistle-blowing   Action taken by a person who goes outside the organization for the public's best interest when the organization is unresponsive after a danger is reported through the organization's proper channels.

Workforce management   A comprehensive system that includes patient classification, scheduling, staffing, and budgeting systems.

Index